CRACK the Final FRCR Part A Exam
Modules 4, 5, 6

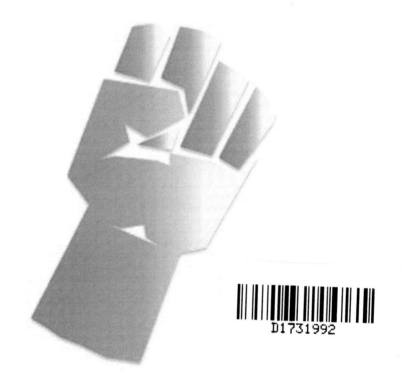

—PROMETHEUS LIONHART, M.D.

CRACK the Final FRCR PART A Exam - Modules 4,5,6

Disclaimer:

Readers are advised - this book is **NOT to be used for clinical decision making**. Human error does occur, and it is your responsibility to double check all facts provided. To the fullest extent of the law, the Author assumes no responsibility for any injury and/or damage to persons or property arising out or related to any use of the material contained in this book.

Copyright © 2015 by Prometheus Lionhart

All rights reserved - Under International and Pan-American Copyright Conventions. This book, or parts thereof, may not be reproduced in any form without permission from the Author.

Published by: Prometheus Lionhart

Title ID: 5708706

ISBN-13: 978-1517122379

Cover design, texts, and illustrations: copyright © 2015 by Prometheus Lionhart

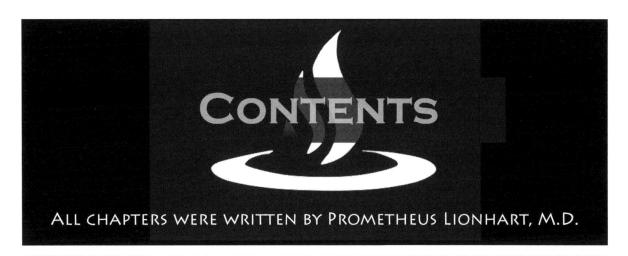

CONTENTS

All chapters were written by Prometheus Lionhart, M.D.

VOLUME 1

 MODULE 1: CARDIOTHORACIC AND VASCULAR

 MODULE 2: MUSCULOSKELETAL AND TRAUMA

 MODULE 3: GASTRO-INTESTINAL

 STRATEGY & GAMESMANSHIP

VOLUME 2

 MODULE 4: GENITO-URINARY, ADRENAL, OBSTETRICS & GYNAECOLOGY AND BREAST (9-156)

 MODULE 5: PAEDIATRIC (157-230)

 MODULE 6: CENTRAL NERVOUS AND HEAD & NECK (231-372)

 STRATEGY & GAMESMANSHIP (373-391)

Introduction

The Final FRCR (Part A) is a single best answer exam ("multiple choice test" - we call it in the states). The candidates are grilled on all aspects of clinical radiology plus some physics and anatomy. The "Specialty Training Curriculum for Clinical Radiology" is referenced by the RCR as the source - but it is nothing more than a vague laundry list of radiology diagnoses and skills. The exam is held over three consecutive days. Success is measured by the ability to pass all 6 modules.

What makes this book unique?

Dr. Prometheus Lionhart is the premier Radiology board review expert in the United States. He is the sole author, illustrator, and publisher of the #1 selling and most used board review book series for the American Board of Radiology's CORE Exam (*Crack the CORE Exam Vol 1 & 2*). The "CORE Exam" is essentially the American equivalent to the FRCR Part A.

Dr. Lionhart has turned his attention to the FRCR Exam, remastering his famous American texts for direct use on the FRCR Exam.

The Impetus for this book was to not write a reference text or standard review book, but instead, strategy manual for solving multiple choice questions for Radiology. The author wishes to convey that the multiple choice test is different than an oral exam in that you can't ask the same kinds of open ended essay type questions. *"What's your differential?"*

Questioning the contents of one's differential is the only real question on oral examinations, or real life view-box work. That simple question becomes nearly impossible to format into a multiple choice test. Instead, the focus for training for such a test should be on things that can be asked. For example, anatomy facts - what is it? ... OR... trivia facts - what is the most common location, or age, or association, or syndrome? ... OR... What's the next step in management? In this book, the author tried to cover all the material that could be asked (reasonably), and then approximate how questions might be asked about the various topics. Throughout the book, the author will intimate, "this could be asked like this", and "this fact lends itself well to a question." Included as the last chapter in each volume is a strategy chapter focusing on high yield "buzzwords" that lend well to certain questions.

This is NOT a reference book.
This book is NOT designed for patient care.
This book is designed for studying specifically for multiple choice tests

Legal Stuff

Readers are advised - **this book is NOT to be used for clinical decision making**. Human error does occur, and it is your responsibility to double check all facts provided. To the fullest extent of the law, the Author assumes no responsibility for any injury and/or damage to persons or property arising out or related to any use of the material contained in this book.

I FIGHT FOR THE USERS

-TRON 1982

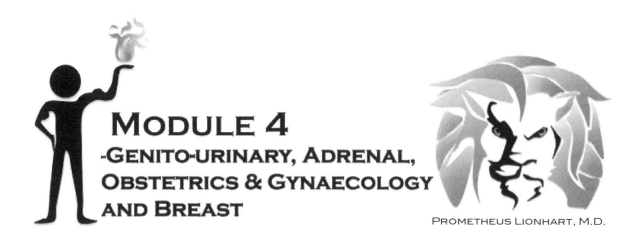

Module 4
-Genito-urinary, Adrenal, Obstetrics & Gynaecology and Breast

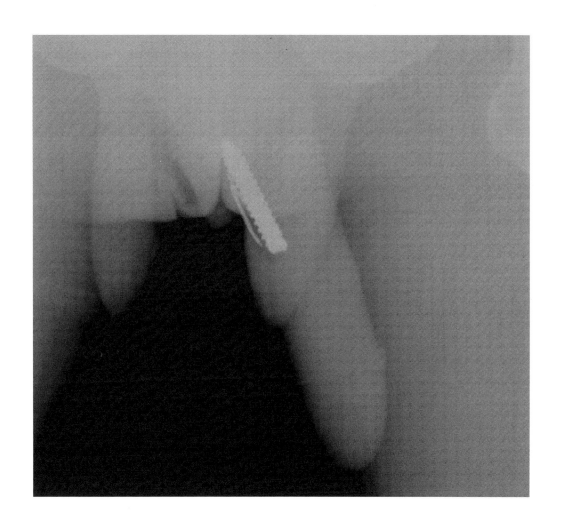

Section 1: Genito-Urinary

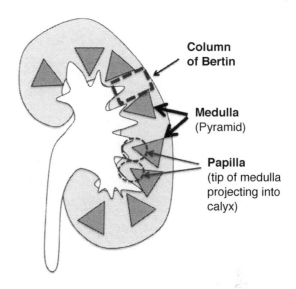

Normal Anatomy: The normal adult kidney is shaped like a bean, with a smooth (often lobulated) outer border. The kidney is surrounded by a thick capsule outlined by echogenic perirenal fat. This echogenic fat is contiguous with the renal sinus, filling the middle of the kidney. The cortex extends centrally into the middle of the kidney, separated by slightly less echogenic medullary pyramids. The normal kidney should be between 9cm and 15cm in length.

The echogenicity of the kidney should be equal to or slightly less than the liver and spleen. If the renal echogencity is greater than the liver, this indicates some impaired renal function (medical renal disease). Liver echogenicity greater than the kidney indicates a fatty liver.

Variant Anatomy

Fetal Lobulation – The fetal kidneys are subdivided into lobes that are separated with grooves. Sometimes this lobulation persists into adult life. The question is always;

Fetal Lobulation vs Scarring:

- **Lobulation** = *renal surface indentations overlie the space between the pyramids*

- **Scarring** = *renal surface indentations overlie the medullary pyramids.*

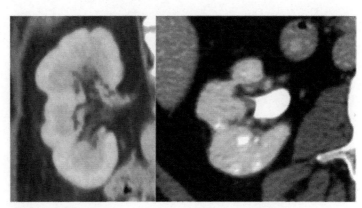

Fetal Lobulation — Indentations Between Pyramids

Renal Scarring — Indentations Over Pyramids

Dromedary Hump – Focal bulge on the left kidney, which forms as the result of adaptation to the adjacent spleen.

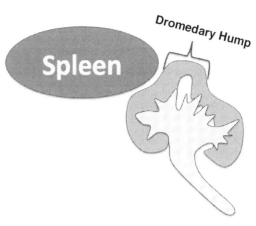

Prominent (or hypertrophied) Column of Bertin – Normal variant in which hypertrophied cortical tissue located between the pyramids results in splaying of the sinus. Other than the hypertrophy it looks totally normal. It will enhance the same as adjacent parenchyma.

Expect this to be shown on ultrasound - looks like a big echogenic cortex.

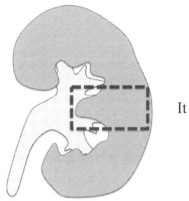

Prominent Column of Bertin

Renal Agenesis – Congenital absence of one or both kidneys. If it's unilateral this can be asymptomatic. If it's bilateral think about the "Potter Sequence." When it's unilateral (it's usually sporadic), but for the purpose of multiple choice think about associated GYN anomalies in women (70% of women with unilateral renal agenesis have associated genital anomalies - **unicornuate uterus**). With regard to men, **20% with renal agenesis have absence of the ipsilateral epididymis and vas deferens or an ipsilateral seminal vesicle cyst.**

Associations: Ipsilateral seminal vesicle cysts, absent ipsilateral ureter, absent ipsilateral hemitrigone and absent ipsilateral vas deferens

- o **Potter Sequence:** Insult (maybe ACE inhibitors) = kidneys don't form, if kidneys don't form you can't make piss, if you can't make piss you can't develop lungs (pulmonary hypoplasia).
- o **Mayer-Rokitansky-Kuster-Hauser.** – Mullerian duct anomalies including absence or atresia of the uterus. Associated with unilateral renal agenesis.
- o **Lying Down Adrenal or "Pancake Adrenal" Sign** – describes the elongated appearance of the adrenal not normally molded by the adjacent kidney. It can be used to differentiate surgical absent vs congenital absent.

Horseshoe Kidney – This is the most common fusion anomaly. The IMA gets hung up on the IMA. Complications include Traumatic Injury (gets crushed against vertebral body), UPJ Obstruction, Recurrent Infection, Recurrent Stones, Wilms Tumor (8x higher), TCC (from all those infections). A rare situation, but known association is the renal carcinoid occurring in horseshoe kidney. Turners syndrome is a classically tested association.

Crossed Fused Renal Ectopia – One kidney comes across the midline and fuses with the other. "The Ectopic Kidney is Inferior." The left kidney more commonly crosses. Complications include stones, infection, and hydronephrosis (50%).

Renal Masses

Renal Cell Carcinoma:

The most common primary renal malignancy. RCC till proven otherwise: (a) Enhances with contrast (> 15 H.U.), (b) calcifications in a fatty mass. Risk factors include tobacco use, syndromes like VHL, chronic dialysis (> 3years), family history. These dudes make hypervascular mets. They are ALWAYS lytic when they met to the bones.

- *Pseudoenhancement:* A less than 10 HU increase in attenuation is considered within the technical limits of the study and is not considered to represent enhancement. More rare once a cyst is larger than 1.5cm.

- *Can RCC have fat in it?* - Oh yeah, for sure -especially clear cell. This leads to the potential sneaky situation of a fat containing lesion in the liver (which can be a RCC met). Now to make this work they'd have to tell you the patient had RCC - or show you one. A helpful hint is that RCCs with macroscopic fat nearly always have some calcification/ossification - if they don't it's probably an AML.

Subtypes:
- **Clear Cell** – Most common subtype. This is the one that is associated with VHL. It is typically more aggressive than papillary, and will enhance equal to the cortex on corticomedullary phase.
- **Papillary** – This is the second most common type. It is usually less aggressive than clear cell (more rare subtypes can be very aggressive). They are less vascular and will not enhance equal to the cortex on corticomedullary phase. They also are in the classic T2 dark differential (along with lipid poor AML, and hemorrhagic cyst).
- **Medullary** – Associated with Sickle Cell Trait. It's highly aggressive, and usually large and already metastasized at the time of diagnosis. Patient's are usually younger.
- **Chromophobe** – All you need to know is that it's associated with Birt Hogg Dube.

Conventional RCC Staging:

Stage 1: Limited to Kidney and < 7cm
Stage 2: Limited to Kidney but > 7cm
Stage 3: Still inside Gerota's Fascia
  A: Renal Vein Invaded
  B: IVC below diaphragm
  C: IVC above diaphragm
Stage 4: Beyond Gerota's Fasica
Ipsilateral Adrenal

Subtype	Syndrome / Association
Clear Cell	Von Hippel-Lindau
Papillary	Hereditary papillary renal carcinoma
Chromophobe	Birt Hogg Dube
Medullary	Sickle Cell Trait

Sneaky Move

Does Adult Polycystic Kidney Disease increase your risk for RCC???? – Well No, but sorta. The genetic syndrome does NOT intrinsically increase your risk. However, dialysis does. Who gets dialysis?? People with APCKD. It would be such a crap way to ask a question - but could happen. If you are asked, I'm recommending you say no to the increased risk, - unless the question writer specifies that the patient is on dialysis.

Renal Masses That Are Not RCC

Renal Lymphoma – This can literally look like anything. Having said that the most common appearance is bilateral, enlarged kidneys, with small, low attenuation cortically based solid nodules or masses. A solitary mass is seen in about 1/4 of the cases.

Trivia: Out of all the renal masses - lymphoma is the most likely to preserve the normal reniform shape.

Renal Leukemia: The kidney is the most common visceral organ involved. Typically the kidneys are smooth and enlarged. Hypodense lesions are cortically based only, with little if any involvement of the medulla.

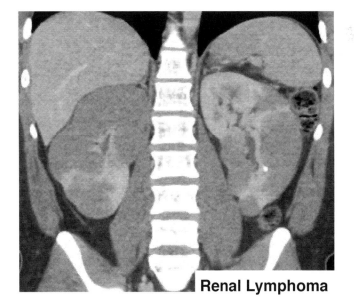

Renal Lymphoma

Oncocytoma - This is the second most common benign tumor (after AML). It looks a lot like a RCC, but has a **central scar** 33% of the time (and 100% of the time on multiple choice). There will be no malignant features (such as vessel infiltration). They cannot be distinguished from RCC on imaging and must be treated as RCC till proven otherwise.

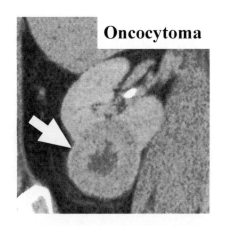

It they want to ask about an Oncocytoma they can show it 3 ways: (1) Solid Mass with central scar - CT or MRI, (2) On Ultrasound "spoke wheel" vascular pattern, (3) on PET CT it will be hotter than surrounding renal cortex.

Gamesmanship: I have encountered two types of GU radiologists in my life. The first type is the practical type - he/she doesn't EVER even mention oncocytoma, because enhancing renal masses have to come out. Even if you biopsy it and get oncocytes, it doesn't matter because RCCs can have oncocytic features.

The second type is more of your classic academic type. To try and sound impressive this person will often include this (and other rare entities) in the differential. Another common psychopathology in these types is excessive word nazism ("don't say that, say this"). I'm fairly certain you have met this person - there is usually one in every section.

The PET Trick:

RCC is typically COLDER than surrounding renal parenchyma on PET,

Oncocytoma is typically HOTTER than surrounding renal parenchyma on PET,

So if you are shown an enhancing renal mass with a central scar how do you decided if it's a RCC or an oncocytoma? The way to figure it out is simple - just read the mind of the person who wrote the question. If it's a practical type then all enhancing renal masses are RCC till proven otherwise. If it's the academic type then central scar = oncocytoma. You may also think… which of these two people is more likely to volunteer to write board questions?

Trivia: A syndrome associated with bilateral oncocytomas is <u>Birt Hogg Dube</u> (they also get chromophobe RCC).

Multilocular Cystic Nephroma – "Non-communicating, fluid-filled locules, surrounded by thick fibrous capsule." By definition these things are characterized by the absence of a solid component or necrosis.

Buzzword is "protrudes into the renal pelvis."

The question is likely the bimodal occurrence (4 year old boys, and 40 year old women).

I like to think of this as the *Michael Jackson lesion – it loves young boys and middle aged women.*

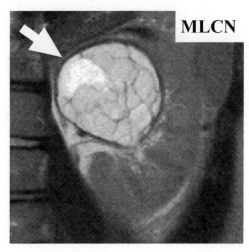

Cystic Disease

Bosniak Cyst Classification:
- Class 1: Simple – less than 15 H.U. with no enhancement
- Class 2: Hyperdense (< 3cm). Thin calcifications, Thin septations
- Class 2F: Hyperdense (>3cm). Minimally thickened calcifications (5% chance cancer)
- Class 3: Thick Septations, Mural Nodule (50% chance cancer)
- Class 4: Any enhancement (>15 H.U.)

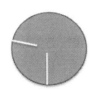
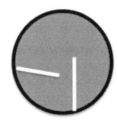
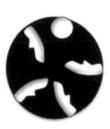
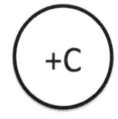

Class 1:
-Simple Anechoic
- 0% chance of CA

Class 2:
-Hyperdense (<3cm)
-Thin Calcifications
-Thin Septations
- 0% chance of CA

Class 2F:
-Hyperdense (>3cm)
-Thin Calcifications
- < 5% chance of CA

Class 3:
-Thick Calcifications
-Mural Nodule
-50% chance of CA

Class 4:
-Any Enhancement
-100% chance of CA

Hyperdense cysts: Basically, if the mass is _greater than 70 H.U._ and homogenous it's benign (hemorrhagic or proteinaceous cyst) 99.9% of the time.

Autosomal Dominant Polycystic Kidney Disease (ADPKD) – Kidneys get progressively larger and lose function (you get dialysis by 5th decade). Hyperdense contents & calcified wall are frequently seen due to prior hemorrhage. What you need to know is: (1) it's **A**utosomal **D**ominant "**AD**ult", (2) They get cysts in the liver 70% of the time, and (3) they get Berry Aneurysms. As mentioned before they don't have an intrinsic risk of cancer, but do get cancer once they are on dialysis.

Autosomal Recessive Polycystic Kidney Disease (ARPKD) – These guys get HTN, and renal failure. The liver involvement is different than the adult form. Instead of cysts they have abnormal bile ducts and fibrosis. This **congenital hepatic fibrosis is ALWAYS present in ARPKD**. The ratio of liver and kidney disease is inversely related. _The worse the liver is the better the kidneys do. The better the liver is the worse the kidneys are._ On ultrasound the kidneys are smoothly enlarged and diffusely echogenic, with a loss of corticomedullary differentiation.

Uremic Cystic Kidney Disease – About 40% of patients with end stage renal disease develop cysts. This rises with duration of dialysis in about 90% in patients after 5 year of dialysis. The thing to know is: **Increased risk of malignancy with dialysis (3-6x).**

Trivia: The cysts will regress after renal transplant

Von Hippel Lindau – Autosomal dominant multi-system disorder. 50-75% have renal cysts. 25-50% develop RCC (clear cell)

- Pancreas: - Cysts, Serous Microcystic Adenomas, Neuroendocrine (islet cell) tumor
- Adrenal: Pheochromocytoma (often multiple)
- CNS: Hemangioblastoma of the cerebellum, brain stem, and spinal cord

Tuberous Sclerosis – Autosomal dominant multi-system disorder. You have hamartomas everywhere (brain, lung, heart, skin, kidneys). The renal findings are bilateral multiple angiomyolipomas. They also have renal cysts, and occasionally RCC (same rate as general population, but in younger patient population). With regard to other organ systems:

- Lung – LAM – thin walled cysts and chylothorax
- Cardiac – Rhabdomyosarcoma (typically involve cardiac septum)
- Brain – Giant Cell Astrocytoma, Cortical and subcortical tubers, subependymal nodules
- Renal – AMLs, RCC (in younger patients)

Lithium Nephropathy – Occurs in patients who take lithium long term. Can lead to diabetes insipidus and renal insufficiency. The kidneys are normal to small in volume with multiple (innumerable) tiny cysts, usually 2-5mm in diameters. These "microcysts" are distinguishable from larger cysts associated with acquired cystic disease of uremia. They are probably going to show this on MRI with the history of bipolar disorder.

ADPKD	Cysts in Liver	Kidneys are BIG
VHL	Cysts in Pancreas	
Acquired (Uremic)		Kidneys are small

Multicystic Dsyplastic Kidney This is a peds thing, where you have multiple tiny cysts forming in utereo. What you need to know: (1) that there is "no functioning renal tissue," (2) contralateral renal tract abnormalities occur like 50% of the time.

MCDK vs Bad Hydro?

- In hydronephrosis the cystic spaces are seen to communicate.
- In difficult cases renal scintigraphy can be useful. MCDK will show no excretory function.

Peripelvic Cyst vs Parapelvic Cyst-

- Peri: Originates from renal sinus, mimics hydro
- Para: Originates from parenchyma, may compress the collecting system

T2 Dark Renal Cyst

Cysts are supposed to T2 bright. If you see the "T2 Dark Cyst" then you are dealing with the classic differential of:

(1) Lipid Poor AML
- A small percentage of AMLs are lipid poor in the general population.
- For the purpose of multiple choice - If you see a lipid poor AML (especially if your see a bunch of them) you need to think about Tuberous Sclerosis - about 30% of their AMLs are lipid poor.

(2) Hemorrhagic Cyst
- These will likely be T1 bright

(3) Papillary Subtype RCC
- Remember that clear cells (the most common sub-type) are T2 HYPER Intense.
- Both Clear Cell and Papillary will enhance, - but the clear cell enhances more avidly (equal to cortex on cortico-medullary phase).

Renal Infection

Pyelonephritis – This is a clinical diagnosis. However since ED doctors are universally stupid, you do end up diagnosing it. It's associated with stones. The most common organism is E. Coli. In acute bacterial nephritis, alternating bands of hypo and hyperattenuation (striated nephrogram) are seen. These wedge shaped areas are related to decreased perfusion. Perinephric stranding is also commonly seen.

> ***Striated Nephrogram DDx:***
>
> - Acute ureteral obstruction
> - Acute pyelonephritis
> - Medullary sponge kidney
> - Acute renal vein thrombosis
> - Radiation nephritis
> - Acutely following renal contusion
> - Hypotension (bilateral)
> - Infantile polycystic kidney (bilateral)

Abscess – Pyelo may be complicated by abscess, which can present on CT as round or geographic low attenuation collections that do not enhance centrally, but do have an enhancing rim. Bigger than 3cm and these guys might visit the IR section for drainage.

Chronic Pyelonephritis – Sort of a controversial entity. It is not clear whether the condition is an active chronic infection, arises from multiple recurrent infections, or represents stable changes from a remote single infection. The imaging findings are characterized by renal scarring, atrophy and cortical thinning, with hypertrophy of residual normal tissue. Basically, you have a small deformed kidney, with a bunch of wedge defects, and some hypertrophied areas.

Emphysematous Pyelonephritis – This is a life threatening necrotizing infection characterized by gas formation within or surrounding the kidney. What you need to know (1) it's really bad, (2) diabetics almost exclusively get it, (3) echogenic foci with dirty shadowing on ultrasound,

Emphysematous Pyelitis – This is less bad relative to emphysematous pyelonephritis. The gas is localized to the collecting system. It's more common in women, diabetics, and people with urinary obstruction. Radiographic finding is gas outlining the ureters and dilated calices.

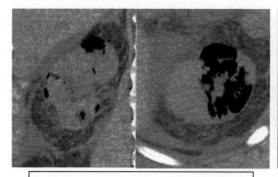

Emphysematous Pyelonephritis

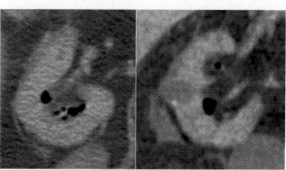

Emphysematous Pyelitis

Pyonephrosis – An infected or obstructed collecting system (which is frequently enlarged). Can be from a variety of causes; stones, tumor, sloughed papilla secondary to pyelonephritis. Can totally jack your renal function if left untreated. Fluid-Fluid level in the collecting system can be seen on US. CT has trouble telling the difference between hydro and pyonephrosis.

Xanthogranulomatous Pyelonephritis (XGP) – chronic destructive granulomatous process that is basically always seen with a staghorn stone acting as a nidus for recurrent infection. You can have an associated psoas abscess with minimal perirenal infection. It's an Aunt Minnie, with a very characteristic "Bear Paw" appearance on CT. The kidney is not functional, and sometimes nephrectomy is done to treat it.

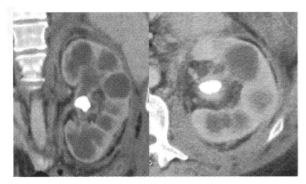

Xanthogranulomatous Pyelonephritis - *Bear Paw*

Papillary Necrosis: This is ischemic necrosis of the renal papillae, most commonly involving the medullary pyramids.

Diabetes is the most common cause.

Other important causes include; pyelonephritis (especially in kids), sickle cell, TB, analgesic use, and cirrhosis.

Filling defects might be seen in the calyx

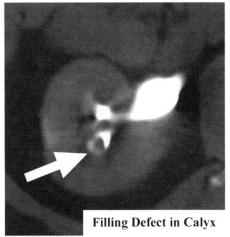

Filling Defect in Calyx

The appearance of a necrotic cavity in the papillae with linear streaks of contrast inside the calyx has been called a "lobster claw sign."

Trivia: 50% sickle cell patient's develop papillary necrosis

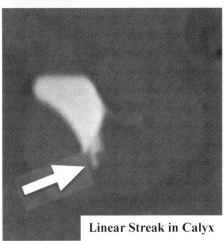

Linear Streak in Calyx

TB- The most common extrapulmonary site of infection is the urinary tract. There are features of papillary necrosis and parenchymal destruction. You can have extensive calcification. Basically you end up with a shrunken calcified kidney "putty kidney." This end stage appearance is essentially an auto nephrectomy. The "Kerr Kink" is a sign of renal TB with scarring leading to a sharp kink at the pelvi-ureteric junction.

HIV Nephropathy – Normal sized (or **big) kidneys that are echogenic on US**. Loss of the renal sinus fat appearance has also been described (it's edema in the fat, rather than loss of the actual fat).

Disseminated PCP in HIV patients can result in punctate (primarily cortical) calcifications.

Contrast Induced Nephropathy (CIN)

The more you read about this the more you realize it's probably complete (or at least near complete) bullshit. But, some academic people have made a career on it so we have to treat it like it's a real thing.

In your abundant free time, read this paper and become enlightened. I will warn you if you are a follower of conventional wisdom (you think books need to be published under a conventional publisher to be legitimate, you think screening mammography improves mortality, or you think the NSA is protecting you by recording all your cell phone conversations) this paper may make you cry.

Davenport, Matthew S., et al. "The challenges in assessing contrast-induced nephropathy: where are we now?." American Journal of Roentgenology 202.4 (2014): 784-789.

Trivia to know:
- Allergic reactions are a NOT considered a risk factor for CIN.
- "Risk Factors" for CIN include pre-existing renal insufficiency, diabetes mellitus (even more so with pre-existing renal insufficiency), cardiovascular disease with CHF, dehydration, and myeloma
- Hydration via IV with 1/2 normal saline 12 hours before and after contrast administration supposedly decreases the incidence of CIN in patients with chronic renal insufficiency (true mechanism is diluting Cr levels).

Renal Calcification / Misc:

Nephrolithiasis (kidney stones) – They are very common.

- *Calcium Oxalate* – by far the most common type (75%)
- *Struvite Stone* – More common in women, and associated with UTI
- *Uric Acid* – "Unseen" on x-ray
- *Cystine* – rare, and associated with congenital disorders of metabolism
- *Indinavir* – Stones in HIV patients, which are **the ONLY stones NOT seen on CT.**

Cortical Nephrocalcinosis – This is typically the sequella of cortical necrosis, which can be seen with an acute drop in blood pressure (shock, postpartum, burn patients, etc…). It starts out as a hypodense non-enhancing rim that later develops thin calcifications. Mimic is disseminated PCP.

Medullary Nephrocalcinosis – Hyperechoic renal papilla / pyramids which may or may not shadow. There are multiple causes, the most common of which is probably hyper PTH (*a few texts say medullary sponge kidney is most common*). Other things to think about include Lasix use (in a child), Renal Tubular Acidosis (distal subtype – or type 1), medullary sponge kidney (if asymmetric). RTA and Hyperparathyroid usually cause a more dense calcification than medullary sponge kidney.

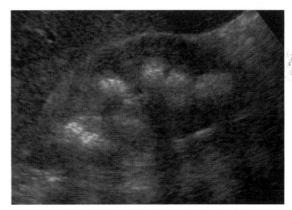

Medullary Nephrocalcinosis
-Hyperechoic Pyramids that shadow-

Medullary Sponge Kidney – A congenital cause of medullary nephrocalcinosis (usually asymmetric). The underlying mechanism is a cystic dilation of the collecting tubules of the kidney - so the testable association with Ehler Danlos makes sense. The association with Carolis sorta makes sense. The association with Beckwith-Weidman doesn't really make sense (and therefore is the most likely to be tested).

Think about medullary sponge kidney with unilateral medullary nephrocalcinosis.

Page Kidney – Sequella of long standing compression of the kidney by some kind of subcapsular collection (hematoma or seroma). The classic scenario is post lithotripsy subcapsular hematoma, with follow up showing a shrunk up kidney.

This vs That: Delayed vs Persistent Nephrogram

Delayed Nephrogram – One kidney enhances and the other doesn't (or does to a lesser degree). Basically this is happening from pressure on the kidney (either extrinsic from a Page kidney situation), or intrinsic from an obstructing stone.

Persistent Nephrogram – This is seen with hypotension/shock, and ATN. They can show this several ways, one would be on a plain film of the abdomen (with dense kidneys), the second would be on CT. The tip offs are going to be that they tell you the time (3 hours etc…), and it's gonna be bilateral.

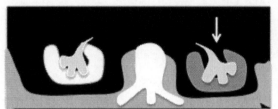
Delayed Nephrogram

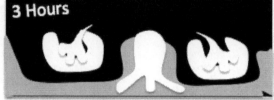
Persistent Nephrogram

Renal Infarct - So wedge shaped hypodensities in the kidney can be seen with lots of stuff (infarct, tumor, infection, etc…). Renal infarcts are most easily identified on post contrast imaging in the cortical phase. If the entire renal artery is out, well then it won't enhance (duh). Two tricks that they could pull are the (1) "Cortical Rim Sign" – which is absent immediately after the insult, but is seen 8 hours to days later. You have a dual blood supply, which allows the cortex to stay perfused. (2) "Flip Flop Enhancement" can be seen where a region of hypodensity / poor enhancement on early phases becomes relatively hyperdense on delayed imaging.

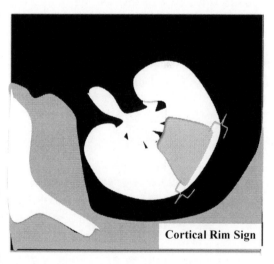
Cortical Rim Sign

Renal Vein Thrombosis – Numerous causes including dehydration, indwelling umbilical venous catheters (most common in neonates), and nephrotic syndrome (most common in adults). This can mimic a renal stone; presenting with flank pain, an enlarged kidney, and a delayed nephrogram. On Doppler they are going to show you Reversed arterial diastolic flow, and absent venous flow. *This is discussed again below - in the transplant section.*

Renal Trauma

Obviously the kidney can get injured in trauma (seen in about 10%). Injury can be graded based on the presence of hematoma -> laceration -> involvement of the vein, artery, or UPJ obstruction.

Gamesmanship: A good "Next Step" type question in the setting of renal trauma (or pelvic fracture) would be to prompt you to get delayed imaging - this is helpful to demonstrate a urine leak.

Terminology:

- *"Fractured Kidney"* - A laceration, which extends the full length of the renal parenchyma. By definition the laceration *must connect two cortical surfaces* - so think about it going all the way through.

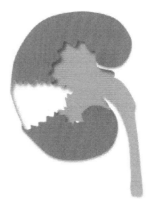

- *"Shattered Kidney"* - This is a more severe form of a fractured kidney. A kidney with 3 or more fragments - this is the most severe form of renal fracture.

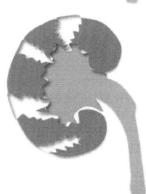

Renal Trauma - Rapid Pearls

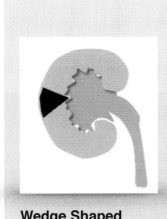

Wedge Shaped Perfusion Abnormality
- Think Segmental Artery Injury

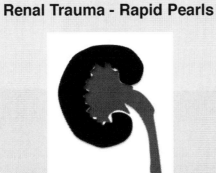

Diffuse NonPerfusion— Think Devascularized Kidney

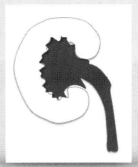

Persistent Nephrogram — Think Renal Vein Injury / Thrombosis

Renal Transplant

Renal transplant is the best treatment for end stage renal disease, and the quality of life is significantly better that of a long term dialysis patient. The transplanted kidney is most commonly placed in the extraperitoneal iliac fossa so that the allograft can be anastomosed with the iliac vasculature and urinary bladder.

Normal: A transplant kidney is just like a native kidney. It should have low resistance (it's always "on"). The upstroke should be brisk, and the flow in diastole forward (remember it's always "on").

Significance of RIs: If the meat of the kidney becomes "sick" from whatever the cause might be (rejection, infection, inflammation, etc…) it starts to increase resistance. This increased resistance raises you RI - the higher the RI the sicker the kidney. This is why RIs are useful, and this is why an upward trend in RI is worrisome. RI's should stay below 0.7, higher than that should trigger you to think something is wrong.

You can think of complications in 3 main flavors (a) Urologic, (b) Vascular, (c) Cancer.

Urologic Complications:

Urinoma – This is usually found in the first 2 weeks post op. Urine leak or urinoma will appear as an anechoic fluid collection with no septations, that is rapidly increasing in size. MAG 3 nuclear medicine scan can be used to demonstrate this (or the cheaper ultrasound).

Hematoma – Common immediately post op. Usually resolves spontaneously. Large hematoma can produce hydro. Acute hematoma will be echogenic, and this will progressively become less echogenic (with older hematomas more anechoic and septated).

Lymphocele – Lymphoceles typically occur **1-2 months after transplant**. They are caused by leakage of lymph from surgical disruption of lymphatics. The fluid collection is usually medial to the transplant (between the graft and the bladder).

Acute Rejection / ATN: Up to 20% of transplant patients will have some early rejection. Both ATN and Acute rejection tend to occur in the first week or so. On ultrasound the pyramids become prominent, the transplant itself gets bigger, and the RIs go up. ATN vs Acute Rejection is best distinguished on MAG-3; where the ATN has normal perfusion and the Rejection does not (both will have delayed excretion).

Chronic Rejection – This occurs one year post transplant. The kidney may enlarge, and you can lose corticomedullary differentiation. The RIs will elevate (>0.7) which is nonspecific.

Calculus Disease – Compared with the general population, transplant kidneys are at increased risk of stone formation.

Vascular Complications:

Renal Artery Thrombosis – Occurs in 1% of renal transplants within the 1st week. Typically caused by kinking, hypercoagulation, or hyperacute rejection.

Renal Artery Stenosis – Occurs in 5-10% renal transplants. This usually occurs at the anastomosis. Criteria include:
- PSV > 200-300 cm/s.
- PSV ratio > 3.0 (External Iliac Artery /RA)
- Tardus Parvus: Measured at the Main Renal Artery Hilum (NOT at the arcuates)
- Anastomotic Jetting

Renal Vein Thrombosis - This is more common in the 2nd week post transplant. Typically the kidney is swollen. Instead of showing you the Doppler of the renal vein (which would show no flow), they will most likely show you the artery, which classically has reversed diastolic flow.

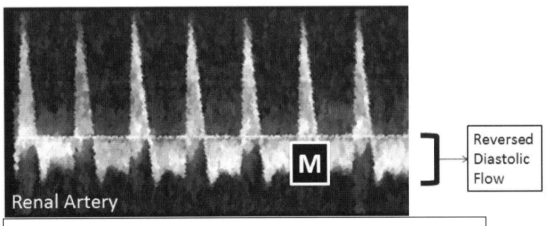

Renal Vein Thrombosis - with the artery showing reversal of diastolic flow. Some people call this the "reverse M sign."

Arteriovenous Fistula (AVF) – These occur secondary to biopsy. They occur about 20% of the time post biopsy, but are usually small and asymptomatic. They will likely show it with **tissue vibration artifact** (Perivascular, mosaic color assignment due to tissue vibration), with high arterial velocity, and pulsatile flow in the vein.

Pseudoaneurysm – These also occur secondary to biopsy, but are less common. They can also occur in the setting of graft infection, or anastomotic dehiscence. They will most likely show you the classic "yin-yang" color picture. Alternatively, they could show Doppler with a biphasic flow at the neck of the pseudoaneurysm.

Cancer in the Transplant

The prolonged immunosuppression therapy that renal transplant patients are on places them at significant (100x) increased risk of developing cancer.

RCC – Increased risk, with most of the cancers (90%) actually occurring in the native kidney. Etiology is not totally understood; maybe it's the immunosuppression or the fact that many transplant patients were on dialysis (a known risk factor) that leads to the cancer risk. In reality it doesn't matter, and is probably both.

Post Transplant Lymphoproliferative Disorder (PTLD) – This is an uncommon complication of organ transplant, associated with B-Cell proliferation. It is most common in the first year post transplant, and often involves multiple organs. The treatment is to back off the immunosuppression.

Cyclophosphamide – As a point of trivia, significant exposure to cyclophosphamide (less common now with the development of cyclosporin A) is associated with increased risk of urothelial cancer.

Renal Transplant Complications			
Week 1	Weeks 1-4	Months 1-6	After 6 Months
Renal Artery Thrombosis	Renal Vein Stenosis (more common)	Drug Toxicity	Chronic Rejection
Renal Artery Stenosis (more common)	Lymphocele	Lymphocele	RCC
Hematoma		Biopsy Related Injury (Pseudoaneurysm, AV Fistula)	Lymphoma
Urinoma			PTLD

Ureters

Normal Anatomy – The ureters run anterior to the psoas muscle, and empty at lateral angles of the bladder trigone. They have 3 layers, with the inner layer being transitional epithelium.

Developmental Ureter Anomalies

Congenital (primary) MEGAureter – This is a "wastebasket" term, for an enlarged ureter which is intrinsic to the ureter (as opposed to the result of a distal obstruction). Causes include (1) Distal adynamic segment (analogous to achalasia, or colonic Hirschsprungs), (2) reflux at the UVJ, (3) it just wants to be big (totally idiopathic). The distal adynamic type "obstructing primary megaureter" can have some hydro, but generally speaking an absence of dilation of the collecting system helps distinguish this from an actual obstruction. Most cases just have dilation of the lower 1/3. It is almost always unilateral (favoring the left side).

Retrocaval Ureter (circumcaval) - Although the name implies that this is the result of a maldeveloped ureter, it's actually a developmental anomaly of the IVC. Most of the time it's asymptomatic, but can cause partial obstruction, and recurrent UTI. IVP will show a "reverse J" or "fishhook" appearance of the ureter.

Duplicated System – The main thing to know about duplicated systems is the so called "Weigert-Meyer Rule" where the upper pole inserts inferior and medially. The upper pole is prone to ureterocele formation and obstruction. The lower pole is prone to reflux.

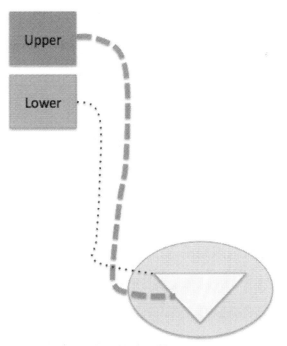

Weigert-Meyer Rule
- *Upper Pole inserts medial and inferior*

Ureterocele – A cystic dilation of the intravesicular ureter, secondary to obstruction at the ureteral orifice. IVP will show the "cobra head" sign, with contrast surrounded by a lucent rim, protruding from the contrast filled bladder. This is associated with a duplicated system (specifically the upper pole). Ureteroceles are best demonstrated during the early filling phase of the VCUG. *There is a picture of this in the Peds chapter (page 197).*

Pseudoureterocele - This is an acquired dilation of the submucosal portion of the distal ureter. A loss of the normal lucent line around the "cobra head" suggests a pseudoureterocele. Causes include an impacted stone, a recently passed stone, and a bladder malignancy.

Ectopic Ureter – The ureter inserts distal to the external spincter in the vestibule. More common in females and associated with incontinence (not associated with incontinence in men).

Vesicoureteral Reflux – Refers to retrograde flow of urine. The supposed malfunction is that the course of the ureter is too short as it crosses the bladder, messing with the ureteral valve mechanism. This is really a Peds thing, and discussed more in the peds chapter.

Congenital UPJ Obstruction – This is the **most common congenital anomaly of the GU tract in neonates**. About 20% of the time, these are bilateral. Most (80%) of these are thought to be caused by intrinsic defects in the circular muscle bundle of the renal pelvis. Treatment is a pyeloplasty. A Radiologist can actually add value by looking for vessels crossing UPJ prior to pyeloplasty, as this changes the management.

Things to know about UPJ Obstruction
- Most common congenital anomaly of the GU tract
- Associated with Crossing Vessels (early branching lower pole vessels compress the ureter)
- Associated with Multicystic Dysplastic Kidney on the other side.

1970 called

They want to know how to tell the difference between a prominent extrarenal pelvis vs a congenital UPJ obstruction.

The Answer is a "Whitaker Test", which is a urodynamics study combined with antegrade pyelogram.

Ureter Infection / Inflammation

Stones – Stones tend to lodge in 3 spots: UPJ, UVJ, pelvic brim.

Ureteral Wall Calcifications – Wall calcifications should make you think about two things: (1) TB, (2) Schistosomiasis.

Ureteritis cystica - Numerous tiny subepithelial fluid filled cysts within the wall of the ureter. The condition is the result of chronic inflammation (from stones, chronic and/or infection). Typically this is seen in diabetics with recurrent UTI. There may be an increased risk of cancer.

Ureteral pseudodiverticulosis – This is similar to ureteritis cystica in that both conditions are the result of chronic inflammation (stones, infection). Instead of being cystic filling defects, these guys are multiple small outpouchings. They are bilateral 75% of the times, and favor the upper and middle third. There is an association with malignancy.

Leukoplakia – This is essentially squamous metaplasia secondary to chronic irritations (stones or infections). The bladder is more commonly involved than the ureter. Imaging findings are unlikely to be shown, but would be mural filling defects. The question is most likely this : Leukoplakia is considered premalignant and the cancer is squamous cell.

Trivia to know: Leukoplakia is associated with squamous cell carcinoma NOT transitional cell

Malacoplakia – This is also an inflammatory condition that occurs in the setting of chronic UTIs (highly associated with E.Coli). It's **often seen in female immunocompromised patients**. This also has plaque-like or nodular intramural lesions, where bugs are incompletely digested. Since malacoplakia most frequently manifests as a mucosal mass involving the ureter or bladder, the most common renal finding is obstruction secondary to a lesion in the lower tract. Step 1 buzzword = Michaelis-Gutmann Bodies. Again, the bladder is more commonly affected. The question is most likely this: Malacoplakia is NOT premalignant, and usually gets better with antibiotics.

Leukoplakia = Premalignant
Malacoplakia = Not Premalignant

Retroperitoneal Fibrosis – This condition is characterized by proliferation of aberrant fibro-inflammatory tissue, which typically surrounds the aorta, IVC, iliac vessels, and frequently traps and obstructs the ureters. It is idiopathic 75% of the time. Other causes include prior radiation, medications (methyldopa, ergotamine, methysergide), inflammatory causes (pancreatitis, pyelonephritis, inflammatory aneurysm), and malignancy (desmoplastic reaction, lymphoma).

Things (trivia) you need to know:
- *Mostly (80%) idiopathic "Ormond Disease"*
- *Associated with IgG4 disorders (autoimmune pancreatitis, riedels thyroid, inflammatory pseudotumor)*
- *Classically shown with medial deviation of ureters*
- *It's more common in men*
- *Malignancy associated RP fibrosis occurs about 10% of the time (some people advocate using PET to find a primary)*
- *The Fibrosis will be Gallium avid, and PET hot in its early stages and cold in its late stages (mirroring its inflammatory stages). Metabolically active RP fibrosis will show increased FDG and Gallium uptake, regardless of a benign or malignant underlying cause*

Subepithelial Renal Pelvis Hematoma: This tends to occur in patients on long term anticoagulation. You are going to have a thickened upper tract wall - which is a classic **mimic for TCC**. They will have to show you pre and post contrast to show you that it's **hyper dense on the pre-contrast and does NOT enhance.**

Lower Tract Cancer

Transitional Cell Carcinoma – This histologic subtype makes up a very large majority (90%) of the collecting system cancers. Imaging buzzword is "goblet" or "champagne glass sign" on CT IVP.

Risk Factors:
- Smoking
- Azo Dye
- Cyclophosphamide
- Aristolochic acid (Balkan Nephropathy – see below)
- Horseshoe Kidney
- Stones
- Ureteral Pseudodiverticulosis
- Hereditary Non-Polyposis Colon Cancer (type 2)

Some high yield statistical trivia (seriously this is high yield):
- Ureter is the least common location for TCC of the urinary tract
- TCC of the renal pelvis is 2x -3x times more common than ureter
- TCC of the bladder is 100x times more common than ureter
- In the ureter 75% of the TCCs are in the bottom 1/3
- If you have upper tract TCC there is a 40% chance of developing a bladder TCC
- If you have bladder TCC there is a 4% chance of developing a Renal Pelvis or Ureteral TCC
- Ureteral TCC is bilateral 5%

Balkan Nephropathy – This is some zebra degenerative nephropathy endemic to the Balkan States. The only reason I mention it is that it has a super high rate of renal pelvis and upper ureter TCCs. It's thought to be secondary to eating aristolochic acid (AA) in seeds of the Aristolochia clematitis plant.

Squamous cell - This is much less common than TCC (in the US anyway). The major predisposing factor is schistosomiasis (they both start with an "S").

Hematogenous Metastasis – Mets to the ureters are rare but can occur (GI, Prostate, Renal, Breast). They typically infiltrate the periureteral soft tissues, and demonstrate Transmural involvement.

Fibroepithelial Polyp - This is a benign entity, which is usually located in the proximal ureter and produces a smooth, oblong, mobile defect on urography.

Deviation of the Ureters
- Classic This vs That -

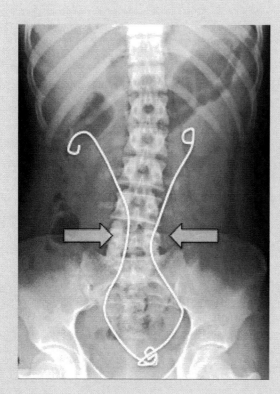
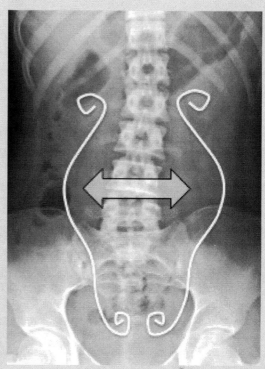

Medial Deviation "Waisting" of the Ureters	Lateral Deviation of the Ureters
Retroperitoneal Fibrosis	Retroperitoneal Adenopathy
Retrocaval Ureter (right side)	Aortic Aneurysm
Pelvic Lipomatosis	
Psoas Hypertrophy *(distal ureter)*	Psoas Hypertrophy *(proximal ureter)*

Bladder

Normal anatomy: Normal bladder is an extraperitoneal structure, with 4 layers. The dome of the bladder has a peritoneal cover. It's lined with transitional urothelium.

Developmental Anomalies

Prune Belly (Eagle Barrett) – This is a malformation triad which occurs in males. This is classically shown with a baby gram with a kid shaped like a pear (big wide belly).

Triad:
- Deficiency of abdominal musculature
- Hydroureteronephrosis
- Cryptorchidism (bladder distention interferes with descent of testes)

Bladder Diverticula – These are more common in boys, and can be seen in a few situations. Most bladder diverticula can also be acquired secondary to chronic outlet obstruction (big prostate). There are a few syndromes (Ehlers Danlos is the big testable one) that you see them in as well.

The "Hutch Diverticulum:" This thing occurs at the UVJ and is NOT associated with posterior urtheral valves, or neurogenic bladder. The Hutch is associated with reflux (because the normal slanted insertion of the ureter is altered).

Things to know:
- Hutch Diverticula are associated with ipsilateral reflux
- Bladder Diverticula typically arise from the lateral walls or near the ureteral orifices
- Diverticula at the anterior / superior bladder are more likely to be urachal diverticula.
- Most Diverticula are acquired (not congenital)
- Ureters more commonly deviate medially adjacent to a diverticula

Bladder Ears – "Transitory extraperitoneal herniation of the bladder" if you want to sound smart. This is not a diverticulum. Instead, it's transient lateral protrusion of the bladder into the inguinal canal. It's very common to see, and likely doesn't mean crap. However, some sources say an inguinal hernia may be present 20% of the time. Smooth walls, and usually wide necks can help distinguish them from diverticula.

Cloacal Malformation – GU and GI both drain into a common opening (like a bird). This only happens in females.

Urachus – The umbilical attachment of the bladder (initially the allantois then urachus) usually atrophies and becomes the umbilical ligament (as the bladder descends into the pelvis). A persistent patent urachus can result in urine flow from the bladder to the umbilicus (and then likely someone's unsuspecting face). There is a spectrum of these things from patent -> sinus -> diverticulum -> Cyst. They can get infected. Really **the main thing to know is that they get adenocarcinoma**. It's midline and they get adenocarcinoma.

Bladder Cancer

Rhabdomyosarcoma – This is the most common bladder cancer in humans less than 10 years of age. They are often infiltrative, and it's hard to tell where they originate. "Paratesticular Mass" is often a buzzword. They can met to the lungs, bones, and nodes. The Botryoid variant produces a polypoid mass, which looks like a bunch of grapes.

Transitional Cell Carcinoma – As stated above, the bladder is the most common site, and this is by far the most common subtype. All the risk factors, are the same as above. If anyone would ask "superficial papillary" is the most common TCC bladder subtype.

Squamous Cell Carcinoma – When I say Squamous Cell Bladder, you say Schistosomiasis. This is convenient because they both start with an "S." The classic picture is a heavily calcified bladder and distal ureters (usually shown on plain film, but could also be on CT).

Adenocarcinoma of the Bladder – This is a common trick question. When I say Adenocarcinoma of the Bladder, you say Urachus. 90% of urachal cancers are located midline at the bladder dome.

Leiomyoma – Benign tumor (not cancer). It's often incidentally discovered (most common at the trigone). If anyone asks it's the most common mesenchymal bladder tumor.

Bladder Cancer

Typical = **T**ransitional Cell
Schistosomiasis = **S**quamous
Urachus = Adenocarcinoma
Kids = Rhabdomyosarcoma

Diversion Surgery

After radial cystectomy for bladder cancer there are several urinary diversion procedures that can be done. People generally group these into incontinent and continent procedures. There are a ton of these (over 50 have been described). I just want to touch on the big points, and focus on complications (the most testable subject matter). The general idea is that a piece of bowel is made into either a conduit or reservoir, and then the ureters are attached to it.

Early Complications:

- *Alteration in bowel function:* **Adynamic ileus is the most common early complication**, occurring in almost 25% of cases. In about 3% of cases you can get SBO, usually from adhesive disease near the enteroenteric anastomosis.

- *Urinary Leakage:* This occurs in about 5% of cases, and usually at the ureteral-reservoir anastomsis. A urinoma can develop when the leaked urine is not collected by urinary drains.

- *Fistula:* This is uncommon and seen more in patients who have had pelvic radiation.

Late Complications (> 30 days)

- *Urinary infection:* This can be early or late.

- *Stones:* Remember to look on the non-contrasted study.

- *Parastomal Herniation:* This occurs about 15% of the time with ileal conduits. Obesity is a contributing factor. Most don't matter, but 10% will need a surgical fix.

- *Urinary stricture:* The **left side is higher risk than the right**, secondary to the angulation (it's brought through or under the mesentery).

- *Tumor Recurrence:* The more advanced the original disease, the higher the risk for recurrence. The incidence is between 3-15%, and can present as a soft tissue mass at the ureter, bladder, or a pelvic lymph node.

Infectious / Inflammation

Emphysematous Cystitis – Gas forming organism in the wall of the bladder. More than half the time it's a diabetic patient. It's usually from E. Coli. It's gonna be very obvious on plain film and CT. Ultrasound would be sneaky, and you'd see dirty shadowing.

TB – The upper GU tract is more commonly effected, with secondary involvement of the bladder. Can eventually lead to a thick contracted bladder. Calcifications might be present.

Schistosomiasis – Common in the third world. Eggs are deposited in the bladder wall which leads to chronic inflammation. Things to know: the entire bladder will calcify (often shown on plain film or CT), and you get squamous cell cancer.

Fistula – This occurs basically in 3 conditions; (1) diverticulitis, (2) Crohns, (3) Cancer. They are more common in men, although women are at significantly increased risk after hysterectomy (the uterus protects the bladder).

> **Most Common Cause**
>
> - Colovesicial Fistula = Diverticular Disease
> - Ileovesical Fistulas = Crohns
> - Rectovesical Fistulas = Neoplasm or Trauma

Neurogenic Bladder – This comes in two flavors: (a) small contracted bladder, (b) atonic large bladder. The buzzword / classic sign is *"pine cone" bladder*, because of its appearance. It can lead to urine stasis, and that stasis can predispose to bladder CA, **stones**, and infection.

Acquired Bladder Diverticula - As mentioned above, these can be acquired mainly via outlet obstruction (just think big prostate). They are most common at the UVJ. They can lead to stasis, and that stasis can predispose to bladder CA, stones, and infection.

Bladder Stones – These guys show up in two scenarios: (1) they are born as kidney stones and drop into the bladder (2) they develop in the bladder secondary to stasis (outlet obstruction, or **neurogenic bladder**). They can cause chronic irritation and are a known risk factor for both TCC and SCC.

"Pear Shaped Bladder" – This is more of a sign than a pathology. Think two things (1) pelvic lipomatosis, and (2) hematoma.

Bladder Trauma

Bladder Rupture – What they want you to know is; extra versus intra peritoneal rupture. CT Cystography (contrast distending bladder) is needed.

- *Extraperitoneal* – This one is **more common (80-90%)**. Almost always associated with pelvic fracture. This can be managed medically.

    o If there is a pelvic fracture, then the chance of a bladder rupture is 10%.
    o If there is a bladder rupture, there is almost always a pelvic fracture

    o Molar Tooth Sign: Contrast surrounding the bladder, in the prevesicle space of Rezius. This indicated extraperitoneal bladder rupture.

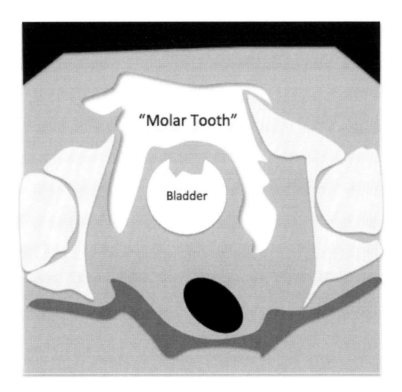

- *Intraperitoneal* This one is less common. Direct blow to a full bladder, basically pops the balloon and blows the top off (bladder dome is the weakest part). The dude will have contrast outlining bowel loops and in the paracolic gutters. This requires surgery.

The Urethra
(the length is variable)

Male:

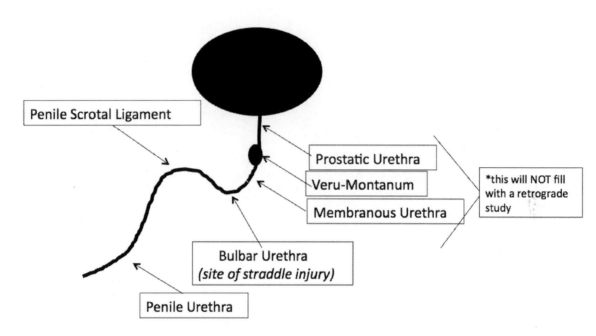

Normal Anatomy (most commonly seen on a RUG), is high yield.

There are really only about three things to know other than anatomy: Urethral Injury, Urethrorectal fistula, Infection, and Diverticulum (with cancer implications).

Trauma: Urethral injuries are graded based on their location (1-5).

- *Type 1: Stretched – periurethral hematoma would be present. This is not well seen on RUG.*
- *Type 2: Rupture ABOVE the UG diaphragm. Extraperitoneal contrast is present.*
- *Type 3: Rupture BELOW the UG diaphragm. Extraperioneal and perineal contrast is present.*
- *Type 4: Injury involves the bladder extending to the urethra.*
- *Type 5: There is injury to the anterior urethra.*

Urethral Strictures -

The Bicycle Crossbar Injury *vs* The Injury From a Woman of Questionable Moral Standard

Straddle Injury: The most common external cause of traumatic stricture is this type of mechanism. The physiology is compression of the urethra against the inferior edge of the pubic symphysis. **The bulbous urethra is the site of injury** (this is the most likely question).

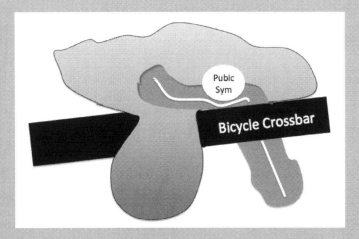

Gonococcal Urethral Stricture: This tends to be a **long irregular stricture** (the straddle stricture was short). It occurs in the **distal bulbous urethra**.

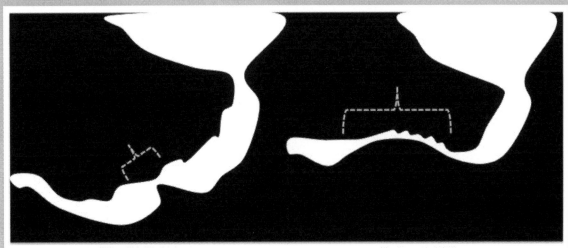

Straddle Injury
Short Segment – Bulbous Urethra

Gonococcal
Long Segment & Irregular – Bulbous Urethra

Other Male Urethral Pathologies:

Pancreatic Transplant: This has been known to cause urethral injury, if the drainage is to the bladder (the old way of doing it). Extravasation from urethral injury is said to occur in about 5% of cases, and is secondary to pancreatic enzymes jacking the urethra.

Condyloma Acuminata – Multiple small filling defects seen on a RUG should make you think this. Although, instrumentation including a retrograde urethrography is actually not recommended because of the possibility of retrograde seeding.

Urethrorectal Fistula: This may occur post radiation, and is classically described with brachytherapy (occurs in 1% of patients).

Urethral Diverticulum: In a man, this is almost always the result of long term foley placement.

Cancer: Malignant tumors of the male urethra are rare. When they do occur **80% are squamous cell cancers** (the *exception is that prostatic urethra actually has transitional cell 90% of the time*).

Urethral Diverticulum Cancer: Cancer in a urethral diverticulum is nearly **ALWAYS adenocarcinoma** (rather than squamous cell).

Female:

Female Urethral Diverticulum: Urethral diverticulum is way more common in females. They are usually the result of repeated infection of the periurethral glands (classic **history is "repeated urinary tract infections"**).

In case books and conferences this is **classically shown as a Sagittal MRI**. It often coexists with stress urinary incontinence (60%) and urinary infection. The **buzzword is "saddle-bag"** configuration, which supposedly is how you tell it from the urethra. Stones can also develop in these things. All this infection and irritation leads to **risk of cancer**, and the very common **high yield factoid is this is most commonly adenocarcinoma (60%).**

Penis:

Anatomy of this thing is cross section:

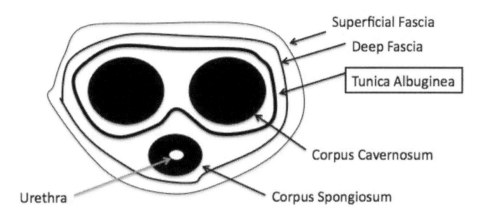

Fractured Penis: This is one of the most tragic situations that can occur in medicine. Can result from a variety of scenarios, but anecdotally seems to be most common in older men having extra-marital sex with dirty strippers (while on viagra and cocaine).

They can show it on ultrasound (look for hematoma) or MRI (look for hematoma). The piece of trivia you should remember is this is **defined by fracture corpus cavernosum and its surrounding sheath, the tunica albuginea.**

Prostate

Cancer: Biopsy of the prostate is a terrible terrible situation, worse than anything you can imagine in a 1000 years of hell. As a result, MRI of the prostate (instead of biopsy) is getting to be a hot topic. You can use prostate MRI for high risk screening (high or rising PSA with negative biopsy), or to stage (look from extracapsular extension).

First lets talk about prostate anatomy: Anatomists like to use "zones" to describe locations, and it actually helps with pathology. The anterior fibromuscular gland is dark on T1 and T2. The central and transitional zones (together called the *"central gland"*) are brighter than the anterior muscular zone, but less bright than the peripheral zone on T2. In other words the **peripheral zone is the most T2 bright**.

Adenocarcinoma:
- Peripheral Zone: 70%
- Transition Zone: 20%
- Central Zone: 10 %

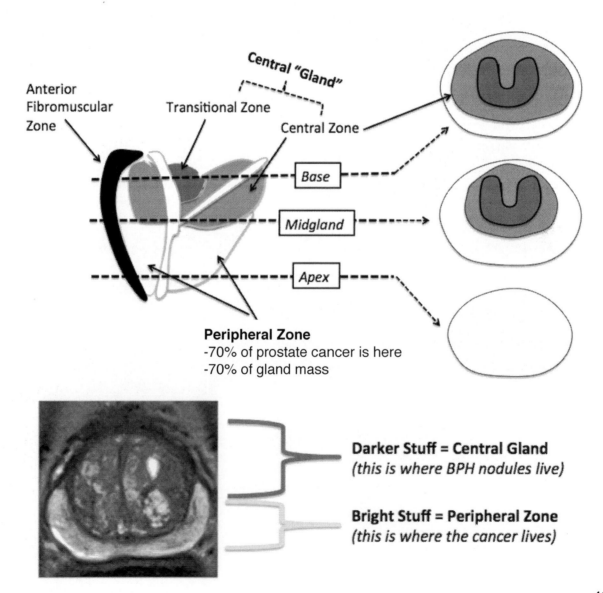

MRI finding for Prostate CA: **Cancer is dark on T2** (background is high), restricts on diffusion (low on ADC), and enhances early and washes out (type 3 curve - just like a breast cancer).

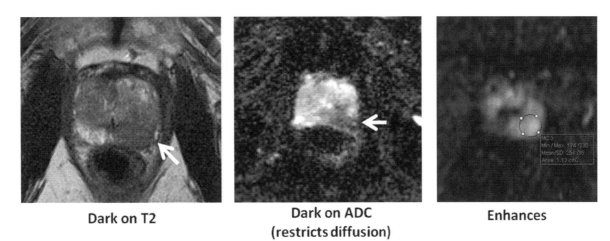

Dark on T2   Dark on ADC (restricts diffusion)   Enhances

Bone scan is the money for prostate mets (vertebral body mets).

Staging: The main thing to know is stage B vs stage C, as extra capsular extension is the most important factor governing treatment.

Stage B	Stage C
Confined by capsule	Extension through capsule
Abutment of the capsule without bulging	Bulging of the capsule, or frank extension through it

Seminal vesicles and the nerve bundle are also right behind the prostate and can get invaded (urologists love to hear about that).

BPH: Obviously this is super common, and makes old men pee a lot. Volume of 30cc is one definition. **Most commonly involves the transitional zone** (cancer is rare in the transition zone – 10%). The **median lobe** is the one that hypertrophies and sticks up into the bladder. It can cause outlet obstruction, bladder wall thickening (detrusor hypertrophy), and development of diverticulum.

The IVP buzzword is "J shaped" or "Fishhook" shaped ureter.

With regard to the BPH nodules you see on MRI, they are usually:
- In the transitional Zone
- T2 Heterogenous
- Can Restrict Diffusion
- May enhance and washout

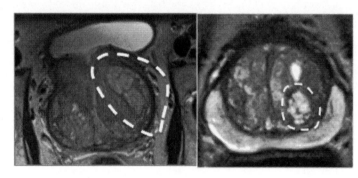

BPH Nodules
- *Bright / Heterogeneous Shit in the Central Gland*

Post Biopsy Changes: This is going to be T1 bright stuff in the gland. It's subacute blood.

Prostate Summary Chart

	T2	ADC	Enhancement
Peripheral Zone Tumor	Dark	Dark	Early Enhancement, Early Washout
Peripheral Zone Hemorrhage *Like after a biopsy*	Dark (sometimes T1 bright)	Dark (less dark)	None
Central Gland / Transitional Tone Tumor	Dark "Charcoal"	Dark	Early Enhancement, Early Washout
BPH	Dark "Well Defined"	Less Dark	Can enhance

Misc Male Reproductive Conditions

Prostatic Utricle Cyst / Mullerian Duct Cyst: Some people try and distinguish between a prostatic utricle, and a mullerian duct cyst. They look very very similar. The Mullerian duct cyst is an anatomic variant of the caudal ends of the mullerian ducts (male equivalent of the vagina / cervix). The prostatic utricle is a focal dilation in the prostatic urethra. This can be shown with multiple imaging modalities. Think about it if you see a **midline cystic structure near the bladder of a man.** A sneaky trick would be to show it on a RUG, where a prostate utricle cyst would look like a focal out-pouching from the prostatic urethra.

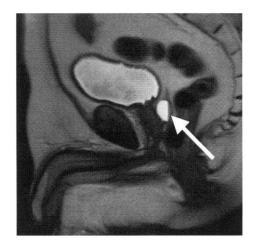

Things to know (prostatic utricle cyst):
 •*Hypospadias is the most common associated condition*
 •*Prune Belly Syndrome, Downs, unilateral renal agenesis, and Imperforate Anus are also associated*
 •*If its large, it can get infected*

Things to know (mullerian duct cyst)
 •*Does not have the same associations as utricle cyst*
 •*Can contain cancer (various types: endometrial, clear cell, squamous).*

Seminal Vesicle Cysts: The classic look is a **unilateral, lateral cyst** (lateral to the prostate). If they get large they can look midline, but if they show you a large one you won't be able to tell it from the utricle cyst. They can be congenital or acquired.

Congenital Trivia:
 •*Associated with renal agenesis*
 •*Associated with vas deferens agenesis*
 •*Associated with ectopic ureter insertion*
 •*Associated with polycystic kidney disease*

Acquired Trivia:
 •*Obstruction often from prostatic hypertrophy, or chronic infection/scarring*
 •*Classic history is prior prostate surgery*

Male Pelvic Cysts	
Midline	*Lateral*
Prostatic Utricle	Seminal Vesicle Cyst
Mullerian Duct Cyst	Diverticulosis of the ampulla of vas deferens
Ejaculatory Duct Cysts	

Testicular Trauma: The big distinction is rupture vs fracture. Surgical intervention is required if there is testicular rupture. Intratesticular fracture, and hematomas (small) do not get surgery.

- *Rupture:* Disrupted tunica albuginia, heterogenous testicle, poorly defined testicular outline
- *Fracture:* Intact tunica albuginia, linear hypoechoic band across the parenchyma of the testicle, well defined testicular outline.

Torsion of the Testicle – Results from the testis and spermatic cord twisting within the serosal space leading to ischemia. If it was 1950 you'd call in your nuclear medicine tech for scintigraphy. Now you just get a Doppler ultrasound. Findings will be absent or asymmetrically decreased flow, asymmetric enlargement and slightly decreased echogenicity of the affected testis.

- *Cause:* The "bell-clapper deformity" which describes an abnormal high attachment of the tunical vaginalis, increases mobility and predisposes to torsion. It is usually a bilateral finding, so the contralateral side gets an orchiopexy.

- *Viability:* The viability is related to the degree of torsion (how many spins), and how long it has been spun. As a general rule, the surgeons try and get them in the OR before 6 hours.

Epididymitis – Inflammation of the epididymis, and the most common cause of acute onset scrotal pain in adults. In sexually active men the typical cause is chlamydia or gonorrhea. In older men its more likely to be e-coli, due to a urinary tract source. The epididymal head is the most affected. Increased size and hyperemia are your ultrasound findings. You can have infection of the epididymis alone or infection of the epididymis and testicle (isolated orichitis is rare).

Orichitis – Typically progresses from epididymitis (isolated basically only occurs from mumps). It looks like asymmetric hyperemia.

Epidermoid Cysts: This is a benign mass of the testicle (no malignant potential), with an Aunt Minnie "**onion skin**" look, - alternating hypoechoic and hyperechoic rings. It's relatively non-vascular relative to the rest of the testicle.

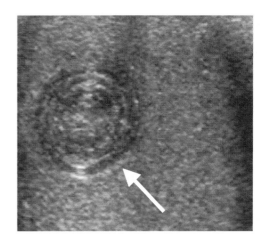

Tubular Ectasia of the Rete Testis: This is a common benign finding, resulting from obliteration (complete or partial) of the efferent ducts. It's usually bilateral - and in older men. The location of the cystic dilation is next to the mediastinum testis. Think about this as a normal variant. It requires no follow up or further evaluation.

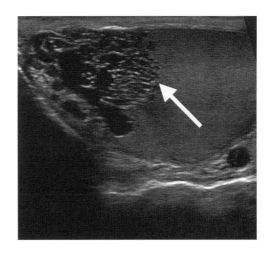

Calcified Vas Deferens: You see this all the time in bad **diabetics.**

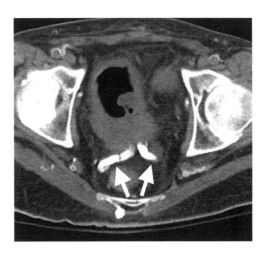

Testicular Cancer:

Testicle Cancer in the pediatric setting is discussed in the pediatric chapter. This discussion will focus of the adult subtypes (with some overlap).

In general, hypoechoic solid intratesticular masses should be thought of as cancer until proven otherwise. Doppler flow can be helpful only when it is absent (can suggest hematoma - in the right clinical setting). If it's extratesticular and cystic it's probably benign. The step 1 trivia is that cryptorchidism increases the risk of cancer (in both testicles), and is not reduced by orchiopexy. Most testicular tumors met via the lymphatics (retroperitoneal nodes at the level of the renal hilum). The testable exception is choriocarcinoma, which mets via the blood. Most testicular cancers are germ cell subtypes (95%) - with seminomas making up about half of those.

Risk Factors: Cryptorchidism (for both testicles), Gonadal Dysgenesis, Klinefelters, Trauma, Orchitis, and testicular microlithiasis (maybe).

Testicular Mircolithiasis – This appears as multiple small echogenic foci within the testes. Testicular microlithiasis is usually an incidental finding in scrotal US examinations performed for unrelated reasons. It <u>might</u> have a relationship with Germ Cell Tumors (controversial). Follow-up in 6 months, then yearly is probably the recommendation - although this recommendation is controversial.

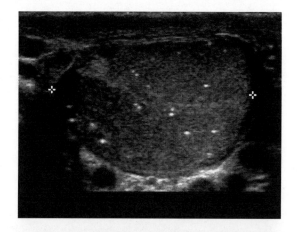

Seminoma: This is the most common testicular tumor, and has the best prognosis as they are very radiosensitive. They are much more common (9x) in white people. The classic age is around 25. It usually looks like a homogenous hypoechoic round mass, which classically replaces the entire testicle. On MRI they are usually homogeneously T2 dark (non-seminomatous GCTs are often higher in signal).

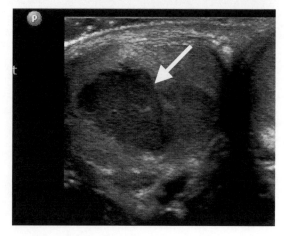

Non-Seminomatous Germ Cell Tumors: Basically this is not a seminoma. We are talking about mixed germ cell tumors, teratomas, yolk sac tumors, and choriocarcinoma. They typically occur at a young age relative to seminomas (think teenager). They are more heterogenous and have larger calcifications.

Testicular Lymphoma – Just be aware that lymphoma can "hide" in the testes because of the blood testes barrier. Immunosuppressed patients are at increased risk for developing extranodal/ testicular lymphoma. Almost all testicular lymphomas are non-hodgkin B-cell subtypes. On US, the normal homogeneous echogenic testicular tissue is replaced focally or diffusely with hypoechoic vascular lymphomatous tissue **Buzzword = multiple hypoechoic masses of the testicle.**

Burned Out Testicular Tumor - If you see large dense calcifications with shadowing in the testicle of an old man this is probably what you should be thinking. The idea is that you've had spontaneous regression of a germ cell testicular neoplasm, that is now calcified. An important pearl is that there can still be viable tumor in there. Management is somewhat controversial and unlikely to be asked (most people pull them out).

Staging Pearl

Testicular mets should spread to the para-aortic, aortic, caval region. It's an embryology thing.

If you have mets to the pelvic, external iliac, and inguinal nodes - this is considered "non-regional" i.e. M1 disease. The exception is some kind of inguinal or scrotum surgery was done before the cancer manifested - but I wouldn't expect them to get that fancy on the test.

Just remember inguinal / pelvic nodes are non-regional and a higher stage (M1).

High Yield Testicle Tumor Trivia
Seminoma is the most common, and has the best prognosis (it melts with radiation)
Multiple hypoechoic masses = Lymphoma
Homogenous and Microcalcifications = Seminoma
Cystic Elements and Marcocalcifications= Mixed Germ Cell Tumor/ Teratoma
Most testicular tumors met via the lymphatics (choriocarcinoma mets via the blood - and tends to bleed like stink)
Gynecomastia can be seen with Sertoli Leydig Tumors
Sertoli Cell Tumors are also seen with Peutz Jeghers

Elevated hCG	Elevated AFP
Seminoma	Mixed Germ Cell
Choriocarcinoma	Yolk Sac

Seminoma

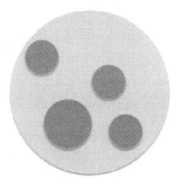
Lymphoma

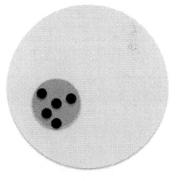
Mixed Germ Cell / Teratoma

Male Infertility

Causes: Can be thought of as obstructive vs non obstructive.

- Obstructive: Congenital bilateral absence of the vas deferens (seen in Cystic Fibrosis), ejaculatory duct obstruction, prostatic cysts. **Think about associated renal anomalies (Zinner Syndrome).**

- Non-Obstructive: Varicocele, Cryptorchidism, Anabolic Steroid Use, Erectile Dysfunction.

Varicocele: This is **the most common correctable cause of infertility**. They can be unilateral or bilateral. Unilateral is much more common on the left. Isolated **right sided should make you think retroperitoneal process** compressing the right gonadal vein.

Cryptorchidism: Undescended testes. The testicle is usually found in the inguinal canal. The testicle has an increased risk of cancer (actually they both will – which is weird). It's **most commonly seen in premature kids** (20%).

Major complication association for cryptorchidism:
- Malignant degeneration - of both the undescended and contralateral testicle
- Infertility
- Torsion
- Bowel Incarceration - related to the association of indirect inguinal hernia

Gamesmanship: A common distractor is "orchitis." Test writers love to try and get you to say that un-descended testicles get orchitis. They can… but not at a higher rate. It's not a reported association - so don't fall for that.

 Zebras and Syndromes associated with male infertility:

- *Pituitary Adenoma* making prolactin
- *Kallmans Syndrome* (can't smell + infertile)
- *Klinefelters Syndrome* (tall + gynecomastia + infertile)
- *Zinner Syndrome* (renal agenesis + ipsilateral seminal vesicle cyst)

GU Cancer Blitz!

Renal Cancer: *(Adenocarcinoma)*

--- Subtypes
- Clear Cell – most common *(enhances more)*
- Papillary – 2nd most common *(enhances less)*
- Medullary – Buzzword for Sick Cell Trait
- Chromophobe – Buzzword for Burt Hogg Dube

--- Syndrome
- Von Hipple Lindau – Multiple Clear Cells

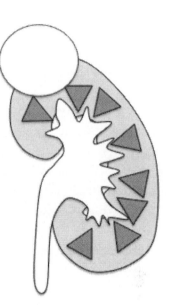

Ureter Cancer *(Transitional Cell):*

---Location --- *think about where you get the most stasis*
- Renal Pelvis– Twice as common as Ureter
- Distal Third of the Ureter – Most common site
- Middle is 2nd, and Proximal is 3rd

--- *Relationship to Bladder CA:*

Bladder CA is way more common (like 100x more). So if you have bladder CA you don't need upper tract CA. Since upper tract CA is not all that common, if you smoked enough Marlboro Reds to get a renal pelvis CA, you probably smoked enough to get multi focal disease including the bladder.

Bladder can be isolated
Ureteral usually has bladder

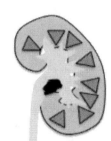

Bladder Cancer

Transitional Cell CA
- The normal kind
- Much more common than the ureter (like 100x)

Squamous Cell CA
- With lots of calcifications,
- In the setting of schistosomiasis

Adenocarcinoma
- Midline CA
- Patent Urachus

Urethral Cancer

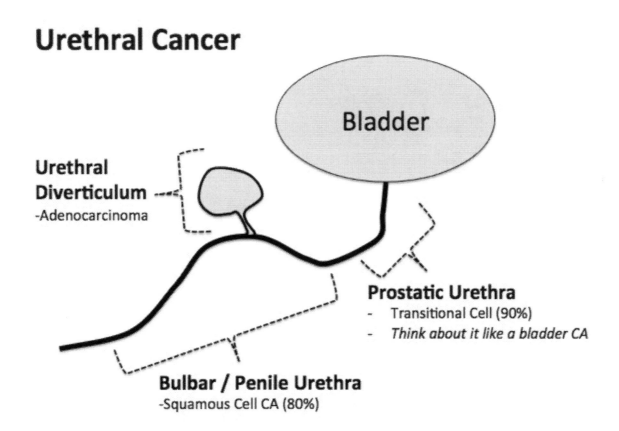

Urethral Diverticulum
- Adenocarcinoma

Prostatic Urethra
- Transitional Cell (90%)
- *Think about it like a bladder CA*

Bulbar / Penile Urethra
- Squamous Cell CA (80%)

Section 2: Adrenal

Anatomy: The adrenal glands are paired retroperitoneal glands that sit on each kidney. The right gland is triangular in shape, and the left gland tends to be more crescent shaped. If the kidney is congenitally absent the glands will be more flat, straight, discoid, or *"pancake"* in appearance. Each gland gets arterial blood from three arteries (superior from the inferior phrenic, middle from the aorta, and inferior from the renal artery). The venous drainage is via just one main vein (on the right into the IVC, on the left into the left renal vein).

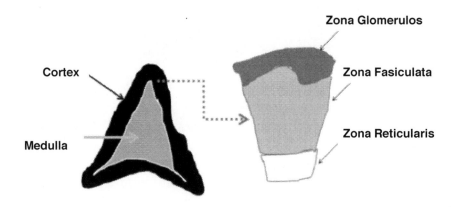

Step 1 Trivia: There are 4 zones to the adrenal, each of which makes different stuff.

- *Zona Glomerulosa*: Makes Aldosterone – prolonged stimulation here leads to hypertrophy.
- *Zona Fasiculata:* More Cortisol
- *Zona Reticularis* – Makes Androgens
- *Medulla* – Makes Catecholamines

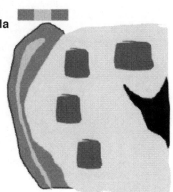

Normal Look on Ultrasound: In babies you can actually seen the adrenal on ultrasound. If they show you a PEDS adrenal case it's gonna be on ultrasound (or MIBG). If it's an adult case it will be CT or MRI. In babies the cortex is hypoechoic, and the medulla is hyperechoic. This gives the adrenal a **triple stripe appearance (dark cortex, bright medulla, dark cortex).**

Hypertrophy:

- **21-Hydroxylase Deficiency:** Congenital adrenal hypertrophy is caused **by 21-hydroxylase deficiency** in > 90% of cases. It will manifest clinically as either **genital ambiguity (girls)** or some salt losing pathology (boys). The salt losing can actually be life threatening. The look on imaging is adrenal limb width greater than 4mm, and loss of the central hyperechoic stripe.

- **Cushing Syndrome:** Too much cortisol. This is most commonly the result of a pituitary adenoma (75%), or ectopic production from a small cell lung cancer. In these cases you are going to see **bilateral adrenal gland hyperplasia**. *Less commonly (20%) it is from an adrenal adenoma*.

Hemorrhage: This occurs most commonly in the setting of trauma, or stress (neonates).

- **Stress:** It's classically seen after a breech birth, but can also be seen with fetal distress, and congenital syphilis. Imaging features change based on the timing of hemorrhage. It will evolve from hyperechoic to isoechoic to hypoechoic. Calcification is often the end result. It should be avascular. This can occur bilaterally, but favors the right side (75%). Serial ultrasounds (or MRI) can differentiate it from a cystic neuroblastoma. The hemorrhage will get smaller (the cancer will not).

- **Trauma:** This is going to be an adult (in the setting of trauma). Most likely it will be shown on CT. It's more common on the right.

- ***Zebra: Waterhouse-Friderichsen Syndrome*** – *Hemorrhage of the adrenal in the setting of fulminant meningitis (from Neisseria Meningitidis).*

Masses (other than adenoma).

- **Pheochromocytoma** – Uncommon in real life (common on multiple choice tests). They are usually large at presentation (larger than 3cm). It's usually a heterogenous mass on CT. On MRI they are **T2 bright**. Both MIBG and Octreotide could be used (but MIBG is better since Octreotide also uptakes in the kidney).

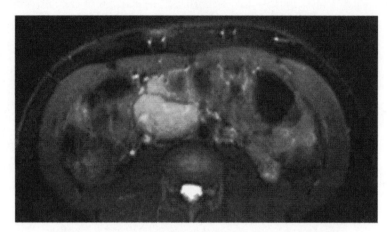

Pheo *at Organ of Zuckerkandl* – T2 Bright

- *Trivia: "Rule of 10s"*
    - 10% are extra adrenal (organ of Zuckerdandl – usually at the IMA), 10% are bilateral, 10% are in children, 10% are hereditary, 10% are NOT active (no HTN).

- *Trivia: "Syndromes"*
    - Associated syndromes: First think **Von Hippel Lindau**, then think **MEN IIa and IIb.** Other things less likely to be tested include NF-1, Sturge Weber, and TS.

- *Trivia: "* *Carney Triad"*
    - Extra-Adrenal Pheo, GIST, and Pulmonary Chondroma (hamartoma).
    - *Don't confuse this with the Carney Complex (Cardiac Myxoma, and Skin Pigmentation).*

- **Neuroblastoma** – *Discussed extensively in the Peds chapter.*

- **Myelolipoma** – Benign tumor that **contains bulk fat**. About ¼ have calcifications. If they are big (> 4cm) they can bleed, and present with a retroperitoneal hemorrhage. Another piece of trivia is the association with endocrine disorders (Cushings, Congenital Adrenal Hyperplasia, Conns). Don't get it twisted, these tumors are NOT functional, they just happen to have associated disorders about 5-10% of the time.

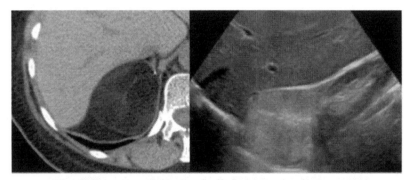

Myelolipoma – Contains bulk fat, Hyperechoic on US

- **Cyst** – You can get cysts in your adrenal. They are often unilateral, and can be any size. The really big ones can bleed. They have a thin wall, and do NOT enhance.

- **Mets:** Think **breast, lung, and melanoma**. They have no specific imaging findings and look like lipid poor adenomas. If the dude has a known primary (especially lung, breast, or melanoma), and it's not an adenoma then it's probably a met.

- **Cortical Carcinoma:** These are **large** (4cm-10cm), maybe functional (Cushings), and **calcify in about 20% of cases**. They are bad news and often met everywhere (direct invasion often first). As a pearl, an adrenal carcinoma is not likely to be less than 5cm and often has central necrosis.

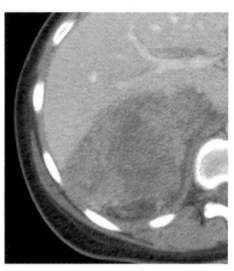

Adrenal Cortical Carcinoma
– *Direct Invasion of the liver*

Adenoma:

These things are super common, and are easily the most common tumor in the adrenal gland. Up to 8% of people have them. Proving it is an adenoma is an annoying problem.

- Non-Contrast: Less than 10 HU

- Contrast: Two options:

    Absolute:

    $$\frac{\text{Enhanced CT} - \text{Delayed CT}}{\text{Enhanced CT} - \text{Unenhanced CT}} \times 100 \quad \text{Greater than 60\% = Adenoma}$$

    Relative:

    $$\frac{\text{Enhanced CT} - \text{Delayed CT}}{\text{Enhanced CT}} \times 100 \quad \text{Greater than 40\% = Adenoma}$$

- MRI: Look for drop out on in and out of phase T1.

Trivia: Although most adenomas are not functional, Cushings (too much cortisol) and Conn (too much aldosterone) can present as a functional adenoma.

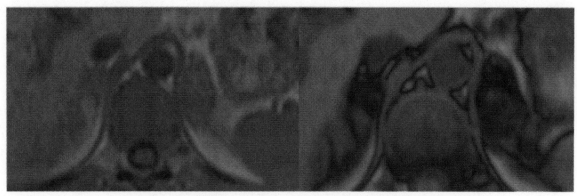

Adrenal Adenoma – Signal drop out In and Out of Phase

Conn's Syndrome: Syndrome of excessive aldosterone production. This is **most commonly caused by a benign adenoma** (70%). Cortical-carcinoma can also do it, but that is much more rare and usually accompanied by hypercortisolism.

Calcifications:

This is often the result of prior trauma or infection (TB). Certain tumors (cortical carcinoma, neuroblastoma) can have calcifications. Melanoma mets are known to calcify.

Wolman Disease: - This is a **total Aunt Minnie** (and massive zebra). **Bilateral enlarged calcified adrenals.** It's a fat metabolism error thing that kills within 6 months. The disease usually kills before the first year of life.

Syndromes:

MEN: "Multiple Endocrine Neoplasia"

There are three of these stupid things, and people who write multiple choice tests love to ask questions about them.

- **MEN 1:** Parathyroid Hyperplasia (90%), Pituitary Adenoma, Pancreatic Tumor (Gastrinoma most commonly)

- **MEN 2:** Medullary Thyroid Cancer (100%), Parathyroid hyperplasia, Pheochromocytoma (33%)

- **MEN 2b:** Medullary Thyroid Cancer (80%), Pheochromocytoma (50%), Mucosal Neuroma, Marfanoid Body Habitus

---

MEN Mnemonic

MEN I *(3 Ps)*
- **P**ituitary, **P**arathyroid, **P**ancreas

MEN IIa *(1M, 2Ps)*
Medullary Thyroid Ca,
Pheochromocytoma, **P**arathyroid

MEN IIb *(2Ms, 1P)*
- **M**edullary Thyroid Ca, **M**arfanoid Habitus /mucosal neuroma,
Pheochromocytoma

SECTION 3: OBSTETRICS AND GYNAECOLOGY

Uterus and Vagina

The Uterus – Changes During Life

- *Neonate* - Uterus is larger than you would think for a baby (maternal / placental hormones are still working). If you look close, the shape is a little weird with the <u>cervix often larger than the fundus.</u>

- *Prepuberty* - The shape of the uterus changes - becoming more <u>tube like</u>, with the <u>cervix and uterus the same size.</u>

- *Puberty* - The shape of the uterus changes again, now looking more like an adult (<u>pear like</u>) - with the <u>fundus larger than the cervix</u>. In puberty, the uterus starts to have a visible endometrium - with phases that vary during the cycle.

The Ovaries – Changes During Life

Just like with the uterus, infants tend to have larger ovaries (volume around 1cc), which then decreases and remains around or less than 1cc until about age 6. The ovaries then gradually increase to normal adult size as puberty approaches and occurs.

Turner Syndrome – The XO kids. Besides often having aortic co-arctations, and horseshoe kidneys they will have a <u>pre-puberty uterus</u> and <u>streaky ovaries.</u>

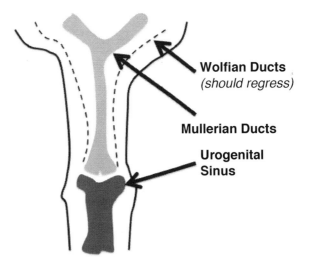

Embryology

The quick and dirty of it is that the mullerian ducts make the uterus and upper 2/3 of the vagina. The urogenital sinus grows up to meet the mullerian ducts and makes the bottom 1/3 of the vagina. Wolfian ducts are the boy parts, and should regress completely in girls.

Mullerian Ducts	**Wolfian Ducts**	**Urogenital Sinus**
Uterus Fallopian Tubes Upper 2/3 of the Vagina	Vas Deferens Seminal Vesicles Epididymis	Prostate Lower 1/3 of the Vagina

My idea for teaching this somewhat confusing topic is to tap into the thought process of embryology to help understand why anomalies happen, and why they happen together. The embryology I'm about to discuss is not strict and doesn't using all the fancy French / Latin words. It's more concept related…

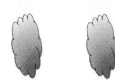

Imagine that the stuff that makes the kidneys and the uterus is all the same soup. You have two bowls of this stuff - half on the left, and half on the right.

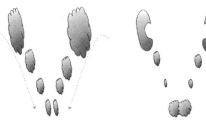

As development occurs, this soup gets poured down with the first part making the kidney, and the bottom part making the uterus.

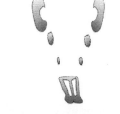

Now because you have two separate pools of soup, they need to fuse to make one uterus.

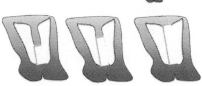

But because they are just mashed together, they don't have a central cavity necessary to carry a baby. So, there is a clean-up operation (cleavage), and this occurs from bottom to top - like zipping up a jacket.

So there are 3 main ways this who process can get screwed up.

(1) You can only have soup on one side. This is a **"failure to form"** As you can imaging, if you don't have the soup on one side you don't have a kidney on that side. You also don't have half of your uterus. This is why a unilateral absent kidney is associated with Unicornuate Uterus (+/- rudimentary horn).

(2) As the soup gets poured down it can **fail to fuse** completely. This can be on the spectrum of mostly not fused - basically separate (Uterus Didelphys) or mostly used except the top part - so it looks like a heart (Bicornus). Because the Bicornus and Didelphys are related pathologies - they both get vaginal septa (Dideplphus more often than Bicornus - easily remembered because it's a more severe fusion anomaly).

(3) The clean up operation can be done sloppy (**"failure to cleave"**). The classic example of this is a "Septate uterus" where a septum remains between the two uterine cavities.

"Failure to Form" -

- *Mullerian Agenesis* (Mayer-Rokitansky-Kuster-Hauser syndrome): Has three features: (1) vaginal atresia , (2) absent or rudimentary uterus (unicornuate or bicornuate) and (3) normal ovaries. The key piece of trivia is that the **kidneys have issues** (agenesis, ectopia) in about half the cases.

- *Unicornuate Uterus* – There are 4 subtypes (basically +/- rudimentary horn, +/- endometrial tissue). Obviously, endometrial tissue in a non-communicating horn is going to cause pelvic pain. Also, Endometrial tissue in a rudimentary horn (communicating or not – increases the risk of miscarriage and uterine rupture). **40% of these chicks will have renal issues (usually renal agenesis) ipsilateral to the rudimentary horn.**

"Failure to Fuse"

> **Vocab**
> *(in case you don't speak French or whatever)*
>
> **Cornus = Uterus**
>
> **Collis = Cervical**

- **Uterus Didelphys** – This is a complete uterine duplication (two cervices, two uteri, and two upper 1/3 vagina). A vaginal septum is present 75% of the time. If the patient does not have vaginal obstruction this is usually asymptomatic.

- **Bicornus** – This comes in two flavors (one cervix "unicollis", or two cervix "bicollis"). There will be separation of the uterus by a deep myometrial cleft - makes it look "heart shaped". Vaginal septum is seen around 25% of the time (less than didelphys). Although they can have an increased risk of fetal loss, it's much less of an issue compared to Septate. Fertility isn't as much of a "size thing" as it is a blood supply thing. Remember you can have 8 babies in your belly at once and have them live… live long enough to take part in your reality show.

- **T- Shaped** – This is the **DES related anomaly**. It is historical trivia, and therefore extremely high yield for the "exam of the future." DES was a synthetic estrogen given to prevent miscarriage in the 1940s. The daughters of patients who took this drug ended up with vaginal clear cell carcinoma, and uterine anomalies – classically the "T-Shaped Uterus."

"Failure to Cleave"

- **Septate** – This one has two endometrial canals separated by a fibrous (or muscular) septum. Fibrous vs Muscular can be determined with MRI and this distinction changes surgical management (different approaches). There is an increased risk of infertility and recurrent spontaneous abortion. The septum has a shitty blood supply, and if there is implantation on it - it will fail early. They can resect the septum - which improves outcomes.

- **Arcuate Uterus** – Mild smooth concavity of the uterine fundus (instead of normal straight or convex) This is not really a malformation, but more of a normal variant. It is **NOT associated with infertility or obstetric complications**.

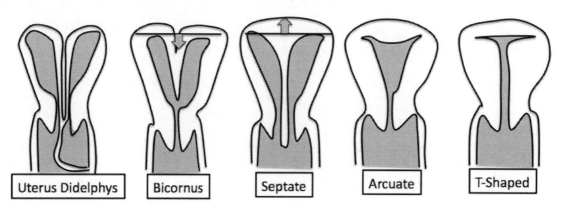

The Classic This vs That - *Bicornuate vs Septate*

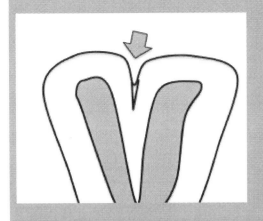

Bicornuate

- ***"Heart Shaped"*** - Fundal contour is <u>less</u> than 5mm above the tubal ostia

- No significant infertility issues

- Resection of the "septum" results in poor outcomes

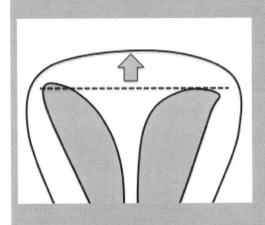

Septate

- Fundal contour is **Normal**; <u>more</u> than 5mm above the tubal ostia

- Legit infertility issues - implantation fails on the septum (it's a blood supply thing)

- Resection of the septum can help

Hysterosalpingogram (HSG)

If you haven't seen (or done one) before - this is a procedure that involves cannulation of the cervix and injecting contrast under fluoro to evaluate the cavity of the uterus.

Testable trivia:
- HSGs are performed on days 7-10 of menstrual cycle, (after menstrual bleeding complete - i.e. "off the rag")
- Contraindications: infection (PID), active bleeding ("on the rag"), pregnancy, and contrast allergy.
- Bicornuate vs Septate is tough on HSG - you need MRI or 3D Ultrasound to evaluate the outer fundal contour

Acquired Pathology

Salpingitis Isthmica Nodosa (SIN): This a nodular scarring of the fallopian tubes that produces an Aunt Minnie Appearance. As trivia, it usually involves the proximal 2/3 of the tube. This is of unknown etiology, but likely post inflammatory / infectious. It's strongly **associated with infertility and ectopic pregnancy** and that is likely the question.

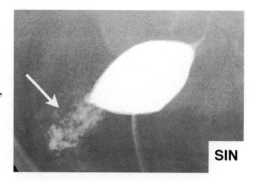

Uterine AVM – These can be congenital or acquired, with acquired types being way more common. They can be serious business and you can totally bleed to death from them. The typical ways to acquire them include: **previous dilation and curettage,** therapeutic abortion, caesarean section, or just multiple pregnancies. Doppler ultrasound is going to show: serpiginous and/or tubular anechoic structures within the myometrium with **high velocity color Doppler flow**.

Intrauterine Adhesions (Ashermans) – This is scarring in the uterus, that occurs secondary to injury: prior dilation and curettage, surgery, pregnancy, or infection (classic GU TB). This is typically shown on HSG, with either (a) non filling of the uterus, or (b) multiple irregular linear filling defects (lacunar pattern), with inability to appropriately distend the endometrial. MRI would show a bunch of T2 dark bands. Clinically, this results in infertility.

Endometritis – This is in the spectrum of PID. You often see it 2-5 days after delivery, especially in women with prolonged labor or premature rupture. You are going to have fluid and a thickened endometrial cavity. You can have gas in the cavity (not specific in a post partum women). It can progress to pyometrium, which is when you have expansion with pus.

Masses and Tumors and Stuff

Fibroids (Uterine Leiomyoma): These benign smooth muscle tumors are the most common uterine mass. They are more common in women of African ancestry. They like estrogen and are most common in reproductive age (rare in prepubertal females). Because of this estrogen relationship they tend to grow rapidly during pregnancy, and involute with menopause. Their location is classically described as submucosal (least common), intramural (most common), or subserosal.

Typical Appearance: The general rule, is they **can look like anything**. Having said that, they are usually hypoechoic on ultrasound, often with peripheral blood flow and shadowing in the so called "Venetian Blind" pattern. On CT, they often have peripheral calcifications ("popcorn" as seen on plain film). On MRI, **T1 dark** (to intermediate), **T2 dark**, and variable enhancement. The fibroids with higher T2 signal are said to respond better to IR treatment. A variant subtype is the lipoleiomyoma, which is fat containing.

Degeneration: 4 types of degeneration are generally described. *What they have in common is a lack of / paucity of enhancement (fibroids normally enhance avidly).*

- *Hyaline – This is the most common type.* The fibroid outgrows its blood supply, and you end up getting the accumulation of proteinaceous tissue. They are T2 dark, and do not enhance post Gd.

- *Red (Carneous) –* This one **occurs during pregnancy.** This is the cause of venous thrombosis. The classic imaging finding is a **peripheral rim of T1 high signal**. The T2 signal is variable.

- *Myxoid –* Uncommon type of degeneration. This is suggested by T1 dark, **T2 bright** and minimal gradual enhancement.

- *Cystic –* Uncommon type -

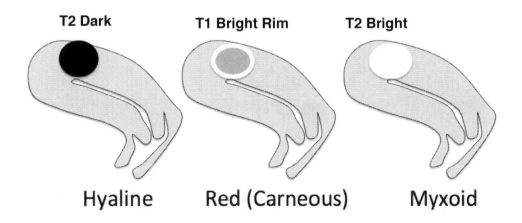

Hyaline   Red (Carneous)   Myxoid

Uterine Leiomyosarcoma – The risk of malignant transformation to a leiomyosarcoma is super low (0.1%). These look like a fibroid, but rapidly enlarging. Areas of necrosis are often seen.

Adenomyosis - This is endometrial tissue that has migrated into the myometrium. You see it **most commonly in multiparous women of reproductive age, especially if they've had a history of uterine procedures** (Caesarian section, dilatation and curettage).

Although there are several types, adenomyosis is usually generalized, favoring large portions of the uterus (especially the **posterior wall**), but **sparing the cervix**. It classically causes marked enlargement of the uterus, with preservation of the overall contour.

They can show it with Ultrasound or MRI. Ultrasound is less specific with findings including a heterogeneous uterus (hyperechoic adenomyosis, with hypoechoic muscular hypertrophy), or just enlargement of the posterior wall. MRI is the way better test with the most classic feature being **thickening of the junctional zone of the uterus to more than 12 mm** (normal is < 5mm). The thickening can be either focal or diffuse. Additionally, the findings of small high T2 signal regions corresponding to regions of cystic change is a classic finding.

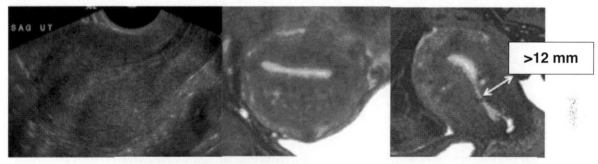

Adenomyosis of the Uterus
- Note the T2 Bright Cystic Foci and thick junctional zone

Thick Endometrium

Remember the stripe is measured without including any fluid in the canal. Focal or generalized thickening in post menopausal women greater than 5mm should get sampled. Premenopausal endometriums can give very thick - up to 20mm can be normal.

Trivia:
- *Estrogen secreting tumors – Granulosa Cell tumors of the ovary will thicken the endometrium.*
- *Hereditary Non-Polyposis Colon Cancer (HNPCC) – have a 30-50x increased risk of endometrial cancer*

Post Menopausal Bleeding:
Is it from atrophy or cancer?

•Endometrium less than 5mm = Probably Atrophy

•Endometrium > 5mm = Maybe cancer and gets a biopsy

Tamoxifen Changes – This is a SERM (acts like estrogen in the pelvis, blocks the estrogen effects on the breast). It's used for breast cancer, but **increases the risk of endometrial cancer**. It will cause subendometrial cysts, **and the development of endometrial polyps** (30%). Normally post menopausal endometrial tissue shouldn't be thicker than 4mm, but on Tamoxifen the endometrium gets a pass up to 8mm. At >8mm it gets a biopsy. If you are wondering if a polyp is hiding you can get a sonohysterogram (ultrasound after instillation of saline).

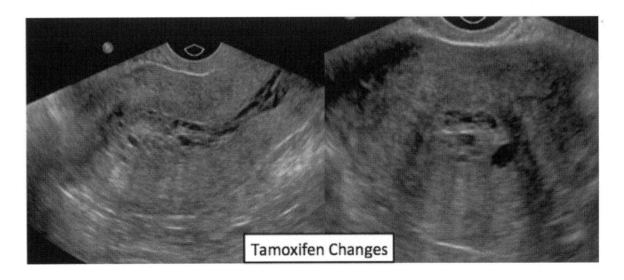

Tamoxifen Changes

Endometrial Fluid – In a premenopausal women this is a common finding. In a post menopausal women it means either cervical stenosis or an obstructing mass (**usually cervical stenosis**).

Cervix

Cancer: It's **usually squamous cell**, related to **HPV** (like 90%). The big thing to know is parametrial invasion (stage IIb). Stage IIa or below is treated with surgery. **Once you have parametrial invasion (stage IIb),** or involvement of the lower 1/3 of the vagina it's gonna get chemo/ radiation. In other words, management changes so that is the most likely test question.

	Cervical Cancer Staging Pearls	
Stage II A	Spread beyond the cervix, but NO parametrial invasion	Surgery
Stage II B	Parametrial involvement but does NOT extend to the pelvic side wall.	Chemo/ Radiation

How can I tell If there is Parametrial Invasion?
I don't even know what the hell the "parametrium" is....

What is this parametrium? The parametrium is a fibrous band that separates the supravaginal cervix from the bladder. It extends between the layers of the broad ligament.

Why is is so important? The uterine artery runs inside the parametrium, hence the need for chemo - once invaded.

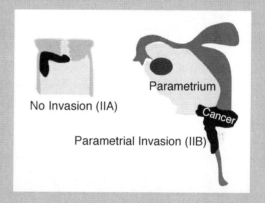

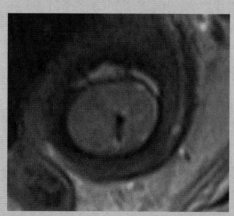

T2 Dark Ring Intact
(no parametrial invasion)

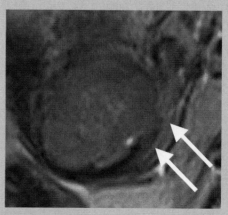

T2 Dark Ring Disrupted (arrow)
Parametrial invasion)

Vagina

Solid Vaginal Masses:

A solid vaginal mass is usually a bad thing. It can be secondary (cervical or uterine carcinoma protruding into the vagina), or primary such as a clear cell adenocarcinoma or rhabdomyosarcoma.

Leiomyoma – Rare in the vagina, but can occur (most commonly in the anterior wall).

Squamous Cell Carcinoma – The most common cancer of the vagina (85%). This is associated with HPV. This is just like the cervix.

Clear Cell Adenocarcinoma - This is the zebra cancer seen in women whose mothers took DES (a synthetic estrogen thought to prevent miscarriage). That plus "T-Shaped Uterus" is probably all you need to know.

Vaginal Rhabdomyosarcoma - This is the most common tumor of the vagina in children. There is a bimodal age distribution in ages (2-6, and 14-18). They usually come off the anterior wall near the cervix. It can occur in the uterus, but typically invades it secondarily. Think about this when you see a solid T2 bright enhancing mass in the vagina / lower uterus in a child.

Mets Trivia: A met to the vagina in the anterior wall upper 1/3 is "always" (90%) upper genital tract. A met to the vagina in the posterior wall lower 1/3 is "always (90%) from the GI tract.

Cystic Vaginal / Cervical Masses:

Nabothian Cysts – These are usually on the cervix and you see them all the times. They are the result of inflammation causing epithelium plugging of mucous glands.

Gartner Ducts Cysts – These are the result of **incomplete regression of the wolffian ducts**. They are classically located along the anterior lateral wall of the upper vagina. If they are located at the level of the urethra, that **can cause mass effect on the urethra** (and symptoms).

Bartholin Cysts – These are the result of obstruction of the Bartholin glands (mucin-secreting glands from the urogenital sinus). They are found below the pubic symphysis (helps distinguish them from Gartner duct).

Skene Gland Cysts – Cysts in these periurethral glands, can cause recurrent UTIs and urethral obstruction.

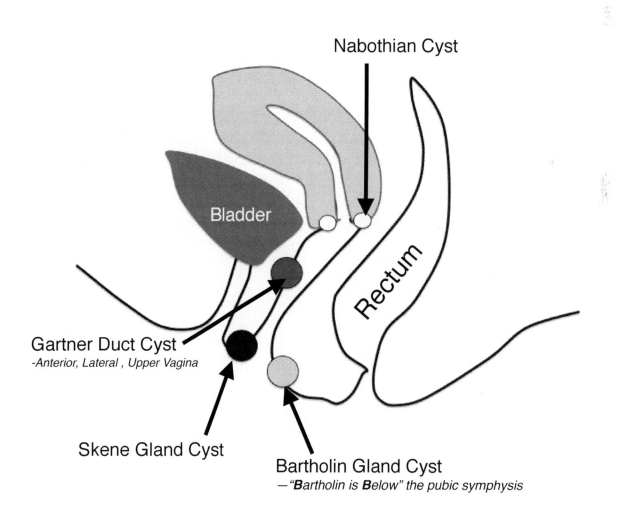

Ovaries / Adnexa

- Before I start, a few general tips (1) never biopsy or recommend biopsy of an ovary, (2) on CT if you can't find the ovary, follow the gonadal vein, and (3) hemorrhage in a cystic mass usually means it's benign.

- A quick note on ovarian size, the maximum ovarian volume can be considered normal up until 15ml (some say 20ml). The post menopausal ovary should NOT be larger than 6cc.

Let's talk about ovulation, *to help understand the normal variation in the ovary.*

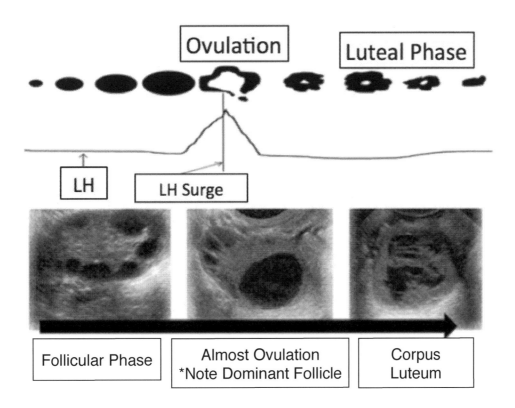

Follicles seen during the early menstrual cycle are typically small (< 5mm in diameter). By day 10 of the cycle, there is usually one follicle who has emerged as the dominant follicle. By mid cycle, this dominant follicle has gotten pretty big (around 20mm). Its size isn't surprising because it contains a mature ovum. The LH surge causes the dominant follicle to rupture releasing the egg. The follicle then regresses in size forming a Corpus Luteum. A small amount of fluid can be seen in the cul-de-sac. Occasionally, a follicle bleeds and re-expands (hemorrhagic cyst) – more on this later.

Cumulus Oophorus – this is a piece of anatomy trivia. It is a collection of cells in a mature dominant follicle that protrudes into the follicular cavity, and **signals imminent ovulation** (its absence means nothing).

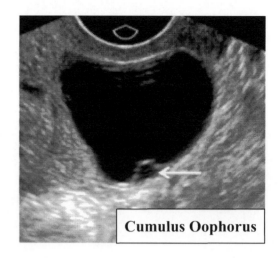

Cumulus Oophorus

Let's speak briefly about fertility meds

Medications such as a Clomiphene Citrate (Clomid), force the maturation of multiple bilateral ovarian cysts. It is not uncommon for the ovaries of women taking this drug to have multiple follicles measuring more than 20mm in diameter by mid cycle.

Theca Lutein Cysts – this is a type of functional cyst (more on that below), related to overstimulation from b-HCG. What you see are large cysts (~ 2-3 cm) and the **ovary has a typical multilocular cystic "spoke-wheel" appearance**.

Think about 3 things:

- *Multifetal pregnancy,*
- *Gestational trophoblastic disease (moles),*
- *Ovarian Hyperstimulation syndrome.*

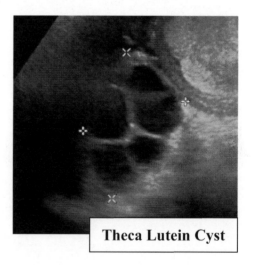

Theca Lutein Cyst

Ovarian Hyperstimulation Syndrome – This is a complication associated with fertility therapy (occurs in like 5%). They will show you the ovaries with **theca lutein cysts**, then ascites, and **pleural effusions**. They may also have pericardial effusions. Complications include increased risk for ovarian torsion (big ovaries), and hypovolemic shock.

Old vs Young

Premenstrual: The ovaries of a pediatric patient stay small until around age 8-9. Ovaries may contain small follicles.

Premenopausal: A piece of trivia; premenopausal ovaries **may be HOT on PET** (depending on the menstrual cycle). This is why you do a PET in the first week of the menstrual cycle.

Postmenopausal *(one year after menses stops):* Considered **abnormal** if it exceeds the upper limit of normal, or is **twice the size of the other ovary (even if no mass is present).** Small cysts (< 3cm) are seen in around 20% of post menopausal women. In general, postmenopausal ovaries are atrophic, lack follicles, and can be difficult to find with ultrasound. The ovarian volume will decrease from around 8cc at age 40, to around 1cc at age 70. The **maximum ovarian volume in a post menopausal woman is 6ml.** Unlike premenopausal ovaries, **post menopausal ovaries should NOT be hot on PET.**

Cyst in Postmenopausal Woman
WTF Do I Do Now?

If the cyst is simple, regardless of age it's almost certainly benign.

Having said that, the rule is:

- Greater than 1cm gets yearly follow up
- Less than 5cm (still likely benign) 3-6 month followup
- Greater than 7cm gets either an MRI or a surgeon.

If it's first seen on another modality (CT), I would get an Ultrasound first to confirm its totally cystic - without suspicious features like papillary projections, nodules, thick septations etc.... Then follow the rules as above.

The Big 6

(The Sinister Six – For You Spiderman Fans)

In most clinical practices, the overwhelming majority of ovarian masses are benign (don't worry I'll talk about cancer too).

- Physiologic and functioning follicles
- Corpora lutea
- Hemorrhagic cysts
- Endometriomas
- Benign cystic teratomas (dermoids)
- Polycystic ovaries

Functioning Ovarian Cysts: Functioning cysts (follicles) are affected by the menstrual cycle (as I detailed eloquently above). These cysts are benign and usually 25mm or less in diameter. They will usually change / disappear in 6 weeks. If a cyst persists and either does not change or increases in size, it is considered a nonfunctioning cyst (not under hormonal control).

Simple cysts that are > 7cm in size may need further evaluation with MR (or surgical evaluation). Just because it's hard to evaluate them completely on US when they are that big, and you risk torsion with a cyst that size.

Corpus Luteum: The normal corpus luteum arises from a dominant follicle (as I detailed eloquently above). These things can be large (up to 5-6cm) with a variable appearance (solid hypoechoic, anechoic, thin walled, thick walled, cyst with debris). The most common appearance is solid and hypoechoic with a "ring of fire" (intense peripheral blood flow).

Corpus Luteum vs Ectopic Pregnancy

They both can have that "ring of fire" appearance, but please don't be an idiot about this. Most ectopic pregnancies occur in the tube (the corpus luteum is an ovarian structure). If you are really lucky, a "hint" is that the corpus luteum should move with the ovary, where an ectopic will move separate from the ovary (you can push the ectopic away from it). Also, the tubal ring of an ectopic pregnancy is usually more echogenic when compared to the ovarian parenchyma. Whereas, the wall of the corpus luteum is usually less echogenic. A specific (but not sensitive) finding in ectopic pregnancy is a RI of <0.4 or >0.7.

	Ectopic	Corpus Luteum
	RI < 0.4, or > 0.7	RI 0.4 – 0.7
	Thick echogenic rim	Thin Echogenic Rim
	"Ring of Fire"	"Ring of Fire"
	Moves Separate from the Ovary	Moves with the Ovary

Endometrioma: This affects young women during their reproductive years and can cause chronic pelvic pain associated with menstruation. The traditional clinical history of endometriosis is the triad of infertility, dysmenorrhea, and dyspareunia. The buzzword classic appearance is **rounded mass with homogeneous low level internal echoes and increased through transmission (seen in 95% of cases)**. Fluid-fluid levels and internal septations can also be seen. It can look a lot like a hemorrhagic cyst (sometimes). As a general rule, the more unusual or varied the echogenicity and the more ovoid or irregular the shape, the more likely the mass is an endometrioma. Additionally, and of more practical value, they are not going to change on follow up (hemorrhagic cysts are). In about 30% of cases you can get small echogenic foci adhering to the walls (this helps make the endometrioma diagnosis more likely). Obviously, you want to differentiate this from a true wall nodule. The complications of endometriosis (bowel obstruction, infertility, etc...) are due to a fibrotic reaction associated with the implant. The most common location for solid endometriosis is the uterosacral ligaments

Do Endometriomas Ever Become Cancer? About 1% of endometriomas undergo malignant transformation (usually endometrioid or **clear cell carcinoma**). How do you tell which one is which??? Malignancy is very rare in endometriomas smaller than 6 cm. They usually have to be bigger than 9 cm. Additionally, the majority of women with carcinoma in an endometrioma are older than 45 years. So **risk factors for turning into cancer: (a) older than 45, (b) bigger than 6-9cm.**

Q: What is the most sensitive imaging feature on MRI for the diagnosis of malignancy in an endometrioma ?

A: An enhancing mural nodule

Pregnancy Trivia: There is a thing called a *"decidualized endometrioma."* This is a vocab word used to describe a solid nodule with blood flow in an endometrioma of a pregnant girl. Obviously this is still gonna get followed up - but is a mimic of malignancy. The thing never to forget is that if the patient is NOT pregnant and you see a solid nodule with blood flow - that is malignant degeneration - period - no hesitation, next question.

Endometrioma on MRI: Will be T1 bright (from the blood). Fat saturation will not suppress the signal (showing you it's not a teratoma). Will be T2 dark! (from iron in the endometrioma). The shading sign is a buzzword for endometriomas on MR imaging. On T2 you should look for "shading." **The shading sign, describes T2 shortening (getting dark) of a lesion that is T1 bright.**

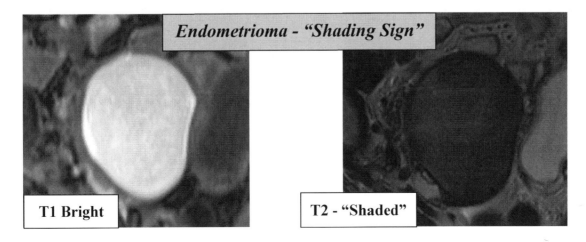

Endometrioma - "Shading Sign"

T1 Bright

T2 - "Shaded"

Hemorrhagic Cysts: As mentioned above, sometimes a ruptured follicle bleeds internally and re-expands. The result is a homogenous mass with **enhanced through transmission** *(tumor won't do that)* with a very similar look to an endometrioma. A lacy **"fishnet appearance"** is sometimes seen and is considered classic. Doppler flow will be absent. The traditional way to tell the difference between a hemorrhagic cyst vs endometrioma, is that the **hemorrhagic cyst will go away in 1-2 menstrual cycles** (so repeat in 6-12 weeks).

Hemorrhagic Cyst on MRI – Will be T1 bright (from the blood). Fat saturation will not suppress the signal (showing you it's not a teratoma). The lesion should NOT enhance.

Hemorrhagic cysts in old ladies? Postmenopausal women may occasionally ovulate, so you don't necessarily need to freak out (follow up in 6-12 weeks). Now, late postmenopausal women should NEVER have a hemorrhagic cyst and if you are shown something that looks like a hemorrhagic cyst in a 70 year old – it's cancer till proven otherwise.

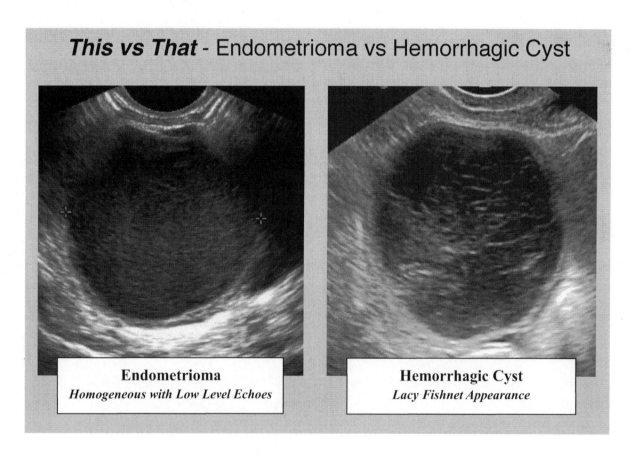

This vs That - Endometrioma vs Hemorrhagic Cyst

Endometrioma — *Homogeneous with Low Level Echoes*

Hemorrhagic Cyst — *Lacy Fishnet Appearance*

Dermoid: These things typically occur in young women (20s-30s), and are the most common ovarian neoplasm in patients younger than 20. The "Tip of the Iceberg Sign" is a classic buzzword and refers to absorption of most of the US beam at the top of the mass. The typical ultrasound appearance is that of a cystic mass, with a hyperechoic solid mural nodule, (Rokitansky nodule or dermoid plug). Septations are seen in about 10%.

Dermoid on MRI: Will be bright on T1 (from the fat). There will be fat suppression (not true of hemorrhagic cysts, and endometriomas).

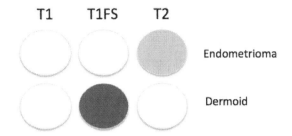

Do Dermoids Ever Become Cancer? About 1% of dermoids can undergo malignant transformation (**almost always to squamous cell CA**). Again, risk factors are size (usually larger than 10cm), and age (usually older than 50).

Rare Cancer Transformation Subtypes	
Endometrioma	Clear Cell
Dermoid	Squamous

Polycystic Ovarian Syndrome: Typically an overweight girl with infertility, acne, and a mustache

The imaging criteria is:

- **Ten or more peripheral simple cysts** *(typically small <5mm)*
- Usually Characteristic 'string-of-pearls' appearance.
- **Ovaries are typically enlarged (>10cc),** although in 30% of patients the ovaries have a normal volume.

Ovarian Cancer

Ovarian cancers often present as complex cystic and solid masses. They are typically intra-ovarian (most extra-ovarian masses are benign). The role of imaging is not to come down hard on histology (although the exam may ask this of you), but instead to distinguish benign from malignant and let the surgeon handle it from there.

Think Cancer if:

- Unilateral (or bilateral) complex cystic adnexal masses with thick (>3mm) septations, and papillary projections (nodule with blood flow).
- Solid adnexal masses with variable necrosis

Knee Jerks:

- Multiple thin or thick septations = Call the Surgeon
- Nodule with Flow = Call the Surgeon
- Solid Nodules Without Flow =
    - Get an MR to make sure it's not a dermoid plug,
    - If it's not a dermoid, then call the surgeon

Serous Ovarian / Cystadenocarcinoma / Cystadenoma

Serous tumors are the **most common type of ovarian malignancy**. About 60% of serous tumors are benign, and about 15% are considered borderline (the rest are malignant). They favor women of childbearing age, with the malignant ones tending to occur in older women. They typically are unilocular with few septations. They are frequently bilateral (especially when malignant). Papillary projections are a common finding, which suggests malignancy. If you see ascites they have mets (70% have peritoneal involvement at the time of diagnosis).

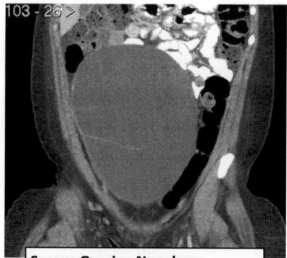

Serous Ovarian Neoplasm
- Large, Unilocular, Few Septations

Mucinous Ovarian Cystadenocarincoma

Often a large mass. They are **typically multiloculated** (although septa are often thin). **Papillary projections are less common** with serous tumors. You can see low level echos (from mucin). These dudes can get Pseudomyxoma peritonei with scalloping along solid organs. Smoking is a known risk factor (especially for mucinous types).

This vs That: Serous vs Mucinous	
Serous:	**Mucinous:**
Unilocular (fewer septations)	Multi-locular (more septations)
Papillary Projections Common	Papillary Projections Less Common

Endometroid Ovarian Cancer: This is the second most common ovarian cancer (serous number one, mucinous number three). These things are bilateral about 15% of the time.

What to know:

- 25% of women will have concomitant endometrial cancer. The endometrial cancer is the primary (ovary is met).
- Endometriomas can turn into endometroid cancer
- 15% are bilateral

> **Gamesmanship: Ovarian Mass + Endometrial Thickening**
>
> This is a way to show both <u>Endometroid CA</u> (which often has both ovarian and endometrial CA), and <u>Granulosa-Theca Cell Tumor</u> (which produce estrogen - and cause endometrial hyperplasia)

B.F.M's - for Adults

It's useful to have a differential for a **B.F.M.** (**B**ig **F**ucking **M**ass) in an adult and a child. I discuss the child version of this in the Peds chapter. For adults think about 3 main things:

(1) Ovarian Masses - Mucinous and Serous
(2) Desmoids - *Remember Gardner Syndrome*
(3) Sarcomas

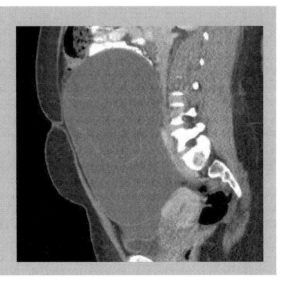

Fibroma / Fibrothecoma:

The ovarian fibroma is a benign ovarian tumor, most commonly seen in middle aged women. The fibrothecoma / thecoma spectrum has similar histology. It's **very similar to a fibroid**. On ultrasound it's going to be hypoechoic and solid. On MRI its going to be T1 and T2 dark, with the **band of T2 dark signal around the tumor on all planes. Calcifications are rare**

Similar or Related Conditions:

- **Meigs Syndrome:** This is the triad of ascites, pleural effusion, and a benign ovarian tumor (most commonly fibroma).

- **Fibromatosis:** This is a zebra. You have tumor-like enlargement of the ovaries due to ovarian fibrosis. It typically hits girls around the age of 25. It's associated with omental fibrosis, and sclerosing peritonitis. You are going to get dark T1 and T2 signal. **The buzzword for that T2 signal is "black garland sign."** The condition is benign, and sometimes managed with surgical removal of the ovaries.

- **Brenner Tumor:** Epithelial tumor of the ovary seen in women in their 50s-70s. It's fibrous and T2 dark. Unlike Fibromas, calcifications are common (80%).

  They are also called *"Ovarian Transitional Cell Carcinoma"* for the purpose of fucking with you.

Struma ovarii: These things are actually a subtype of ovarian teratoma. On imaging you are looking for a multilocular, predominantly cystic mass with an INTENSELY enhancing solid component. On MRI - the give away is very low T2 signal in the "cystic" areas which is actually the thick colloid. These tumors contain THYROID TISSUE, and even though it's very rare (like 5%) I would expect that the question stem will lead you to this diagnosis by telling you the patient is hyperthyroid or in a thyroid storm.

Metastatic Disease to the Ovary

Around 10% of malignant ovarian tumors are mets. The primary is most common from colon, gastric, breast, lung, and contralateral ovary. The most common look is bilateral solid tumors.

Krukenburg Tumor – This is a metastatic tumor to the ovaries from the GI tract (usually stomach).

Miscellaneous Topics:

Ovarian Torsion

Rotation of the ovarian vascular pedicle (partial or complete) can result in obstruction to venous outflow and arterial inflow. Torsion is typically associated with a cyst or tumor (any thing that makes it heavy, so it flops over on itself). Critical point = the most constant finding in ovarian torsion is a large ovary.

Features:

- *Unilateral enlarged ovary (greater than 4cm)*
- ***Mass on the ovary***
- *Peripheral Cysts*
- *Free Fluid*
- *Lack of arterial or venous flow*

The Ovary is Not a Testicle: The ovary has a dual blood supply. Just because you have flow, does NOT mean there isn't a torsion. You can torse and de-torse. In other words, big ovary + pain = torsion. *Clinical correlation recommended.*

Hydrosalpinx

Thin (or thick in chronic states) elongated tubular structure in the pelvis. The buzzword is **"cogwheel appearance"**, referring to the normal longitudinal folds of a fallopian tube becoming thickened. Another buzzword is **"string sign"** referring to the incomplete septae. The **"waist sign"** describes a tubular mass with indentations of its opposing walls (this is suppose to help differentiate hydrosalpinx from an ovarian mass).

There are a variety of causes, the most common is being a skank, infidel, or free spirit (PID). Additional causes include endometriosis, tubal cancer, post hysterectomy (without oophorectomy), and tubal ligation.

Rare and late complication is tubal torsion.

Pelvic Inflammatory Disease (PID)

Infection or inflammation of the upper female genital tract. It's usually secondary to skank like behavior (Gonorrhea, or Chlamydia). On ultrasound you are gonna get Hydrosalpinx. The margin of the uterus may become ill defined ("indefinite uterus" – is a buzzword). Later on you can end up with tubo-ovarian abscess or pelvic abscess. You can even get bowel or urinary tract inflammatory changes.

Paraovarian Cyst

This is a congenital remnant that arises from the Wolffian duct. They are more common than you think with some texts claiming these account for 10-20% of adnexal masses. They are classically round or oval, simple in appearance, and **do NOT distort the adjacent ovary** (key finding). They can indent the ovary and mimic an exophytic cyst, but a good sonographer can use the transducer to separate the two structures.

Ovarian Vein Thrombophlebitis

This is seen most commonly in **postpartum women**, often presenting with acute pelvic pain and <u>fever</u>. For whatever reason, **80% of the time it's on the right**. It's most likely to be shown on CT (could be ultrasound) with a tubular structure with an enhancing wall and low-attenuation thrombus in the expected location of the ovarian vein. A dreaded sequella is pulmonary embolus.

Peritoneal Inclusion Cyst

This is an inflammatory cyst of the peritoneal cavity, that occurs when adhesions envelop an ovary. Adhesions can be thought of as diseased peritoneum. Whereas the normal peritoneum can absorb fluid, adhesions cannot. So, you end up with normal secretions from an active ovary confined by adhesions and resulting in an expanding pelvic mass. The classic history is patient with prior pelvic surgery (they have to tell you that, to clue you in on the presence of adhesions), now with pain. Alternatively, they could get tricky and say history of PID or endometriosis (some kind of inflammatory process to piss off the peritoneum). Then they will show an ultrasound (or MR) with a complex fluid collection occupying pelvic recesses and containing the ovary. It's not uncommon to have septations, loculations and particulate matter within the contained fluid.

Key features:

- *(1) Lack of walls. They have a "passive shape" that conforms to and is defined by surrounding structures*
- *(2) Entrapment of an ovary. Ovary will be either in the collection, or at the periphery.*

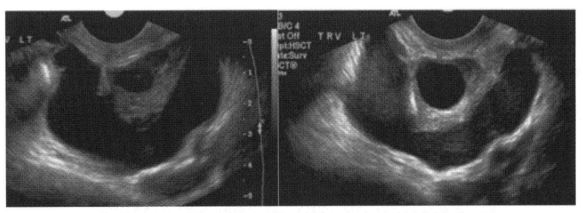

Peritoneal Inclusion Cyst – Adhesions around an ovary

Gestational Trophoblastic Disease

Think about this with marked elevation of B-hCG. They will actually trend betas for tumor activity. Apparently, elevated B-hCG makes you vomit – so hyperemesis is often part of the given history. Another piece of trivia is that age over 40, and prior moles makes you more likely to get another mole.

Hydatidiform Mole

This is the most common form, and the benign form of the disease. There are type subtypes:

- *Complete mole* (classic mole) (70%): This one involves the entire placenta. There will be no fetus. The worthless trivia is that the karyotype is diploid. A total zebra scenario is that you have a normal fetus, with a complete mole twin pregnancy (if you see that in the wild, write it up). The pathogenesis is fertilization of an egg that has lost its chromosomes (46XX).
    - *First Trimester US:* Classically shows the uterus to be filled with an echogenic, solid, highly vascular mass, often described as **"snowstorm"** in appearance.
    - *Second Trimester US*: Vesicles that make up the mole enlarge into individual cysts (2-30mm) and produce your **"bunch of grapes"** appearance.
- *Partial mole* (30%): This one involves only a portion of the placenta. You do have a fetus, but it's all jacked up (triploid in karyotype). The pathogenesis is fertilization of an ovum by two sperm (69XXY). Mercifully, it's lethal to the fetus.
    - *US:* The placenta will be enlarged, and have areas of multiple, diffuse anechoic lesions. You may see fetal parts.

Remember that I mentioned that **Theca Lutein cysts are seen in molar pregnancies**. The piece of trivia is that they are actually most commonly seen in the second trimester, and are bilateral.

Invasive Mole

This refers to invasion of molar tissue into the myometrium. You typically see it after the treatment of a hydatidiform mole (about 10% of cases). US may show echogenic tissue in the myometrium. However, MRI is way better at demonstrating muscle invasive. MRI is going to demonstrate focal myometrial masses, dilated vessels, and areas of hemorrhage and necrosis.

Choriocarcinoma

This is a very aggressive malignancy that forms only trophoblasts (no villous structure). The typical attacking pattern of choriocarcinoma is to spread locally (into the myometrium and parametrium) then to spread hematogenous to any site in the body. It's very vascular and bleeds like stink. The classic clinical scenario is serum β-hCG levels that rise in the 8 to 10 weeks following evacuation of molar pregnancy. On ultrasound, choriocarcinoma (at any site) results in a highly echogenic solid mass. Treatment = methotrexate.

OB

Early Pregnancy:

Vocab:

- Menstrual Age: Embryologic Age + 14 days
- Embryo: 0-10 weeks (menstrual age)
- Fetus: > 10 weeks (menstrual age)
- Threatened Abortion – Bleeding with closed cervix
- Inevitable Abortion – Cervical dilation and/or placental and/or fetal tissue hanging out
- Incomplete Abortion – Residual products in the uterus
- Complete Abortion – All products out
- Missed Abortion – Fetus is dead, but still in the uterus.

Intradecidual Sign: This is the early gestational sac. When seen covered by echogenic decidua is very characteristic of early pregnancy. You can see it around 4.5 weeks. You want to see the thin echogenic line of the uterine cavity pass by (not stop at) the sac to avoid calling a little bit of fluid in the canal a sac.

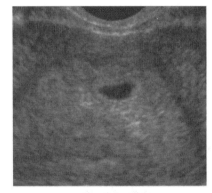

Intradecidual Sign

Double Decidual Sac Sign: This is another positive sign of early pregnancy. It's produced by visualizing the layers of decidua.

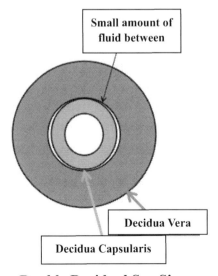

Double Decidual Sac Sign

Yolk Sac: This is the first structure visible within the GS. The classic teaching was you should always see it when the GS measures 8mm in diameter. The thing should be oval or round, fluid filled, and smaller than 6mm.

The yolk sac is located in the chorionic cavity, and hooked up to the umbilicus of the embryo by the vitelline duct.

Yolk Sac Gone Bad: The yolk sac shouldn't be too big (> 6mm), shouldn't be too small (< 3mm), and shouldn't be solid or calcified.

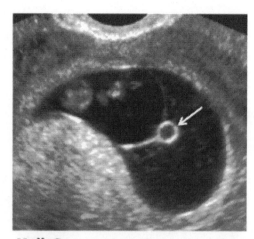

Yolk Sac – in the chorionic cavity

The Amnion: The membranes of the amniotic sac and chorionic space typically remain separated by a thin layer of fluid, until about 14-16 weeks at which point fusion is normal. If the amnion gets disrupted before 10 weeks the fetus might cross into the chorionic cavity and get tangled up in the fibrous bands. This is the etiology of **amniotic band syndrome**, which can be terrible (decapitation, limb amputation, etc…).

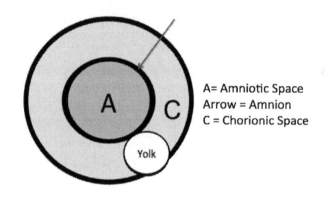

Double Bleb Sign: This is the earliest visualization of the embryo. This is two fluid filled sacs (yolk and amniotic) with the flat embryo in the middle.

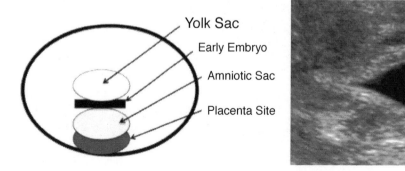

Double Bleb Sign

Crown Rump Length – This is typically used to estimate gestational age, and is more accurate then menstrual history. *Embryo is normally visible at 6 weeks.

Anembryonic Pregnancy – A gestational sac without an embryo. When you see this, the choices are (a) very early pregnancy, or (b) non-viable pregnancy. The classic teaching was you should see the yolk sac at 8mm (on TV). Just remember that a large sac (> 8-10 mm) without a yolk sac, and a distorted contour is pretty reliable for a non-viable pregnancy.

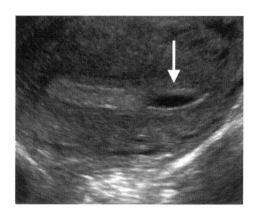

Pseudogestational Sac – This is not the same thing as an anembryonic pregnancy. This is seen in the presence of an ectopic pregnancy. What you are seeing is a little bit of blood in the uterine cavity with surrounding bright decidual endometrium (charged up from the pregnancy hormones).

Old criteria for fetal demise vs new criteria for fetal demise – They have recently (very recently) redone the numbers for calling it non-viable and I'm not sure which version will be tested so I'm presenting both. For the most part, the new ones give more wiggle room.

Most Recent Guideline for Fetal Demise		Old School (Traditional) Guidelines for Abnormal Pregnancy
Diagnostic of Pregnancy Failure	**Suspicious for Pregnancy Failure**	
Crown–rump length of ≥7 mm and no heartbeat	No embryo ≥6 wk after last menstrual period	Absent Yolk Sac with MSD > 8mm
Mean sac diameter of ≥25 mm and no embryo	Mean sac diameter of 16–24 mm and no embryo	Absent Embryo when MSD > 16mm
No embryo with heartbeat ≥11 days after a scan that showed a gestational sac with a yolk sac	No embryo with heartbeat 13 days after a scan that showed a gestational sac without a yolk sac	No Cardiac Activity when Embryo can be seen on Transabdominal (or >5mm on TV). "5 Alive".
No embryo with heartbeat ≥2 wk after a scan that showed a gestational sac without a yolk sac	No embryo with heartbeat 10 days after a scan that showed a gestational sac with a yolk sac	** Always give 1-2mm as the benefit of doubt.

Doubilet, Peter M., et al. "Diagnostic criteria for nonviable pregnancy early in the first trimester." New England Journal of Medicine 369.15 (2013): 1443-1451.

Subchorionic Hemorrhage: These are very common. The thing to know is that the percentage of placental detachment is the prognostic factor most strongly associated with a fetal demise; hematoma greater than 2/3 the circumference of the chorion has a 2x increased risk of abortion. Other trivia, women older than 35 have worse outcomes with these.

Implantation Bleeding: This is a nonspecific term referring to a small subchorionic hemorrhage that occurs at the attachment of the chorion to the endometrium.

Ectopic:

High Risk for Ectopic: Hx of PID, Tubal Surgery, Endometriosis, Ovulation Induction, Previous Ectopic, Use of an IUD.

The majority of ectopic pregnancies (nearly 95%) occur in the fallopian (usually the isthmic portion). A small percentage (around 2%) are "interstitial" developing in the portion of the tube which passes through the uterine wall. These interstitials are high risk, as they can grow large before rupture causing a catastrophic hemorrhage. It is also possible (although very rare) to have implantation sites in the abdominal cavity, ovary, and cervix.

Always start down the ectopic pathway with a positive BhCG. At around 2000 IU/L you should see a gestational sac. As a general rule, a normal doubling time makes ectopic less likely.

> **The Big 3 to Remember with Ectopics (positive BhCG)**
>
> (1) Live Pregnancy / Yolk Sac outside the uterus = Slam Dunk
> (2) Nothing in the uterus + anything on the adnexa (other than corpus luteum) = 75-85% PPV for ectopic
>   a. A moderate volume of free fluid increases this to 97% PPV
> (3) Nothing in the uterus + moderate free fluid = 70% PPV
>   a. More risk if the fluid is echogenic

Tubal Ring Sign: An echogenic ring, which surrounds an un-ruptured ectopic pregnancy. This is an excellent sign of ectopic pregnancy – and has been described as 95% specific.

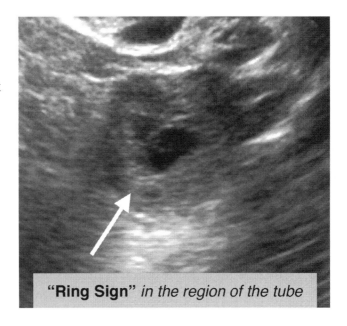

"Ring Sign" in the region of the tube

Heterotopic Pregnancy: This is a baby in the uterus and a baby in the tube (or other ectopic location). This is pretty rare, and typically only seen in women taking ovulation drugs, or prior bad PID.

Fetal Biometry and Fetal Growth:

In the second and third trimesters, four standard measurements of fetal growth are made (Biparietal, Head Circumference, Abdominal Circumference, and Femur Length). The testable trivia seems to include what level you make the measurement, and what is and is not included (see chart).

Fetal Measurement For Growth			
	Measurement Made	**NOT including**	**Trivia**
Biparietal Diameter "BPD"	Recorded at the level of the thalamus from the outermost edge of the near skull to the inner table of the far skull		Affected by the shape of the fetal skull (false large from brachycephaly, false small from dolichocephaly)
Head Circumference	Recorded at the same slice as BPD	Does NOT include the skin	Affected less by head shape
Abdominal Circumference	Recorded are the level of the junction of the umbilical vein and left portal vein	Does NOT include the subcutaneous soft tissues	
Femur Length	Longest dimension of the femoral shaft	Femoral epiphysis is NOT included	

Estimated Fetal Weight: This is calculated by the machine based or either (1) BPD and AC, or (2) AC and FL.

Gestational Age (GA): Ultrasound estimates of gestation age are the most accurate in an early pregnancy (and become less precise in the later portions). Age in the first trimester is made from crown rump length. Second and third trimester estimates for age are typically done using BPD, HC, AC, and FL – and referred to as a "composite GA."

Gestation Age (Less good later in the pregnancy)	
First Trimester – Crown Rump Length	Accurate to 0.5 weeks
2nd and 3rd Trimester – "Composite GA"	Accurate to 1.2 weeks (between 12 and 18 weeks)
	Accurate to 3.1 weeks (between 36 and 42 weeks)

Intrauterine Growth Retardation:

Readings Suggestive of IUGR:

- Estimated Fetal Weights Below 10th percentile
- Femur Length / Abdominal Circumference Ratio (F /AC) > 23.5
- Umbilical Artery Systolic / Diastolic Ratio > 4.0

Not All is lost: If the kid is measuring small, he might just be a little guy. If he has normal Doppler studies – most of the time they are ok.

Maybe All is lost: If the kid is measuring small, suggesting IUGR and he has oligohydramnios (AFI < 5) or polyhydramnios he/she is probably toast.

Trivia: Most common cause for developing oligohydramnios during the 3rd trimester = Fetal Growth Restriction associated with Placental Insufficiency.

Symmetrical vs Asymmetrical:

- *Asymmetrical:* Think about this as a restriction of weight followed by length. It is the more common of the two types. The head will be normal in size, with the body being small. Some people call this "**head sparing**," as the body tries to protect the brain. You **see this mainly in the third trimester**, as a result of extrinsic factors.

    The classic scenario would be normal growth for the first two trimesters, with a normal head / small body in the third trimester - with a mom having chronic high BP / pre-eclampsia.

    There are a bunch of causes. I recommend remembering these three: **High BP, Severe Malnutrition, Ehler-Danlos.**

- *Symmetric:* This is a global growth restriction, that **does NOT spare the head**. This is **seen throughout the pregnancy** (including the first trimester). The head and body are both small. This has a **much worse prognosis**, as the brain doesn't develop normally.

    There are also a bunch of causes. I recommend remembering these: **TORCH infection, Fetal Alcohol Syndrome / Drug Abuse, Chromosomal Abnormalities, and Anemia.**

Biophysical Profile: This thing was developed to look for acute and chronic hypoxia. Points are assigned (2 for normal, 0 for abnormal). A score of 8-10 is considered normal. To call something abnormal, technically you have to be watching for 30 mins.

Components of Biophysical Profile		
Amniotic Fluid	At least one pocket that measures 2cm or more in a vertical plane	Assess Chronic Hypoxia
Fetal Movement	3 discrete movements	Assess Acute Hypoxia
Fetal Tone	1 episode of fetal extension from flexion	Assess Acute Hypoxia
Fetal Breathing	1 episode of "Breathing motion" lasting 30 seconds	Assess Acute Hypoxia
Non-stress Test	2 or more fetal heart rate accelerations of at least 15 beats per minute and or 30 seconds or longer	Assess Acute Hypoxia

Umbilical Artery Systolic / Diastolic Ratio: The resistance in the umbilical artery should progressively decrease with gestational age. **The general rule is 2-3 at 32 weeks**. The ratio should not be more than 3 at 34 weeks. An elevated S/D ratio means there is high resistance. High resistance patterns are seen in pre-eclampsia and IUGR. Worse than an elevated ratio, is absent or reversed diastolic flow – this is associated with a very poor prognosis.

Macrosomia: Babies that are too big (above the 90th percentile). **Maternal diabetes** (usually gestational, but could be type 2 as well), is the most common cause. As a point of trivia, type 1 diabetic mothers can also have babies that are small secondary to hypoxia from microvascular disease of the placenta. The big issue with being too big is **complications during delivery** (shoulder dystocia, brachial plexus injury) and **after delivery** (neonatal hypoglycemia, meconium aspiration).

Erb's Palsy: Injury to the upper trunk of the brachial plexus (C5-C6), most commonly seen in shoulder dystocia (which kids with macrosomia are higher risk for).

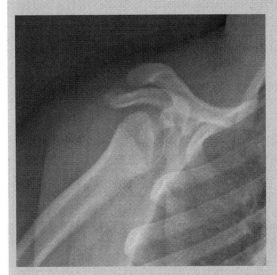

If you see an aplastic or hypoplastic humeral head / glenoid in a kid, you should immediately think about an Erbs Palsy.

Clinical Correlation.

Amniotic Fluid: Early on, the fluid in the amnion and chorionic spaces is the result of filtrate from the membranes. After 16 weeks, the fluid is made by the fetus (urine). The balance of too much (polyhydramnios) and too little (oligohydramnios) is maintained by swallowing of the urine and renal function. In other words, if you have too little fluid you should think kidneys aren't working. If you have too much fluid you should think swallow or other GI problems. Having said that, a common cause of too much fluid is high maternal sugars (gestational diabetes). Fine particulate in the fluid is normal, especially in the third trimester.

Amniotic Fluid Index: Made by measuring the vertical height of the deepest fluid pocket in each quadrant of the uterus then summing the 4 measurements. **Normal is 5-20. Oligohydramnios is defined as AFI < 5cm. Polyhydramnios is defined as AFI > 20cm, or a single fluid pocket > 8cm.**

Normal Development:

I'm going to briefly touch on what I think is testable trivia regarding normal development.

Brain: Choroid plexus is large and echogenic. There should be less than 3mm of separation of the choroid plexus from the medial wall of the lateral ventricle (if more it's ventriculomegaly). The cisterna magna should be between 2mm-11mm (too small think Chiari II, too large think Dandy Walker).

Face / Neck: The "fulcrum" of the upper lip is normal, and should not be called a cleft lip.

Lungs: The lungs are normally homogeneously echogenic, and similar in appearance to the liver.

Heart: The only thing to know is that a papillary muscle can calcify "Echogenic Foci in the ventricle", and although this is common and can mean nothing – it's also associated with an increased risk of Downs (look hard for other things).

Abdominal: If you only see one artery adjacent to the bladder, you have yourself a two vessel cord. Bowel should be less than 6mm in diameter. Bowel can be moderately echogenic in the 2nd and 3rd trimester but should never be more than bone. The adrenals are huge in newborns, and are said to be 20x their relative size.

Two Vessel Cord - Gamesmanship

There are two main ways to show a two vessel cord. The first one is a single vessel running lateral to the bladder down by the cord insertion. The second is to show the cord in cross section with two vessels.

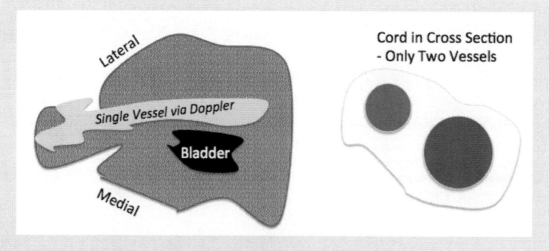

More on the 2 vessel cord in a few pages.

Classic Normal Pictures That Look Scary

Cystic Rhombencephalon: The normal rhombencephalon is present as a cystic structure in the posterior fossa around 6-8 weeks. *Don't call it a Dandy-Walker malformation*, for sure that will be a distractor.

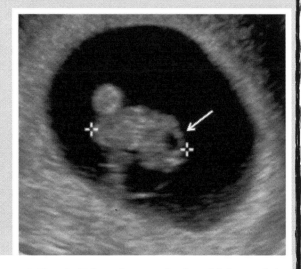

Normal Cystic Rhombencephalon (6-8 weeks)

Physiologic Mid Gut Herniation: The midgut normally herniates into the umbilical cord around 9-11 weeks. *Don't call it an omphalocele*, for sure that will be a distractor.

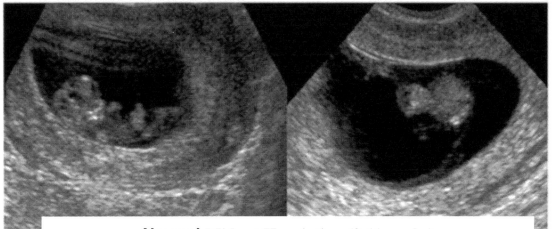

Normal Midgut Herniation (9-11 weeks)

Placenta and Umbilical Cord

Placenta

Normal: You can first start to see the placenta around 8 weeks (focal thickening along the periphery of the gestational sac). It should be shaped like a disc around 12 weeks. The normal sonographic appearance is "granular" with a smooth cover (the chorion). Underneath the basal surface there is a normal retroplacental complex of decidual and myometrial veins.

Normal Placenta Aging: As the placenta ages it gets hypoechoic areas, septations, and randomly distributed calcifications.

Venous Lakes: These are an incidental finding of no significance. They look like focal hypoechoic areas under the chorionic membrane (or within the placenta). You can sometimes see slow flow in them.

Placental Thickness	
Too Thin (< 1cm)	Too Thick (> 4cm)
Placental Insufficiency, Maternal Hypertension, Maternal DM, Trisomy 13, Trisomy 18, Toxemia of Pregnancy	Fetal Hydrops, Maternal DM, Severe Maternal Anemia, Congenital Fetal Cancer, Congenital Infection, Placental Abruption

Variant Placental Morphology:

Bilobed Placenta	Two near equal sized lobes	Increased risk of type 2 vasa previa, post partum hemorrhage from retained placental tissue, and velamentous insertion of the cord
Succenturiate Lobe	One or more small accessory lobes	Increased risk of type 2 vasa previa, post partum hemorrhage from retained placental tissue
Circumvallate Placenta	Rolled placental edges with smaller chorionic plate	High risk for placental abruption and IUGR

Placenta Previa: This is a low implantation of the placenta that covers part of or all of the internal cervical os. The clinical buzzword is "painless vaginal bleeding in the third trimester." A practical pearl is that you need to have an empty bladder when you look for this (full bladder creates a false positive).

Placental Abruption: This is a premature separation of the placenta from the myometrium. The step 1 history was always "mother doing cocaine", but it also occurs in the setting of hypertension. Technically subchorionic hemorrhage (marginal abruption) is in the category – as previously discussed. Retroplacental Abruption is the really bad one. The hematoma will appear as anechoic or mixed echogenicity beneath the placenta (often extending beneath the chorion). Buzzword is "disruption of the retroplacental complex."

Placental Abruption vs Myometrial Contraction / Fibroid	
Placental Abruption will **disrupt** the retroplacental complex of blood vessels	Myometrial Contractions / Fibroids will **displace** the retroplacental complex

Placenta Creta: This is an abnormal insertion of the placenta, which invades the myometrium. The severity is graded with fancy sounding Latin names. The risk factors include prior C-section, placenta previa, and advanced maternal age. The sonographic appearance varies depending on the severity, but generally speaking you are looking for a "moth-eaten" or "Swiss cheese" appearance of the placenta, with vascular channels extending from the placenta into the myometrium (with turbulent flow on Doppler). Thinning of the myometrium (less than 1mm) is another sign. This can be serious business, with life threatening bleeding sometimes requiring hysterectomy. The **big risk factor is prior c-section, and placenta previa.**

Placenta Accreta	Most common (75%) and mildest form. The villi attach to the myometrium, without invading.
Placenta Increta	Villi partially invade the myometrium
Placenta Percreta	The really bad one. Villi penetrate through the myometrium or beyond the serosa. Sometimes there is invasion of the bladder or bowel.

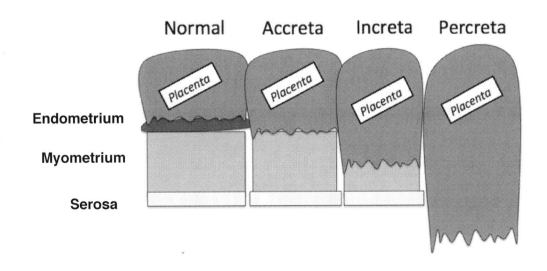

Placenta Chorioangioma: This is basically a **hamartoma** of the placenta, and is the most common benign tumor of the placenta. These are usually well circumscribed hypoechoic masses **near the cord insertion**. Flow within the mass pulsating at the fetal heart rate is diagnostic (they are perfused by the fetal circulation). They almost always mean nothing, but if they are large (> 4cm) and multiple ("choriangiomatosis") they can sequester platelets, and cause a high output failure (hydrops).

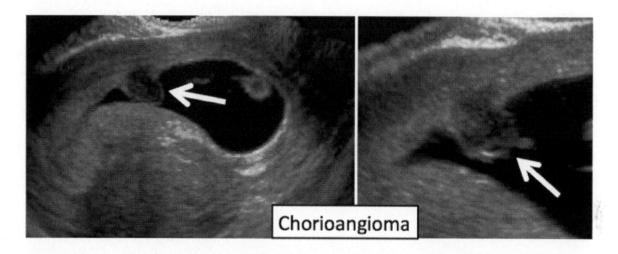

Placental Chorioangioma vs Placental Hematoma	
Chroriangioma has pulsating Doppler flow	Hematoma does NOT have pulsating Doppler flow.

Umbilical Cord

Normal Cord: Should have 3 vessels (2 arteries, 1 vein).

Two Vessel Cord: This is a normal variant – seen in about 1% of pregnancies. Usually the left artery is the one missing. This tends to occur more in twin pregnancies and maternal diabetes. There is an increased association with chromosomal anomalies and various fetal malformations (so look closely). Having said that, in isolation it doesn't mean much.

Velamentous Cord Insertion: This is the term for when the cord inserts into the fetal membranes outside the placental margin, and then has to travel back through the membranes to the placenta (between the amnion and the chorion). It's more common with twins, and increases the risk of intra-uterine growth restriction and growth discordance among twins.

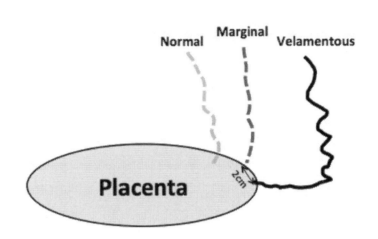

Marginal Cord Insertion: This is basically almost a velamentous insertion (cord is within 2cm of the placental margin). It's also seen more in twin pregnancies.

Vasa Previa: Fetal vessels that cross (or almost cross) the internal cervical os. It's seen more in twin pregnancies, and variant placental morphologies. There are two types:

- Type 1: Fetal vessels connect to a velamentous cord insertion within the main body of the placenta
- Type 2: Fetal vessels connect to a bilobed placenta or succenturiate lobe.

Nuchal Cord: This is the term used to describe a cord wrapped around the neck of the fetus. Obviously this can cause problems during delivery.

Umbilical Cord Cyst: These are common (seen about 3% of the time), and are usually single (but can be multiple). As a point of completely irrelevant trivia you can divide these into false and true cysts. True cysts are less common, but have fancy names so they are more likely to be tested. Just know that the omphalomesenteric duct cyst is usually peripheral, and the allantoic cyst is usually central. If the cysts persist into the 2nd or 3rd trimester then they might be associated with trisomy 18 and 13. You should look close for other problems.

Congenital Fetal Anomalies

Downs:

Ultrasound Findings Concerning for Downs Syndrome	
Congenital Heart Disease	More than half of fetuses (or feti, if you prefer) with Downs have congenital heart issues, - most commonly AV canal and VSD
Duodenal Atresia	Most common intra abdominal pathology associated with Downs (hard to see before 22 weeks)
Short Femur Length	Not Specific
Echogenic Bowel	Not Specific (can be seen with obstruction, infection, CF, ischemia, and lots of other stuff)
Choroid Plexus Cyst	Not Specific, and actually seen more with Trisomy 18. It should prompt a close survey for other findings (normal if in isolation)
Nuchal Translucency	Translucency > 3mm in the first trimester,
Nuchal Fold Thickness	Thickness > 6mm in the second trimester- nonspecific and can also be seen with Turners
Echogenic Focus in Cardiac Ventricle	Not Specific, but increased risk of Downs x 4

Nuchal Lucency: Measured between 9-12 weeks, this anechoic area between the neck/ occiput and the skin **should be less than 3mm**. Measurements > 3mm are associated with Downs (trisomy 21) or other chromosomal abnormalities. Positioning of the neck is critical to avoid false positives.

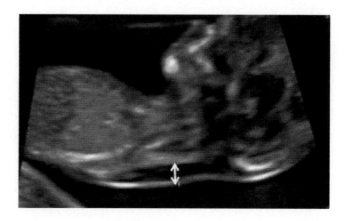

Amniotic Band Syndrome: The fetus needs to stay in the amniotic cavity, and stay the hell out of the chorionic cavity. If the amnion gets disrupted and the fetus wonders / floats into the chorionic cavity he/she can get caught in the sticky fibrous septa. All kinds of terrible can result ranging from decapitation, to arm/leg amputation. This is most likely to be shown in one of two ways: (1) a x-ray of a hand or baby gram showing fingers amputated or a hand/arm amputated – with the remaining exam normal, or (2) a fetal ultrasound with the bands entangling the arms or legs of a fetus.

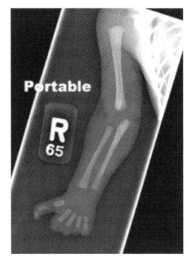

Amniotic Bands Syndrome
-Amputated Fingers

Hydrops: Fetal hydrops is bad news. This can be from immune or non-immune causes. The most common cause is probably Rh sensitization from prior pregnancy. Some other causes include; TORCHS, Turners, Twin Related Stuff, and Alpha Thalassemia. Ultrasound diagnosis is made by the presence of two of the following: **pleural effusion, pericardial effusion**, and Subcutaneous Edema. A sneaky trick is to instead show you a thickened placenta (> 4-5cm), although I think it's much more likely to show a pleural effusion and pericardial effusion.

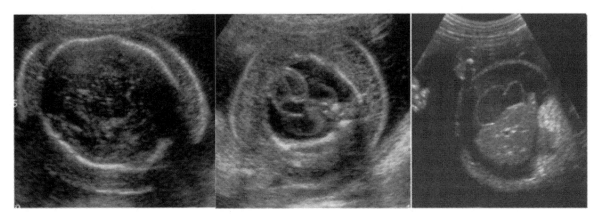

Hydrops - Body Wall Edema, Pleural Effusion, Ascites

Lemon Sign – The appearance of an indented frontal bone, **classically seen as a sign of Chiari II,** although **also seen a lot in spina bifida** (like 90% of the time). You typically see this before 24 weeks (it often **disappears after 24 weeks**).

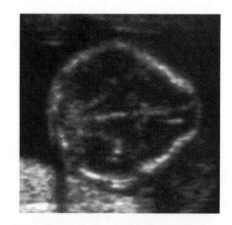

Lemon Sign - Indented Frontal Bone

Banana Sign – The way the cerebellum wraps around the brainstem as the result of spinal cord tethering (and downward migration of the posterior fossa) looks like a banana. In other words, the cisterna magna is obliterated and the cerebellum looks like a banana. Just like the lemon sign this is seen with **Chiari II and Spinal Bifida**.

Anterior curving of the cerebellar hemispheres with simultaneous obliteration of the cisterna magna is the so called "banana sign." Supposedly, the idea is that you have a neural tube defect, which lets you leak CSF from the spinal defect. Once you leak enough, you get hypotension in the subarachnoid space, with prolapse of the cerebellum into the foramen magnum.

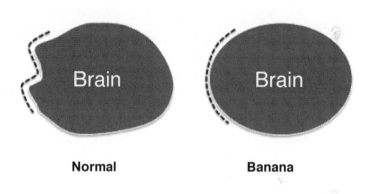

Other findings of spina bifida include a small biparietal diameter and ventricular enlargement.

Choroid Plexus Cyst – This is one of those incidental findings that in isolation means nothing. Having said that, the incidence of this finding is increased in trisomy 18, trisomy 21, Turner's Syndrome, and Klinefelter's.

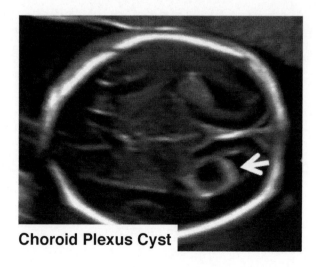

Choroid Plexus Cyst

Facial Clefts – This is the most common fetal facial anomaly. About 30% of the time you are dealing with a chromosome anomalies. Around 80% of babies is cleft lips have cerebral palsy. You can see cleft lips, but cleft palate (in isolation) is very hard to see.

Cystic Hygroma – If they show you a complex cystic mass in the posterior neck, in the antenatal period, this is the answer. The follow up is the association with Turners and Downs.

Ventriculomegaly - There are multiple causes including; hydrocephalus (both communicating and non-communicating), and cerebral atrophy. Obviously this is bad, and frequently associated with anomalies.

Things to know:
- Aquaductal Stenosis is the most common cause of non-communicating hydrocephalus in a neonate
- Ventricular atrium diameter > 10mm = too big
- "Dangling choroid" hanging off the wall more than 3mm = too big

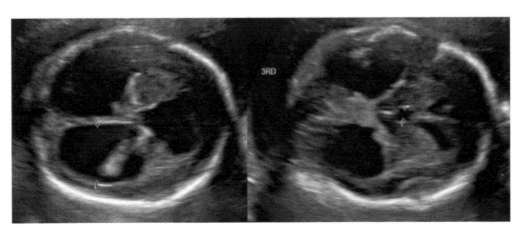

Ventriculomegaly - Shows dangling choroid

Anencephaly - This is the most common neural tube defect. You have total **absence of the cranial vault and brain above the level of the orbits**. Obviously this is not compatible with life.

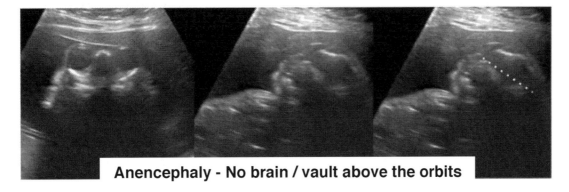

Anencephaly - No brain / vault above the orbits

Pleural Effusion – There are multiple causes of pleural effusion in the neonate, but when you see it I want you to think **Hydrops**. *The way they show hydrops in case conference / case books and very likely multiple choice is pleural effusions, pericardial effusions, and ascites.*

Congenital Diaphragmatic Hernia – Abdominal contents pushing into the chest. Nearly all are on the left (85%). The things to know is that it (1) causes a high mortality because of the association with **pulmonary hypoplasia**, and (2) that all the kids are **malrotated** (it messes with normal gut rotation). If they show this it will either be (a) a newborn chest x-ray, or (b) a 3rd trimester MRI.

Echogenic Intracardiac Focus (EIF) - This is a calcification seen in a papillary muscle (usually in the left ventricle). You see them all the time, they don't mean that much but are seen at a higher rate Trisomy 21 (12%) and Trisomy 13. So you are supposed to look for more features.

If they ask you a question about this they will be testing one of two facts :

(1) *it occurs in the normal general population - around 5%,*
(2) *it occurs more in Downs patients around - 12%.*

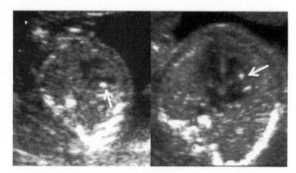

Echogenic Intracardiac Focus (EIF)

Abnormal Heart Rate: Tachycardia is defined as a rate > 180 bpm. Bradycardia is defined as a rate < 100 bpm.

Double Bubble: This is described in detail in the Peds Chapter. Just realize this can be shown with antenatal ultrasound, or MRI. It's still duodenal atresia.

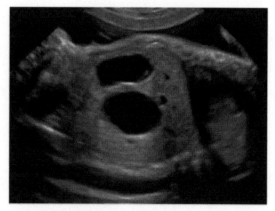

Double Bubble - Duodenal Atresia

Echogenic Bowel: This can be a normal variant but can also be associated with significant badness. Normally bowel is isoechoic to the liver. If it's equal to the iliac crest bone then it's too bright. The DDx includes CF, Downs and other Trisomies, Viral Infections, and Bowel Atresia.

Sacrococcygeal Teratoma: This is the most common tumor of the fetus or infant. These solid or cystic masses are typically large and found either on prenatal imaging or birth. They can cause mass effect on the GI system, hip dislocation, nerve compression causing incontinence, and high output cardiac failure. Additionally, they may cause issues with premature delivery, dystocia, and hemorrhage of the tumor. They are usually benign (80%). Those presenting in older infants tend to have a higher malignant potential. The location of the mass is either external to the pelvis (47%), internal to the pelvis (9%), or dumbell'd both inside and outside (34%).

Autosomal Recessive Polycystic Disease - The classic look is massively enlarged bilateral kidneys with oligohydramnios. Additional details in the Peds chapter.

Posterior Urethral Valves: The classic look is bilateral hydro on either fetal US or 3rd Trimester MRI.

Short Femur: A short femur (below the 5th percentile), can make you think of a skeletal Dysplasia.

Maternal Disorders in Pregnancy

Incompetent Cervix: When shortened the cervix is associated with high risk of premature delivery. You call it short when the endocervical canal is < 2.5cm in length.

Hydronephrosis occurs in 80% of pregnancy (mechanical compression of the ureters is likely the cause). It tends to affect the right more than the left (dextrorotation of the pregnant uterus).

Fibroids: Fibroids tend to grow in the early pregnancy secondary to elevated estrogen. Progesterone will have the opposite effect, inhibiting growth, in later pregnancy. Stretching of the uterus may affect the arterial blood supply and promote infarcts and cystic degeneration.

Things That Grow During Pregnancy:

- *Babies,*
- *Splenic Artery Aneurysms,*
- *Renal AMLs,*
- *Fibroids.*

Uterine Rupture: You see this most commonly in the **3rd trimester at the site of prior c-section**. Other risk factors worth knowing are the unicornuate uterus, prior uterine curettage, "trapped uterus" (persistent retroflexion from adhesions), and interstitial implantation.

HELLP Syndrome: Hemolysis**, E**levated **L**iver Enzymes**, L**ow **P**latelets. This is the most severe form of pre-eclampsia, and favors young primigravid women in their 3rd trimester. It's bad news and 20-40% end up with DIC. If they are going to show this, it will be as a subcapsular hepatic hematoma in pregnant (or recently pregnant) women.

Peripartum Cardiomyopathy: This is a dilated cardiomyopathy that is seen in the last month of pregnancy to 5 months post partum. The cardiac MRI findings include a global depressed function, and non-vascular territory subepicardial late Gd enhancement – corresponding to cellular lymphocyte infiltration.

Sheehan Syndrome: This is pituitary apoplexy seen in post-partum female who suffer from large volume hemorrhage. The pituitary grows during pregnancy, and if you have an acute hypotensive episode you can stroke it out. The look on MR is variable depending on the time period, acute it will probably be **T1 bright** (if they show a picture). Ring enhancement around an empty sella is a late look.

Ovarian Vein Thrombophlebitis – This can be a cause of postpartum fever. Risk factors include C-section, and endometritis. The right side is affected five times more often than the left. They could show you an enlarged ovary and a thrombosed adjacent ovarian vein.

Retained Products of Conception: The typical clinical story is continued bleeding after delivery (or induced abortion). The most common appearance is an echogenic mass within the uterine cavity. The presence or absence of flow is variable, you can have lots or you can have none. A sneaky way to show this is irregular thickening of the endometrium (>10mm) with some reflective structures and shadowing – representing the fetal parts. You can also think about RPOC when the endometrial thickness is > 5mm following dilation and curettage. Testable associations include: medical termination of pregnancy (abortion), second trimester miscarriage, and placenta accreta.

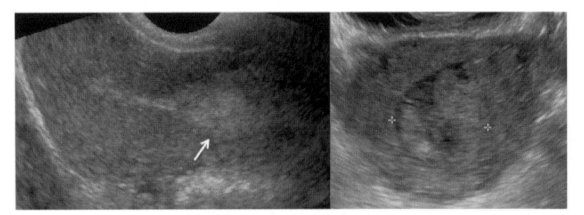

Retained Products of Conception

Endometritis - Broadly speaking it is an inflammation or infection of the endometrium. The history will be (if you are given one) fever and uterine tenderness and c-section (or prolonged labor). On ultrasound you will see a thickened, heterogenous endometrium, with or without fluid / air.

Multiple Gestations

Placentation Terminology: So you can have monozygotic twins (identical), or dizygotic twins (not-identical). The dizygotics are always dichorionic and diamniotic. The placenta of the monozygotics is more variable and depends of the timing of fertilized ovum splitting (before 8 days = diamniotic, after 8 days = monoamniotic). As a point of trivia, a late splitting (after 13 days) can cause a conjoined twin. As a general rule the later the split the worse things do (monoamniotics have more bad outcomes – they get all tangled up, and the conjoined ones have even more problems).

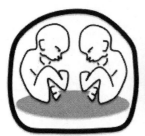
Monochorionic
Monoamniotic

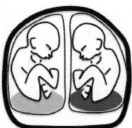
Monochorionic
Diamniotic

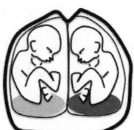
Dichorionic
Diamniotic
Fused Placenta

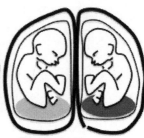
Dichorionic
Diamniotic
Separate Placenta

Monochorionic vs Dichorionic

Membrane Thickness: To differentiate the different types, some people use a method classifying thin and thick membranes. Thick = "easy to see" 1-2 mm, Thin = "hard to see." Thick is supposed to me there are 4 layers (dichorionic). Thin is supposed to be 2 layers (monochorionic). Obviously this method is very subjective

Twin-Peak Sign: A beak-like tongue between the two membranes of a dichorionic diamniotic fetuses. This **excludes a monochorionic pregnancy**.

T Sign: Think about this as basically the absence of the twin peak sign. You don't see chorion between membrane layers. **T sign = monochorionic pregnancy**.

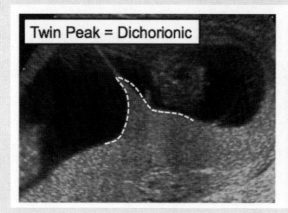
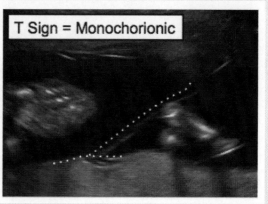

Twin Growth – You can use normal growth charts in the first and second trimester (but not the third). The femur length tends to work best for twin age in the later pregnancy. More than 15% difference in fetal weight or abdominal circumference between twins is considered significant.

Twin- Twin Transfusion - This occurs in monochorionic twins when a vascular communication exists in the placenta. You end up with one greedy fat twin who takes all the blood and nutrients, and one skinny wimpy looking kid who gets the scraps. The somewhat counter intuitive part is that the skinny kid actually does better, and the fat one usually gets hydrops and dies. You are going to have unequal fluid in the amniotic sacs, with the donor (skinny) twin having severe oligohydramnios and is sometimes **(*buzzword) "stuck to the wall of the uterus"**. The fat twin floats freely in his polyhydramniotic sac. The donor (skinny) twin will also have a high resistance umbilical artery spectrum.

Twin Reversed Arterial Perfusion Syndrome – You can get intraplacental shunting that results in a "pump twin" who will pump blood to the other twin. The other twin will not develop a heart and is typically referred to as an "acardiac twin." The acardiac twin will be wrecked (totally deformed upper body). The "pump twin" is usually normal, and does ok as long as the strain on his/her heart isn't too much. If the acardiac twin is really big (> 70% estimated fetal weight of the co-twin) then the strain will usually kill the pump twin. They could show this as a Doppler ultrasound demonstrating umbilical artery flow toward the acardiac twin, or umbilical vein flow away from the acardiac twin.

One Dead Twin – At any point during the pregnancy one of the twins can die. It's a bigger problem (for the surviving twin) if it occurs later in the pregnancy. "**Fetal Papyraceous**" is a fancy sounding Latin word for a pressed flat dead fetus.

"**Twin-Twin Embolization Syndrome**" is when you have embolized necrotic dead baby being transferred to the living fetus *(soylent green is people!)*. This can result in DIC, tissue ischemia, and infarct. By the way, a testable point is that this transfer can only occur in a monochorionic pregnancy.

Section 4: Breast

Anatomy:

Nipple: The nipple is a circular smooth muscle that overlies the 4th intercostal space. There are typically 5-10 ductal openings. *Inversion* is when the nipple invaginates into the breast. *Retraction* is when the nipple is pulled back slightly. They can both be normal if chronic. If they are new, it should make you think about underlying cancers causing distortion. The nipple is suppose to be in profile, so you don't call it a mass. The areola will darken normally with puberty and parity. Nipple enhancement on contrast enhancement breast MRI is normal , don't call it pagets.

Fibroglandular Tissue: The breast mound is fibrous tissue with fat, ducts, and glands laying on top of the anterior chest wall. The axillary extension is called the *"tail of Spence."* The upper outer quadrant is more densely populated with fibroglandular tissue, which is why most breast cancers start there. There is usually no dense tissue in the medial/ inferior breast and retroglandular regions. These are considered "danger zones" and are often where the cancer hides.

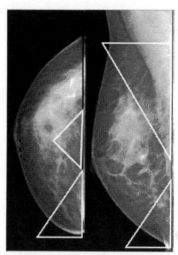

Danger Zones – *where there is usually no dense fibroglandular tissue*

Cooper Ligaments: These are thin sheets of fascia that holds the breasts up. They are the tiny white lines on mammography and the echogenic lines on US. Straightening and tethering of the ligaments manifests as "architectural distortion" which occurs in the setting of surgical scars, radial scars, and IDC.

Breast Asymmetry: This is common and normal (usually), as long as there are no other findings (lumps, bumps, skin thickening, etc..). *For multiple choice, an asymmetric breast should make you think about the "shrinking breast" of invasive lobular breast cancer.* If the size difference is new or the parenchyma looks asymmetrically dense think cancer.

Lobules: The lobules are the flower shaped milk makers of the breast. The terminal duct and lobule are referred to as a "terminal duct lobule unit" or TDLU. This is where most breast cancers start.

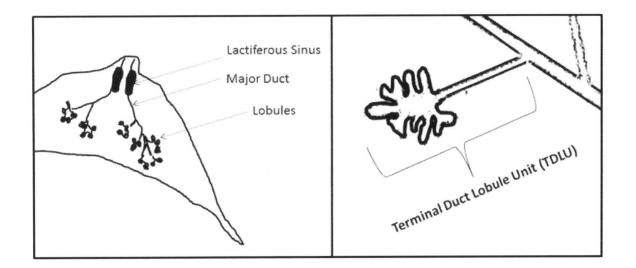

Ducts: The ductal system branches like the roots or branches of a tree. The branches overlap wide areas and are not cleanly segmented like slices of pie. The calcifications that appear to follow the duct ("linear or segmental") are the ones you should worry about cancer with.

Lactiferous Sinus: Milk from the lobules drains into the major duct under the nipple. The dilated portion of the major duct is sometimes called the lactiferous sinus. This thing is normal (not a mass).

Blood Supply / Lymphatic Drainage: The majority (60%) of blood flow to the breast is via the internal mammary. The rest goes to the lateral thoracic and intercostal perforators. Nearly all (97%) of lymph drains to the axilla. The remaining 3% goes to the internal mammary nodes.

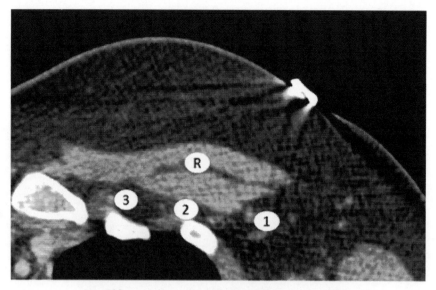

Axillary Lymph Node Levels:

Level 1: Lateral to Pec Minor
Level 2: Under Pec Minor
Level 3: Medial to Pec Minor
Rotter Node: Between Pec Major and Minor

Metastasis to the Internal Mammary Nodes: If you can see them on ultrasound they are abnormal. Isolated mets to these nodes is not a common situation (maybe 3%). When you do see it happen it's from a medial cancer.

Sternalis Muscle: This is an Aunt Minnie. It's a non-functional muscle next to the sternum that can simulate a mass. It is **ONLY SEEN ON THE CC VIEW**. It's usually unilateral more than half of the time. Handling this in real life is all about the old gold. Find that thing on the priors (even better is a CT), CC only, **never on the MLO**.

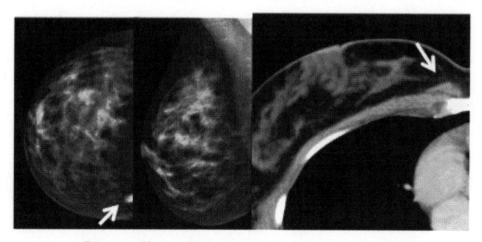

Sternalis – Only on CC, Never on MLO

Breast Development / Physiology: The "milk streak" is the embryologic buzzword to explain the location of the normal breast and location of ectopic breast tissue. Just know that the **most common location for ectopic breast tissue is in the axilla** (second most common is the inframammary fold). Extra nipples are most commonly in the same locations (but can be anywhere along the "milk streak"). At birth both males and females can have breast enlargement and produce milk (maternal hormones). As girls enter puberty their ducts elongate and branch (estrogen effects), then their lobules proliferate (progesterone effects). If you biopsy a breast bud (why would you do that?) you can damage it and affect breast development.... and then get sued.

- *Follicular Phase (day 7-14):* Estrogen Dominates. Best time to have both mammogram and MRI.

- *Luteal Phase (day 15-30):* Progesterone Dominates. This is when you get some breast tenderness (max at day 28-30). Breast density increases slightly.

- *Pregnancy:* Tubes and Duct Proliferate. The breast gets a lot denser (more hypoechoic on US), and ultrasound may be your best bet if you have a mass.

- *Perimenopausal:* Shortening of the follicular phase means the breast gets more progesterone exposure. More progesterone exposure means more breast pain, more fibrocystic change, more breast cyst formation.

- *Menopause:* Lobules go down. Ducts stay but may become ectatic. Fibroadenomas will degenerate (they like estrogen), and get their "popcorn" calcifications. Secretory calcifications will develop (*but not for 15-20 years post menopause).

- *Hormone Replacement Therapy:* Breast get more dense (even more so estrogen-progesterone combos). Breast pain can occur, typically peaking the first year. Fibroadenoma (who like to drink estrogen) can grow.

High Yield Trivia Regarding Breast Anatomy / Physiology

- The nipple can enhance with contrast on MRI. This is normal (not Pagets).
- Most cancers occur in the upper outer quadrant.
- Most cancers start in the terminal duct lobule unit (TDLU).
- Majority (60%) of blood flow is via the internal mammary.
- Mets to the Internal Mammary Nodes are uncommon (3%) – seen in medial cancers.
- Axillary Node Levels (3, 2, 1 – medial to lateral -)
- Sternalis is usually unilateral, and only on the CC, NEVER on MLO.
- Breast Tenderness is max around day 27-30.
- Mammography and MRI are best performed in the follicular phase (days 7-14).
- Don't Biopsy a prepubescent breast – you can affect breast development
- Perimenopause (50s) is the peak time for breast pain, cyst formation
- Fibroadenomas will degenerate (buzzword popcorn calcification) in menopause

What You Know About Lactation?

Density: As mentioned above the breast gets a lot denser in the 3rd trimester. Mammograms might be worthless, and ultrasound could be your only hope. In other words, ultrasound has greater sensitivity than mammo in lactating patients.

Density Trick: Pituitary Prolactinoma, or meds (classically antipsychotics) can create a similar bilateral increased density.

Biopsy: You can biopsy a breast that is getting ready to lactate / lactating - you just need to know there is **the risk of creating a milk fistula**. If you make one, they will have to stop breast feeding to stop the fistula. The fistula can get infected, but that's not very common.

Galactocele: This is one of those "benign fat containing lesions" that you can call benign. This is typically seen on cessation of lactation. The location is typically sub-areolar. The appearance is variable, but can have an **Aunt Minnie look with a fat-fluid level**. It's possible to breast abscess these things up.

Lactating Adenoma: These things look like fibroadenomas, and may actually be a charged up fibroadenoma (they like to drink estrogen). Usually these are **multiple.** If you get pressed on follow up recommendation for these I would say 4-6 months postpartum, post delivery or after cessation of lactation -via ultrasound. They usually **rapidly regress after you stop lactation**.

Technique

Basics: A screening mammogram starts with two standard views; a cranial caudal view and a medial lateral oblique view.

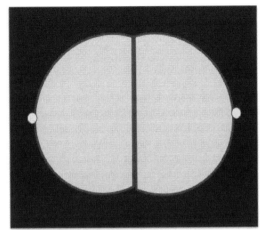
Cranial Caudal View "CC"

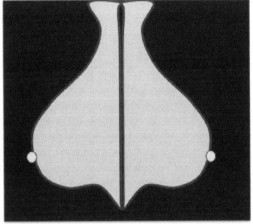
Medial Lateral Oblique View "MLO"

When you see a mammogram, the first question you have to asked - Is the technique adequate?

The **Posterior Nipple Line** – is drawn on the MLO from the nipple to the chest wall. You need to touch pectoralis muscle to be adequate.

Then on CC, you draw a line from the nipple back towards the chest wall. To be adequate **you must be within 1 cm of the length of the posterior nipple line.**

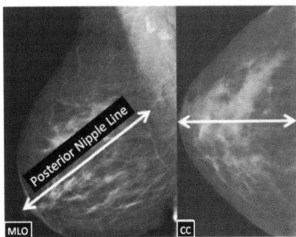

So other points and trivia:

- Ideally, the inframammary fold should be visualized
- "Camel Nose" is the buzzword used to describe a breast on MLO that has not be pulled "up and out" by the tech
- The nipple should be in profile in one of two views (to avoid missing the subareolar cancer).
- Relaxed pectoralis muscles are preferred (concave, instead of convex) – showing more breast tissue.

When do you get a LMO view ? The MLO is the standard, but sometimes you see a LMO. The answer is women with **kyphosis or pectus excavatum**. Or to **avoid a medial pacemaker / central line**.

MLO View Trivia: The MLO view contains the most breast tissue of all the possible views

When using Spot Compression Views: A big point is the recommendation to **leave the collimator open**, giving you a larger field of view, and helping to ensure that you got what you wanted to get. Small paddles give you better focal compression. Large paddles allow for good visualization of land marks.

When using Magnification Views: A CC and ML (true lateral) are obtained. You **get a ML (as opposed to a MLO) to help catch milk of calcium**.

When using a True Lateral View ML vs LM: Using a true lateral is useful for localizing things seen on a single view only (the CC). A trick I use is whatever I said on the screener, is the last letter I'd use on the call backs. In other words, if it's Lateral on the screener you want an ML on the diagnostic. If it's Medial on the screener then you want a LM on the diagnostic. The reason is that you are moving it closer to the receptor. **If you see the area of interest on the MLO only (not the CC), you should pick ML – because most (70%) of breast cancers occur laterally**. --- This would make a good multiple choice question.

Artifacts:

Blur: Can be from breathing or inadequate compression (typically along the inferior breast on the MLO). It can be tricky to pick up. The strategy I like to use, is to look at the Cooper Ligaments – they should be thin white lines in the fat. If they are thick or fuzzy – it is probably blur (or edema). If there is skin thickening think edema.

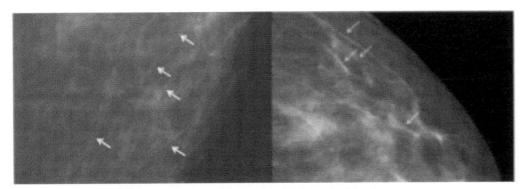

Blur: *Coopers too thick for normal skin*

Grid Lines: Basically mammograms always use a grid (unless it's a mag view). That would make a good multiple choice question actually. No grid on mag views. So, the grid works by moving really fast, and only keeping x-rays that move straight in. You see blur in 3 scenarios (1) patient moved, (2) exposure was too long, (3) exposure was too short.

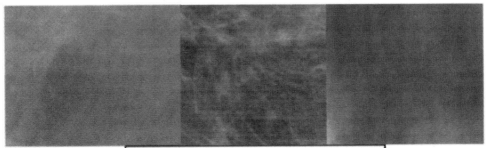

Grid Lines: 3 Examples – horizontal lines

General Tips on Screening Mammograms

You are trying to find **3-8 cancers per 1000 mammograms** – as demanded by the various regulating bodies

Be aware that certain areas can sometimes only be seen on a single view. For example, the **medial breast on a CC may not be seen on MLO**, and the **Inferior Posterior Breast on MLO may be excluded from the CC**. That makes these areas "high risk" for missing a cancer.

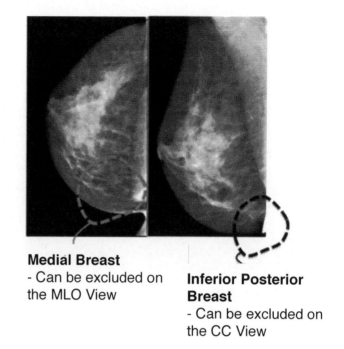

Medial Breast
- Can be excluded on the MLO View

Inferior Posterior Breast
- Can be excluded on the CC View

It's recommended to look at mammograms from 2 years prior (if available) for comparison. Makes it a little easier to see early changes.

Localizing a lesion: This is a very basic skill, but if you had absolutely no interest in mammography or just terrible training a refresher might be useful as this is applicable to multiple choice tests. A lesion that is medial on the CC film, will become more superior on the MLO, and even more superior on the ML. The opposite is true of lateral lesions which become more inferior. The popular mnemonic is *"Lead Sinks, and Muffins Rise"* – L for lateral, and M for medial.

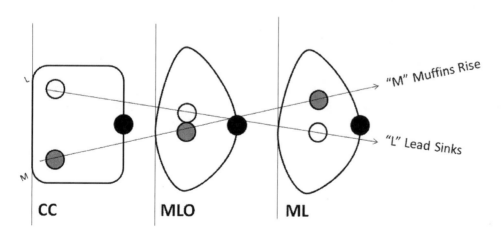

Localizing a lesion (only seen in the CC view): Sometimes you can only see the finding in the CC view. If you want to further characterize it with ultrasound, figuring out if it's in the superior or inferior breast could be very helpful. One method for doing this is a "rolled CC view."

Rolled CC View: This works by positioning the breast for a CC view, but prior to placing the breast in compression you rotate the breast either medial or lateral along the axis of the nipple. Your reference point is the top of the breast.

- If you roll the breast medial; a superior tumor will move medial, an inferior tumor will move lateral.
- If you roll the breast lateral; a superior tumor will move lateral, an inferior tumor will move medial.

In other words, **superior tumors move in the direction you roll** and inferior tumors move in the opposite direction you roll.

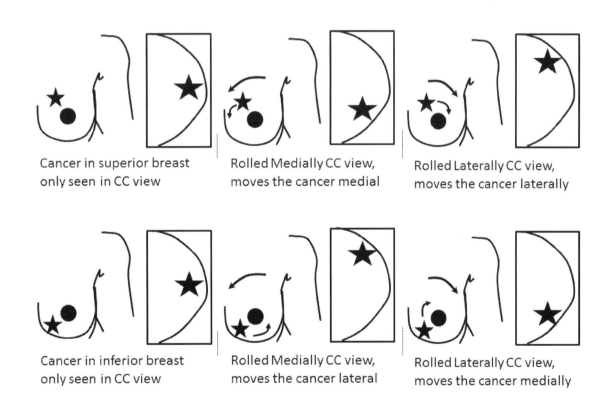

Cancer in superior breast only seen in CC view

Rolled Medially CC view, moves the cancer medial

Rolled Laterally CC view, moves the cancer laterally

Cancer in inferior breast only seen in CC view

Rolled Medially CC view, moves the cancer lateral

Rolled Laterally CC view, moves the cancer medially

BI-RADS / UK System

BI-RADS is an acronym for Breast Imaging-Reporting and Data System. It was developed by the American College of Radiology to keep everyone on the same page. You can't have people just calling stuff "breast nodules". There are "philosophical differences" between the investigation strategies for breast lesions in the UK and the United States that have stippled the applications of the BI-RADS in the UK. As I'm sure you know, the UK uses a 5 point breast imaging scoring system for communication and diagnosis. As an American trained Radiologist, I'm less familiar with this… and don't want to fuck it up. So, I'm going to not get into the mud with this one. I'll leave you to consult the appropriate RCR approved texts on the nomenclature.

Calcifications

Calcifications can be an early sign of breast cancer. "The earliest sign" actually, according to some. Calcifications basically come in three flavors: (1) artifact, (2) benign, and (3) suspicious.

Artifact:

Deodorant: High density material seen in the axilla is the typical appearance. Another trick is to show a speck of high density material that doesn't change position on different views (inferring that it's on the image receptor).

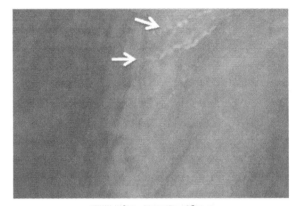

Deodorant Artifact

Zinc Oxide: This is in an ointment old ladies like to put on their floppy sweaty breasts. It can collect on moles and mimic calcifications. If it disappears on the follow up it was probably this (or another dermal artifact).

Metallic Artifact: It's possible for the electrocautery device to leave small metallic fragments in the breast. These will be very dense (metal is denser than calcium). It will also be adjacent to a scar.

Benign vs Suspicious:

The distinction between benign and suspicious is made based on morphology and distribution. Since most breast cancers start in the ducts (a single duct in most cases), a linear or segmental distribution is the most concerning. The opposite of this would be bilateral scattered calcifications.

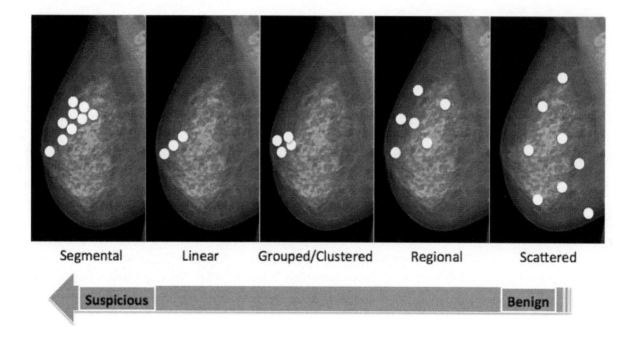

Benign:

Dermal Calcifications: These are found anywhere women sweat (folds, cleavage, axilla). Just think folds. They are often grouped like the paw of a bear, or the foot of a baby. The trick here is that these **stay in the same place on CC, and MLO view**. This is the so called **"tattoo sign."** If you are asked to confirm these are dermal calcs, I'd ask for a "tangential view."

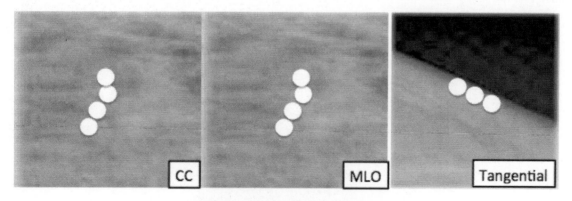

Dermal Calcifications

Vascular Calcifications: These are parallel linear calcifications. It's usually obvious, but not always.

Popcorn Calcifications: This is an immediate buzzword for degenerating fibroadenoma. The typical look is they begin around the periphery and slowly coalescent over subsequent images.

Secretory (Rod-Like) Calcifications: These are big, easily seen, and point toward the nipple. They are typically bilateral. The buzzword is *"cigar shaped with a lucent center."* Another buzzword is *"dashes but no dots."* The buzz age is *"10-20 years after menopause."* **Don't be an idiot and call these in a premenopausal patient,** they happen because the duct has involuted.

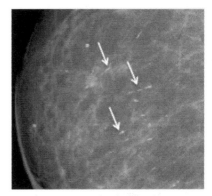

Secretory Calcifications

Eggshell Calcifications: "Fat necrosis" I call them. It can be from any kind of trauma (surgical, or accident - play ground related). If they are really massive you may see the word **"liponecrosis macrocystica."** As I've mentioned many times in this book, anything that sound Latin or French is high yield for multiple choice. *"Lucent Centered" is a buzzword.*

Dystrophic Calcifications: These are also seen after radiation, trauma, or surgery. These are usually big. *The buzzword is "irregular in shape."* They can also have a lucent center.

Milk of Calcium: This has a very characteristic look, and because of that questions can only be asked in one of two ways: (1) what is it? - shown as CC then ML, (2) what is it due to ?

(1) On the CC view the calcifications look powdery and spread out, on the MLO view they may layer. I suspect they will show you a **ML** view because they should layer into a more linear appearance, with a curved bottom **"tea-cupped."** *For the purpose of gamesmanship if they show you a ML view on a calcs question - look hard for anything that resembles tea-cupping.*

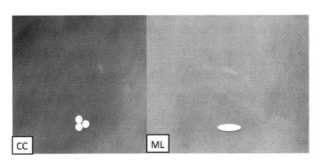

Milk of Calcium – *Tea Cups on ML*

(2) It's fluid-fluid in a lobule - **due to fibrocystic change.**

> **No Calcifications on the Biopsy?**
>
> This is a common trick. Apparently **Milk of Calcium needs to be viewed with polarized light to assess birefringence**. Otherwise, you can't see it. I imagine there are several ways to get at that via multiple choice.

Round: The idea is that these things develop in lobules, are usually scattered, bilateral, and benign. When benign (which is most of the time) they *are going to be due to fibrocystic change* (most of the time). The best way I've heard to think about these is the same as a mass. When masses are bilateral, multiple, and similar they are considered benign. When a mass is by itself or different it's considered suspicious. Round calcifications are the same way. They are usually bilateral and symmetric (and benign). If they are clustered together by themselves, or new they may need worked up (just like a mass).

Suspicious

Amorphous - These things look like powdered sugar, and you should not be able to count each individual calcification. Distribution is key with amorphous calcs (like many other types before). If the calcs are scattered and bilateral they are probably benign, if they are segmental they are probably concerning.

> **DDx Amorphous Ca^{+2}**
>
> Fibrocystic Change *(most likely)*
> Sclerosing Adenosis
> Columnar Cell Change
> DCIS (low grade)

Coarse Heterogeneous - These calcifications are countable, but their tips are dull. If you picked one up it would not be poke you. They are usually **bigger than 0.5mm.** Distribution and comparison to priors is always important. They can be associated with a mass (fibroadenoma, or papilloma).

> **DDx Coarse Heterogeneous Ca^{+2}**
>
> Fibroadenoma
> Papilloma
> Fibrocystic Change
> DCIS *(low - intermediate grade)*

Fine Pleomorphic - These calcifications are countable, and their tips appear sharp. If you picked one up it would poke you. They are usually **smaller than 0.5mm.** *This morphology has the highest suspicion for malignancy (that would make a good multiple choice question huh?).*

> **DDx Fine Pleomorphic Ca^{+2}**
>
> Fibroadenoma *(less likely)*
> Papilloma *(less likely)*
> Fibrocystic Change
> DCIS *(high grade)*

Fine Linear / Fine Linear Branching - This is a distribution that makes fine pleomorphic calcifications even more suspicious. The **DDx narrows to basically DCIS** or an atypical look for secretory calcs or vascular calcs.

Calcifications Associated with Focal Asymmetry/Mass: When you see increased tissue density around suspicious calcifications the chance of an actual cancer goes up. This is sometimes called a **"puff of smoke" sign**, or a "warning shot." This is a situation where ultrasound is useful, for extent of disease.

Calcifications in/near a Lumpectomy Scar: The local recurrence rate is around 6%. New calcifications with a suspicious morphology (not fat necrosis) deserves a biopsy.

Gamesmanship - Next Step:

Ultrasound is NOT typically used to evaluated a pure calcification findings. Exceptions would be (a) if the patient had a mass associated with the calcifications, or (b) if the patient had a palpable finding - then they would get addition evaluation with ultrasound.

Benign Breast Disease

Mondor Disease: This is a thrombosed vein that presents as a tender palpable cord. It looks exactly like you'd expect it to with ultrasound. You don't anticoagulate for it (it's not a DVT). Treatment is just NSAIDS and warm compresses.

Fat Containing Lesions: There are five classic fat containing lesions, all of which are benign. The oil cyst / fat necrosis, hamartoma, galactocele, lymph nodes, and lipoma. Of these 5, only oil cyst/fat necrosis and lipoma are considered "pure fat containing" masses.

- **Hamartoma** – The buzzword is "breast within a breast." They have an Aunt Minnie appearance on mammography, although they are difficult to see on ultrasound (they blend into the background).

- **Galactocele** – Seen in young lactating women. This is typically seen on cessation of lactation. The location is typically sub-areolar. The appearance is variable, but can have an Aunt Minnie look with a fat-fluid level. It's possible to breast abscess these things up.

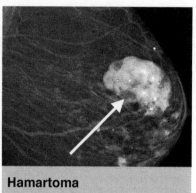

Hamartoma
- "Breast within a Breast"

- **Oil Cyst / Fat Necrosis** – These are areas of fat necrosis walled off by fibrous tissue. You see this (1) randomly, (2) post trauma, (3) post surgery. The peripheral calcification pattern is typically "egg shells." *If you see a ton of them you might think about steatocystoma multiplex* (some zebra with hamartomas).

- **Lipoma** – These are typically radiolucent with no calcifications. Enlargement of a lipoma is criteria for a biopsy.

- **Intramammary Lymph node:** These are normal and typically located in the tissue along the pectoral muscle, often close to blood vessels. They are NOT seen in the fibroglandular tissue.

> **Practice Point:** *Does she need an ultrasound if it's palpable?* Usually a palpable finding is going to get an ultrasound. If you are under 30 most people will skip the mammo and go straight to ultrasound. One of the exceptions is a fat containing lesion a definite benign finding on diagnostic mammography.

Pseudoangiomatous Stromal Hyperplasia (PASH): The is a benign myofibroblastic hyperplastic process (hopefully that clears things up). It's usually big (4-6cm), solid, oval shaped, with well defined borders. Age range is wide and they can be seen between 18-50 years old. Follow up in 12 months (annual) is the typical recommendation.

Pseudoangiomatous Stromal Hyperplasia = Benign thing with a scary sounding name

Fibroadenoma – This is the most common palpable mass in young women. The typical appearance is an oval, circumscribed mass with homogeneous hypoechoic exchotexture, and a central hyperechoic band. If it's shown in an older patient it's more likely to have coarse "popcorn" calcifications – which is a buzzword. On MRI, it's T2 bright with a type 1 enhancement (progressive enhancement).

Phyllodes: Although I clumped this in benign disease, this thing has a malignant degeneration risk of about 10%. They can metastasize - usually hematogenous to the lungs and bone. This is a fast growing breast mass. They need wide margins on resection, as they are associated with a higher recurrence rate if the margin is < 2cm. It occurs in an older age group than the fibroadenoma (40s-50s). Biopsy of the sentinel node is not needed, because mets via the lymphatics are so incredibly rare (if it does met - it's hematogenous).

Distinguishing Features of Phyllodes Tumor
- *Rapid Growth*
- *Hematogenous Mets*
- *Middle-Age to Older Women*
- *Mimics a Fibroadenoma*

Cancer

IDC - Invasive Ductal Carcinoma is by far the most common invasive breast cancer, making up about 80-85% of the cases. This cancer is ductal in origin (duh), but unlike DCIS is not confined to the duct. Instead it "invades" through the duct and if not found by the heroic action of mammographers it will progress to distal mets and certain death. Clinically, the most common story is a hard, non-mobile, painless mass. On imaging, the most common look is an irregular, high density mass, with indistinct or spiculated margins, associated pleomorphic calcifications, and an anti-parallel shadowing mass with an echogenic halo on ultrasound.

Invasive Ductal NOS - By far the most common type of breast cancer is the one that is undifferentiated and has no distinguishing histological features. "Not Otherwise Specified" or NOS they call it. These guys make up about 65% of invasive breast cancer.

IDC Subtypes

IDC Types – (Other than NOS)		
Tubular	Small **spiculated** slow growing mass, with a **favorable prognosis.**	Often conspicuous on ultrasound. **Associated with a Radial Scar.** Contralateral breast will have cancer 10-15% of the time.
Mucinous	**Round** (or lobulated) and circumscribed mass	**Uncommon.** Better outcomes that IDC-NOS
Medullary	**Round** or Oval circumscribed mass, without calcifications.	**Axillary nodes can be large even in the absence of mets.** Typically younger patient (40s-50s). Better outcome that IDC-NOS -25% have BRCA 1 mutation
Papillary	**Complex cystic and solid.**	**Axillary nodes are NOT common.** Typically seen in elderly people, favors people who are not white, and is the 2nd most common (behind IDC-NOS).

Multifocal Breast Cancer	**Multicentric Breast Cancer**
Multiple primaries in the same quadrant (classically same duct system) *Less than 4-5cm apart from one another*	Multiple primaries in different quadrants *Think of this like "multi-center" clinical trial; multiple discrete un-related sites.*

Synchronous Bilateral Breast Cancer – This is seen in 2-3% of women on mammography, with another 3-6% found with MRI. The risk of bilateral disease is increased in infiltrating lobular types, and multi-centric disease.

DCIS - This is the "earliest form of breast cancer." In this situation the "cancer" is confined to the duct. Histologists grade it as low, intermediate, or high. Histologists also use the terms "comedo", and "non-comedo" to subdivide the disease. If anyone would ask, the **comedo type is more aggressive** than than the non-comedo types.

Testable Trivia:
- 10% of DCIS on imaging may have an invasive component at the time biopsy is done
- 25% of DCIS on core biopsy may have an invasive component on surgical excision.
- 8% of DCIS will present as a mass without calcifications
- Most common ultrasound appearance = microlobulated mildly hypoechoic mass with ductal extension, and normal acoustic transmission

If a test writer wants you to come down on this they will show it in 1 of 3 classic ways:
(1) suspicious calcifications (fine linear branching or fine pleomorphic - as discussed above),
(2) non mass like enhancement on MRI, or (3) multiple intraductal masses on galactography.

Lobular (ILC) : This is the second most common type of breast cancer (IDC-NOS being the most common). It makes up about 5-10% of the breast CA cases. This pathophysiology lends itself well to multiple choice questions.

Cell decides to be cancer -> Cells lose "e-cadherin" -> Cells no longer stick to one another and begin to infiltrate the breast "like the web of a spider" -> This infiltrative pattern does not cause a desmoplastic reaction so it gets missed on multiple mammograms -> Finally someone (you) notices some architectural distortion without a central mass, on the CC view only. You get fancy and call it a "dark star."

On Ultrasound: The typical look is an ill-defined area of shadowing without a mass.

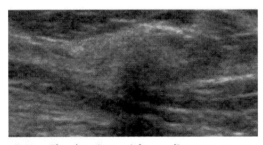

ILC – *Shadowing without discrete mass*

"Shrinking Breast" – This is a buzzword for ILC. The breast isn't actually smaller, it just doesn't compress as much. So when you compare it to a normal breast, it appears to be getting smaller. On physical exam, this breast may actually look the same size as the other one.

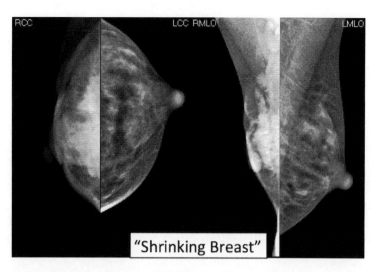

"Shrinking Breast"

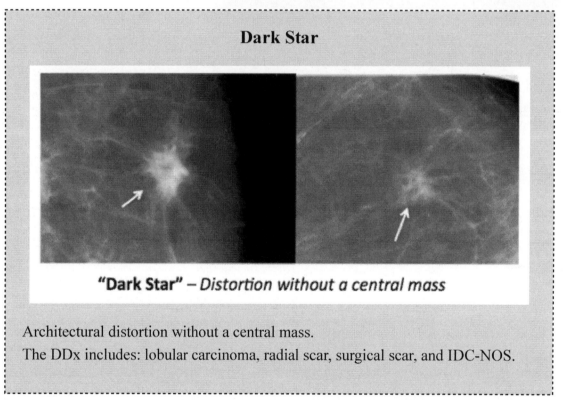

"Dark Star" – *Distortion without a central mass*

Architectural distortion without a central mass.
The DDx includes: lobular carcinoma, radial scar, surgical scar, and IDC-NOS.

ILC vs IDC: ILC is more often multifocal. ILC less often mets to the axilla. Instead, it likes to go to strange places like peritoneal surfaces. ILC more often has positive margins, and more often treated with mastectomy although the prognosis is similar to IDC.

Things to know about ILC:

- It presents later than IDC
- Tends to occur in an older population
- It often is only seen in one view (the CC – as it compresses better)
- Calcifications are less common than with ductal cancers
- Mammo Buzzword = Dark Star
- Mammo Buzzword = Shrinking Breast
- Ultrasound Buzzword = Shadowing without mass
- On MRI – washout is less common than with IDC
- Axillary mets are less common
- Prognosis of IDC and ILC is similar *(unless it's a pleomorphic ILC, - which is very aggressive)*
- More often multifocal and bilateral (compared to IDC) - up to 1/3 are bilateral

Inflammatory Breast Cancer: The prognosis is usually terrible. They will try and do chemotherapy prior to surgery because the chance of a positive margin is so high. The mastectomy is done for "local control", which just sounds awful. A swollen red breast is what you are going to see, and as I'll discuss below under the "symptomatic breast" section your differential is mastitis vs this. "Skin thickening" is a mammography buzzword (non-specific). The inflammation associated with inflammatory breast cancer can actually improve with antibiotics, but does NOT resolve. So, don't be fooled (in the real world or on a multiple choice test). A dermal biopsy is sometimes needed if you can't find an underlying mass.

Pagets - Paget's disease of the breast is a high yield topic. It is basically a carcinoma in situ of the nipple epidermis. About 50% of the time the patient will have a palpable finding associated with the skin changes.

Things to know about Breast Pagets:
- Associated with **high grade DCIS**
- Wedge biopsy should be done on any skin lesion that affect the nipple-areolar complex that doesn't resolve with topical therapy.
- Pagets is NOT considered T4. The skin involvement does not up the stage in this setting.

High Risk Lesions:

There are 5 classic high risk lesions that must come out after a biopsy; Radial Scar, Atypical Ductal Hyperplasia, Atypical Lobular Hyperplasia, LCIS, and Papilloma.

Radial Scar: This is not actually a scar, but does look like one on histology. Instead you have a bunch of dense fibrosis around the ducts giving the appearance of architectural distortion (dark scar).

Things to know:
- *This is high risk and has to come out*
- *It's associated with DCIS and/or IDC 10%-30%*
- *It's associated with Tubular Carcinoma**

Atypical Ductal Hyperplasia (ADH): This is basically DCIS but lacks the quantitative definition by histology (< 2 ducts involved). It comes out (a) because it's high risk and (b) because DCIS burden is often underestimated when this is present. In other words, about 30% of the time the surgical path will get upgraded to DCIS.

Lobular Carcinoma in situ (LCIS): This is classically occult on mammogram. "An incidental finding" is sometimes a buzzword. The best way to think about LCIS is that it can be a precursor to ILC, but isn't obligated to be. The risk of conversion to an invasive cancer is less when comparing DCIS to IDC. Just like pleomorphic ILC is worse than regular ILC, a pleomorphic LCIS is mo' badder than regular LCIS.

Atypical Lobular Hyperplasia (ALH): This is very similar to LCIS, but histologists separate the two based on if the lobule is distended or not (no with ALH, yes with LCIS). It's considered milder than LCIS (risk of subsequent breast CA is 4-6x higher with ALH, and 11x higher with LCIS). For the exam, the answer is excision. In the real world, some people do not cut these out, and it's controversial.

Papilloma: A few most commons come to mind with this one. Most common intraductal mass lesion. Most common cause of blood discharge. You typically see these in women in their late reproductive years / early menopausal years (average around 50). The classic location is the subareolar region (1cm from the nipple in 90% of cases).

—*Mammogram:* Often normal - occasionally just showing calcifications.
—*US:* Well-defined smooth walled hypo-echoic mass. Maybe cystic with solid components. Also, tends to have associated duct dilation.
—*Galactography:* Solitary filling detected, with dilated duct.

Multiple Papillomas: These tend to be more peripheral. On mammography it's gonna be a mass(es) or cluster of calcifications without a mass.

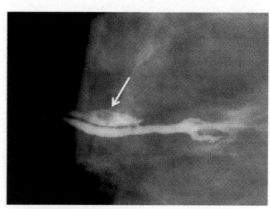

Papilloma — *Solitary filling defect with dilated duct*

Phyllodes: Yes... I mentioned this already under benign disease. I just wanted to bring it up again to make sure you remember that this thing has a malignant degeneration risk of about 10% (some texts say up to 25%). This is a fast growing breast mass. It occurs in an older age group than the fibroadenoma (40s-50s).

Multiple Masses:

To call multiple masses you need to have multiple (at least 3) bilateral well circumscribed masses without suspicious features. At least in America this is considered a benign finding. One common trick is to show multiple unilateral masses, that doesn't fly – they have to be bilateral for you to blow them off.

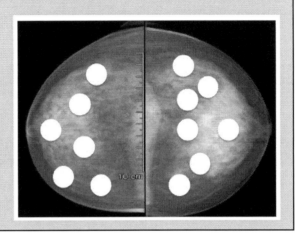

Symptomatic Breasts

Breast Pain: This is super common and typically cyclic (worse during the luteal phase of the menstrual cycle). Pain in both breasts that is cyclical does not need evaluation, it needs a family medicine referral for some "therapeutic communication." Focal non-cyclic breast pain may warrant an evaluation.

Trivia: The negative predictive value of combined mammogram and US for "focal pain" is right around 100%. When breast cancer is found is usually elsewhere in the breast (asymptomatic).

Symptoms that are actually worrisome for cancer include: skin dimpling, focal skin thickening, and nipple retraction.

Non-Focal Skin Thickening / Breast Edema: This is usually the result of benign conditions (congestive heart failure, renal failure). For multiple choice tests it will always be bilateral (in the real world you can sleep on one side and have asymmetric edema). As long as the breast isn't red, you can feel confident that it will be benign. On mammography you will see trabecular thickening (diffuse, and favoring the dependent portions of the breast).

Breast Inflammation: The swollen red breast. This finding has a differential of two things: (1) mastitis / abscess, (2) inflammatory breast cancer.

- **Mastitis / Abscess:** This is a swollen red breast which is painful (Inflammatory breast CA is often painless). Patients are usually sick as a dog. Obviously it's associated with breast feeding, and is more common in smokers and diabetics. Abscess can develop (usually Staph A.).

- **Inflammatory Breast Cancer:** As discussed above, this has a terrible prognosis. The general rule is that a breast that doesn't respond to antibiotics gets a skin biopsy to exclude this. The typical age is 40s-50s. You are going to have an enlarged, red, breast with a "peau d'orange" appearance. The breast is often NOT painful, despite its appearance. Mammogram might show a mass (or masses), but the big finding is diffuse skin and trabecular thickening. The treatment is fair game for multiple choice because it is different than normal breast cancer. Instead of going to surgery first, inflammatory breast cancer gets "cooled down" with chemo and or radiation – then surgery.

Discharge: Women present with nipple discharge all the time, it's usually benign (90%). **The highest yield information on the subject is that; spontaneous, bloody, discharge from a single duct is your most suspicious feature combo. Serous discharge is also suspicious.** The risk of discharge being cancer is directly related to age (very uncommon under 40, and more common over 60).

*Discharge is bad when it's - Spontaneous, Bloody, and from a Single Duct

Milky Discharge: Milky discharge is NOT suspicious for breast cancer but can be secondary to thyroid issues or a pituitary adenoma (prolactinoma). Any medication that messes with dopamine can stimulate prolactin production - (antidepressants, neuroleptics, reglan)

Causes of Discharge (Not Milky)	
Benign Causes	**Worrisome Causes**
Pre-Menopausal Woman = Fibrocystic Change	Intraductal Papilloma (90%) – single intraductal mass near nipple
Post Menopausal Women = Ductal Ectasia	DCIS (10%) – think about multiple intraductal masses

Ductal Ectasia – The most common benign cause of nipple discharge in a post menopausal women. On galactography you will see dilated ducts near the subareolar region, with progressive attenuation more posterior.

Galactography

- Ugh... you take a 27 or 30 gauge blunt tipped canal and attempt to cannulate the duct which is leaking. To determine which duct you want - you'll need to have the patient squeeze breast to demonstrate where it's coming from.

- If you manage to cannulate the duct - gently inject 0.2 - 0.3 cc contrast (rare to need more than 1cc). You then do mammograms (magnification CC and ML). Filling defect(s) get wire localization.

- *Contraindications:* Active infection (mastitis), inability to express discharge at the time of galactogram, contrast allergy, or prior surgery to the nipple areola complex.

Architectural Distortion (AD)

AD: We are talking about distortion of the normal architecture without a visible mass. This manifests in a few ways, including focal retraction, distortion of the edge of the parenchyma, or *radiation of the normal thin lines into a focal point.*

Architectural Distortion vs Summation Artifact: This is the primary differential consideration, with summation of normal vessels, ducts, and ligaments being much more common. The difference is summation should NOT radiate to a central point (AD will).

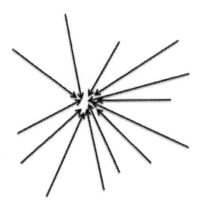 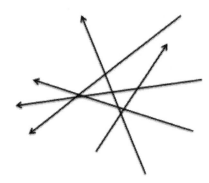

AD – *All lines radiate to a point*   **Summation** – *Lines continue past each other*

Surgical Scar vs Something Bad: Scars should progressively get lighter and harder to see. Some people say that in 5-10 years a benign surgical scar is often difficult to see. Lumpectomy scars tend to stick around longer than a benign biopsy. Basically, look at the priors if it is a surgical scar it better be getting less dense. If it's increasing you gotta stick a needle in it.

Work Up of AD: If you see it on a screener you will want to bring it back for spot compression views. If it persists just know you are either going to have to biopsy it (unless you know it's a surgical scar). You should still ultrasound it for further characterization.

Ultrasound Trivia: The use of harmonic tissue imaging can make it easier to see some lesions. Be aware that compound imaging can make you lose your posterior features, especially when they are soft to start with – like the shadowing of an ILC. Remember, even if you see nothing this gets a biopsy. Harmonics can also make not so simple cysts look simple.

Things to Know for AD:

- Radiating lines to a single point = AD
- AD + Calcifications = IDC + DCIS
- AD without Calcifications = ILC
- Even with no ultrasound or MRI correlate, AD gets a biopsy.
- Even if it has been there a while, it still needs worked up.
- Remember ILC can grow slow.
- Surgical scars should get less dense with time… not more dense. Cancer gets more dense.

Lymph Nodes

You found a breast cancer – now what? Before you make the patient cry, it's time to stage the disease. Ultrasound her arm pit. About 1 in 3 times you are going to find abnormal nodes.

Unilateral vs Bilateral: This can help you if you are thinking this could be systemic. Unilateral adenopathy should make you worry about a cancer (especially if they have a cancer on that side).

Should I Biopsy It? Some people will recommend biopsy if you have the following abnormal features.

- Cortical Thickness greater than 2.3mm (some people say 3mm)
- Loss of Central Fatty Hilum – "most specific sign"
- Irregular Outer Margins.

Staging Trivia: Level 1 and Level 2 nodes are treated the same. Rotter nodes are treated as Level 2. Level 3 and supraclavicular nodes are treated the same.

Special "Sneaky" Situations:

> **Gold Therapy:** Back in the stone ages they treated rheumatoid arthritis with "chrysotherapy." What they can do is show you an "Aunt Minnie" type picture with very dense calcifications within the node.

> **Snow Storm Nodes:** Another Aunt Minnie look is the silicone infiltration of a node from either silicone leaking or rupture.

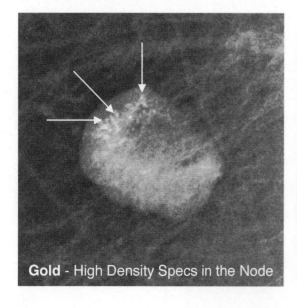
Gold - High Density Specs in the Node

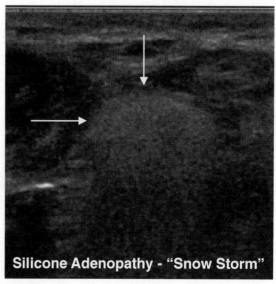
Silicone Adenopathy - "Snow Storm"

The Male Breast

There is no more humiliating way to die for a man than breast cancer. The good news is male breast cancer is uncommon, the bad news is that when it occurs it is often advanced and invasive at the time of diagnosis.

The male breast does NOT have the elongated and branching ducts, or proliferated lobules that women have. This is key because **men do NOT get lobule associated pathology; lobular carcinoma, fibroadenoma, or cysts.**

Gynecomastia: This is a non-neoplastic enlargement of the epithelial and stromal elements in a man's breast. It occurs "physiologically" in adolescents, affecting about 50% of adolescent boys, and men over 65. If you aren't 13 or 65 it's considered embarrassing and you should hit the gym. If you are between 13-65 it's considered pathology and associated with a variety of conditions (spironolactone, psych meds, marijuana, alcoholic cirrhosis, testicular cancer). There are three patterns (nodular is the most common). Just think **flame shaped, behind nipple, bilateral but asymmetric, and can be painful**. Things that make you worry that it's not gynecomastia include not being behind the nipple, eccentric location, and calcification.

Patterns of Gynecomastia	
Nodular (most common)	"Flame Shaped" centered behind the nipple, radiating posterior as it blends into the fat. Breast is often tender. Usually lasts less than 1 year.
Dendritic	Resembles a branching tree. This is a chronic fibrotic pattern. Usually not tender.
Diffuse Glandular	Mammographic pattern looks like a woman's breast (diffuse increase in density). You see this in men receiving estrogen treatment.

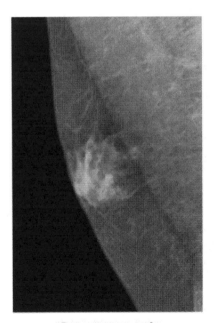
Gynecomastia

Pseudogynecomastia *"Bitch Tits"* – This is an increase in the fat tissue of the breast (not glandular tissue). There will NOT be a discrete palpable finding, and the mound of tissue will not be concentric to the nipple.

Lipoma – After gynecomastia a lipoma is the second most common palpable mass in a man.

Male Breast Cancer: It's uncommon in men, and very uncommon in younger men (average age is around 70). About 1 in 4 males with breast cancer have a BRCA mutation (BRCA 2 is the more common). Other risk factors include Klinefelter Syndrome, Cirrhosis, and chronic alcoholism. The classic description is eccentric but near the nipple. It's almost always an IDC-NOS type. DCIS can occur but is very rare in isolation. On mammography it looks like a breast cancer, if it was a woman's mammogram you'd biopsy the shit out of it. On ultrasound it's the same thing, it looks like a cancer. Having said that nodular gynecomastia can look suspicious on ultrasound.

Things that make you think it's breast cancer:
- *Eccentric to Nipple*
- *Unilateral*
- *Abnormal Lymph nodes*
- *Calcifications*
- *Looks like breast cancer*

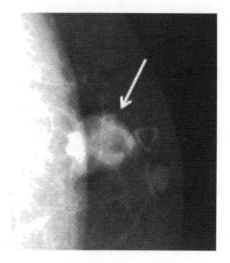

Male Breast CA

Some trivia on calcifications: Micro-calcifications alone are uncommon in men. When you see them they are less numerous, coarser, and associated with a mass (25% of male breast cancers have calcifications).

Should men get screening mammograms? Honestly, women shouldn't even get them (according to the New England Journal of Medicine). This remains controversial, with the bottom line being this; only Klinefelter patients approach the screening range with regards to risk.

As a point of trivia: **males with gynecomastia from gender reassignment on hormone therapy are not high enough risk for screening mammograms**. Obviously, if they have a palpable they can get a diagnostic work up.

Implants

Basic Overview: There are two types, saline and silicone. They both can rupture, but no one really gives a shit if saline ruptures. Saline does not form a capsule, so you can't have intracapsular rupture with saline. There is no additional imaging past mammo for saline rupture, and you just follow up with primary care / plastic surgeon. You can tell it's saline because you can see through it. For silicone you can have both intra and extra capsular rupture. You can only see extra on a mammogram (can't see intra). So, extra creates a dense "snow storm" appearance on US. Intra creates a "step ladder" appearance on US and a "linguine sign" on MRI. MRI is done with FS T2 to look at implants.

Big Points:
- You **CAN** have isolated intracapsular rupture.
- You **CAN NOT** have isolated extra (it's always with intra).
- If you see silicone in a lymph node you need to recommend MRI to evaluate for intracapsular rupture

Implant Location: There are two subtypes:
- *Subglandular (retromammary):* Implant behind breast tissue, anterior to pectoral muscle
- *Subpectoral (retropectoral):* Implant between pectoralis major and minor muscles

Silicone Implants

The body will form a shell around the foreign body (implant), which allows for both intracapsular and extracapsular rupture (an important distinction from saline). About 25% of the time you will see calcifications around the fibrous capsule.

Things to know:
- Implants are NOT a contraindication for a core needle biopsy
- Implants do NOT increase the risk for cancer.

Saline Implants

There are also subglandular and subpectoral subtypes. You can tell the implant is saline because you can see through it. Implant folds and valves can also be seen. If it ruptures no one really cares (other than the cosmetic look). The saline is absorbed by the body, and you have a collapsed implant. A practical point of caution, be careful when performing a biopsy in these patients – even a 25g FNA needle can burst a saline implant.

Trivia: Some sources say that "physical exam" is the test of choice for diagnosing saline implant rupture - this is variable depending on what you read / who you ask.

Implant Complications:

Generally speaking MRI is the most accurate modality for evaluating an implant.

Capsular Contracture: This is the **most common complication of implants**. It occurs secondary to contraction of the fibrous capsule, and can result in a terrible cosmetic deformity. You see it in both silicone and saline implants, but is **most common in subglandular silicone implants**. On mammo it looks like rounding or distortion of the implant (comparisons will show progression).

> **Screening Mammograms in women with Implants:**
>
> You get 4 views of each breast (CC, MLO, implant displaced CC, implant displaced MLO). Obviously sensitivity is decreased in women with implants. Implants are easier to displace if they are subpectorial (so they have better sensitivity than subglandular).

Gel Bleed: Silicone molecules can (and do) pass through the semi-permeable implant shell coating the exterior of the surface. This does NOT mean the implant is ruptured. The classic look is to show you silicone in the axillary lymph nodes *(remember I showed a case of this under the lymph node section)*. Even with axillary lymph nodes, this does NOT mean it has ruptured.

Rupture: As a point of testable trivia the number one risk factor for rupture is age of the implant. Rupture does not have to be post traumatic, it can occur spontaneously. Rupture with compression mammography is actually rare.

- **Saline:** Saline rupture is usually very obvious (deflated boob). It doesn't matter all that much (except cosmetically), as the saline is just absorbed. On mammo, you will see the "wadded up" plastic wrapper. *They could easily write a question asking you what modality you need to see a saline rupture. The answer would be plain mammo (you don't need ultrasound or MRI).*

- **Silicone:** This is a more complicated matter. You have two subtypes; isolated intracapsular and intracapsular with extracapsular.

    - *Isolated Intracapsular:* This will be occult on physical exam, mammography and possibly ultrasound. You might see a stepladder on Ultrasound. MRI is way more sensitive.

    - *Intracapsular with Extracapsular Rupture:* This is usually obvious on mammogram with dense silicone seen outside the capsule. The contour of a normal intact implant is smooth. Silicone outside the implant can go to lymph nodes. On ultrasound you want to know the buzzword **"snow storm" pattern – which is really echogenic with no posterior shadowing.** A sneaky trick is to show a lymph node with a snow storm appearance on ultrasound. On MRI extracapsular silicon is T1 dark, and T2 bright. Lastly, a very important concept is that *you cannot have isolated extracapsular rupture. If it's extracapsular, then it's also intracapsular.*

Radial Folds - The Mimic of Rupture:

Radial folds are the normal in-foldings of the elastomer shell. They are the primary mimic for the linguine sign of intracapsular rupture. To tell them apart ask yourself *"do the folds connect with the periphery of the implant?"* Radial folds should always do this (linguine does not).

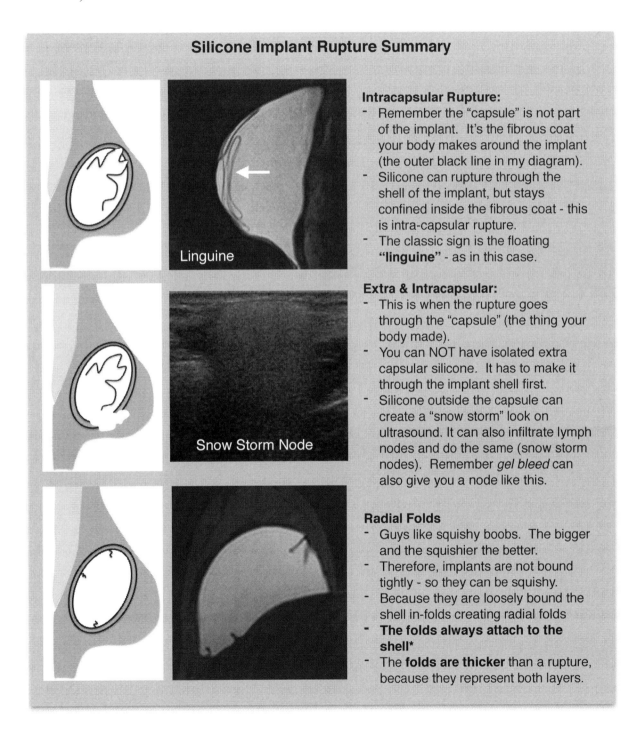

The Post Operative Breast

Reduction Mammoplasty and Mastopexy

Reduction Mammoplasty – Yes, there is actually a subpopulation of women who want SMALLER breasts. I know, it sounds impossible to believe (from a man's prospective). Mammoplasty is done to reduce breast size.

Mastopexy – This is a "breast lift." This is **just a removal of skin**. Women get this done to address floppy "ptotic" boobs.

Normal Findings Post Mastopexy:
- *Swirled Appearance Affecting Inferior Breast*
- *Fat Necrosis / Oil Cysts*
- *Isolated Islands of Breast Tissue*

Keyhole Incision – This is done for both mammoplasty and mastopexy, creating a "swirled" appearance in the inferior aspect of the MLO.

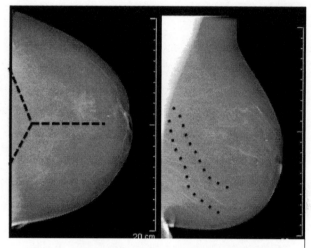
Typical Changes from Mammoplasty

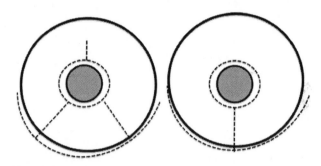
Mammoplasty Keyhole Incision   Mastopexy Keyhole Incision

Surgical Biopsy / Radiation

Terminology:
- **Lumpectomy** – Surgical Removal of Cancer (palpable or not)
- **Excisional Biopsy** – Surgical Removal of **Entire** Lesions
- **Incisional Biopsy** – Surgical Biopsy of a **Portion** of the Lesion

Post Biopsy Changes

The first post operative mammogram is usually obtained around 6-12 months after biopsy. The key is that **distortion and scarring are worst on this film, and should progressively improve.** On ultrasound, scars are supposed to be thin and linear. If they show you a focal mass like thickening in the scar - you've gotta call that suspicious for local recurrence.

Fat necrosis and benign dystrophic calcifications may evolve over the first year or two, and are the major mimics of recurrence. Fat necrosis can be shown on MR (T1 / T2 bright, and then fat sat drops it out).

Risk of Recurrence / Residual Disease:

Numerical Trivia: **Local recurrence occurs 6-8%** of the time, when women have breast conserving therapy. The **peak time for recurrence is 4 years** (most occur between 1-7). **Without radiation local recurrence is closer to 35%.** Tumors that recur early (< 3 years) typically occur in the original tumor bed. Those that occur later are more likely to be in a different location from the original primary.

What gets recurrent disease ? Risk of recurrence is highest in the premenopausal woman (think about them having an underlying genetic issue). Other risks are; having an extensive inarticulate component, a tumor with vascular invasion, multi centric tumors, positive surgical margins, or a tumor that was not adequately treated the first go around.

Residual Calcs: Residual calcifications are not good. Supposedly residual calcifications near or in the lumpectomy bed correlates with a local recurrence rate of 60%.

New Calcs: When it does reoccur, something like 75% of DCIS will come back as calcifications (no surprise). The testable pearl is the **benign calcifications tend to occur early (around 2 years), vs the cancer ones which come back around 4 years.**

Sentinel Node Failure: Sentinel node biopsy works about 95% of the time (doesn't work 5% of the time). So about 5 times in 100 you are going to have a negative SNLB that presents later with an abnormal armpit node.

Tissue Flap: The cancer is not going to start in the belly fat / muscle. The cancer is going to come from either the residual breast tissue or along the skin scar line. Screening of the flaps is controversial - with some saying it's not necessary. The need for screening of tissue flaps is not going to be asked. If you get asked anything it's "where the recurrent is coming from / going to be?"

Specimen Radiography

If the path report says "close margins" or "positive margins" there is a very high chance you are going to have cancer still in the breast. If you are shown a specimen radiograph there are two things you need to look at in real life and on multiple choice: (1) is the mass / calcifications on the sample and (2) is the mass / calcifications near the edge or touching the edge. *If the mass is at the edge, the chance of incomplete excision is going to be near 80%. The "next step" would be to call the surgeon in the OR and tell him/her that.*

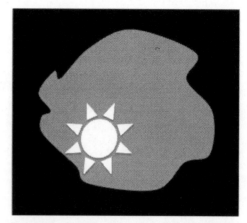
Specimen Radiograph - Cancer at the Margin
-High change of positive margin

Post Radiation Changes:

Practical Point (*the before picture*): The pre-radiation mammogram is very important. If you can identify residual disease on it, the patient has many more treatment options. If you discover the residual disease after the radiation therapy has been given, you've forced the patient to undergo mastectomy.

Radiation Changes: You are going to see skin thickening and trabecular thickening. This is normal post radiation, and should peak on the first post-RT mammogram.

This would be a classic testable scenario:
- Film 1 Post RT: You see skin thickening / trabecular thickening
- Film 2: Skin thickening / trabecular thickening is better
- Film 3: Skin thickening / trabecular thickening is worse * - this is recurrent disease (maybe inflammatory breast CA).

Staging/ Surgical Planning

Breast Cancer Staging: The staging is based on size from T1-T3, then invasion for T4.
- T1 = < 2cm.
- T2 = 2-5cm
- T3 = > 5cm
- T4 = "Any size" with chest wall fixation, skin involvement, or inflammatory breast CA.
Remember that Pagets is NOT T4.

Trivia: Axillary Status is the most important predictor of overall survival in breast cancer

Trivia: Melanoma is the most common tumor to met to the breast.

The contraindications for breast conservation are high yield.

Contraindications for Breast Conservation
Inflammatory Cancer,
Large Cancer Size Relative to Breast,
Multi-centric (multiple quadrants),
Prior Radiation Therapy, to the same breast
Contraindication to Radiation Therapy (collagen-vascular disease).

Breast MRI

Breast MRI can be used for several reasons; High risk screening, extent of disease (known cancer), axillary mets with unknown primary, diagnostic dilemmas, and possible silicone implant rupture. **The big reason is for screening.**

I'll just briefly go over how it's done, and how it's read.

You need a special breast coil and table set up to make it work. The patient lies belly down with her breasts hanging through holes in the table. You have to position them correctly otherwise they get artifact from their breasts rubbing on the coil. Basic sequences are going to include a T2, and pre and post dynamic post contrast fat saturated T1. Remember the breast is a bag of fat - so fat sat is very important. Dynamic imaging is done to generate wash out curves (similar to prostate MRI).

My basic algorithm for reading them is to:

(1) Look at the background uptake. I use this to set my sensitivity when I compare it to prior studies. Ideally you used the same kind of contrast, and imaged at the same time of the month. As I'll mention below, hormone changes with female cycles cause changes in how much contrast gets taken up (less early, and more later).

(2) I look for masses or little dots (foci). MIPS (maximum intensity projections) are helpful just like looking for a lung nodule. If I see a mass or dot I try and characterize it - first by seeing if I can make it T2 bright. Most T2 bright things are benign (lymph nodes, cysts, fibroadenoma). If it's not T2 bright I look at the features - is it a mass? is it spiculated etc? These features are more important than anything else. Is it new? Nipple enhancement is ok - don't be a dumb ass and call it Pagets.

(3) Finally I'll look at the wash out curve, but honestly I've made up my mind before I even look at that. I will never let a benign curve back me off suspicious morphology.

(4) I deal with the findings similar to mammo. New masses get biopsy. NMLE (non-mass like enhancement) get's biopsy if new. T2 bright stuff for the most part (there is one exception of mucinous cancer) get's a benign finding. Anything that needs a biopsy gets a biopsy - via MR guided stereo. I never pussy foot out and hedge around saying I need more imaging in addition to MRI - unless it's a technical problem, (example inadequate fat sat).

Parenchyma Enhancement:

- *Is it normal ?* – Yes
- *Where is it most common ?* – Posterior Breast in the upper outer quadrant, during the lateral part of the menstrual cycle (luteal phase - day 14-28)
- *How do you reduce it?* – Do the MRI during the first part of the menstrual cycle (day 7-14).
- *What does Tamoxifen do?* – Tamoxifen will decrease background parenchyma uptake. **Then it causes a rebound.**

Foci:

- *How is it defined?* Round or oval, circumscribed, and **less than 5mm,**
- *Are they high risk?* Usually not. Usually they are benign (2-3% have a chance of being a bad boy).
- *What would make you biopsy one?* Seemed different than the rest, ill-defined borders, or **suspicious enhancement**.

NMLE (Non-Mass Like Enhancement):

- *What is NMLE ?* It's not a mass - but more like a cloud or clump of tissue enhancement.
- *What are the distributions ?* Segmental (triangular blob pointing at the nipple, indicates a single branch), Regional (a bigger triangle), and Diffuse (sorta all over the place).
- *Which one is more suspicious* - homogenous or heterogenous enhancement of NMLE ? Heterogenous is much more suspicious.

Masses:

- These are defined as being 5mm or larger. They have definable vocabulary for their features (round, oval, indistinct, etc…)
- *When are these bad?* They are bad when you call them bad words. Irregular shape, speculated margins, heterogeneous or rim enhancement. Once you say those words you are going to have to biopsy them, because **morphology trumps kinetics**. It doesn't matter what the kinetics shows, you must biopsy suspicious morphology.
- *When is kinetics helpful?* When you are on the fence. If you have benign morphology and you have suspicious kinetics – you probably are going to need to biopsy that also.

Kinetics:

- Breast kinetics are performed in two portions:
  - (1) Initial upslope phase that occurs over the first 2 minutes. This is graded as slow, medium, or rapid (fast).
  - (2) The washout portion which is recorded sometime between 2 minutes and 6 minutes (around about). These are graded as either continued rise "type 1", plateau "type 2", or rapid washout "type 3".

- Risk of Cancer:
  - Type 1 Curve: 6%
  - Type 2 Curve: 7%-28%
  - Type 3: 29% or more.

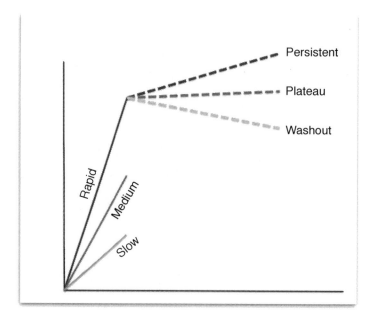

Classic Looks:

- **Fibroadenoma:** These things are classically T2 bright, round, with "non-enhancing septa", and a type 1 curve.
- **DCIS:** Clumped, ductal, linear or segmental **non-mass likely enhancement**. Kinetics are typically not helpful for DCIS.
- **IDC:** Spiculated irregular shaped masses, with heterogeneous enhancement and a type 3 curve.
- **ILC:** Doesn't always show enhancement.

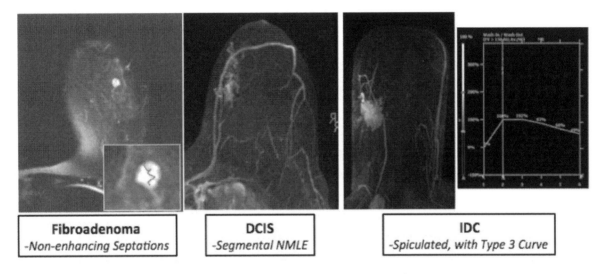

T2 Bright Things:

- Usually T2 Bright = Benign. Things that are T2 Bright include: Cysts, Lymph nodes, fat necrosis, Fibroadenoma.
- The exception *(anytime I say the word "except" you need to think high yield!)*: **Colloid Cancer**, and Mucinous Cancer can be T2 bright.

Pure Trivia:

- *If you have a patient with known breast CA, how often do you find a contralateral breast CA?* - Answer is 0.1-2% via mammogram, and 3-5 % by MRI.

- *Spiculated margins* = 80% malignancy. This is the **single most predictive feature of malignancy.**

Screening Controversy

Recent large heavily powered studies have brought into question the practice of screening mammograms. I highly recommend you read these *"despicable"* papers, but please wait till after the exam, because the people who write multiple choice questions about mammography are definitely not the same people who wrote these papers. For the purpose of multiple choice tests, screening mammography saves lots of lives, you should buy pink ribbons, and low grade DCIS needs a surgical consult.

Bleyer, Archie, and H. Gilbert Welch. "Effect of three decades of screening mammography on breast-cancer incidence." New England Journal of Medicine 367.21 (2012): 1998-2005.

Miller, Anthony B., et al. "Twenty five year follow-up for breast cancer incidence and mortality of the Canadian National Breast Screening Study: randomised screening trial." BMJ: British Medical Journal 348 (2014).

Risk

Estrogen Related: The more exposure to estrogen the higher your risk of breast cancer will be. Anything that prolongs this exposure is said to increase risk. For example, an early age to begin menstruating or a late age to have menopause. Hormone replacement therapy with estrogen alone obviously increases exposure. Early maturation of lobules, which can be achieved by getting pregnant young, reduces your risk. Being fat increases estrogen exposure (more aromatase = more estrogen). Being a drunk increases estrogen exposure – via messing with its normal breakdown in the liver.

Estrogen Related Risks
Early Menstruation
Late Menopause
Late age of first pregnancy / or no kids.
Being Fat
Being a Drunk
Hormone Replacement (with estrogen)

High Risk Lesions: Any of the high risk lesions (ADH, ALH, LCIS, Radial Scar, Papilloma) are associated with an increased risk. These are discussed more in detail later in the chapter.

Density: Density is considered a "medium risk," and is "dose dependent" with the denser you are the more risk you have.

Chest Wall Radiation: Chest wall radiation (usually seen in lymphoma patients) is a big risk, especially at a young age. The risk is supposed to peak around 15 years post treatment. **If the child had more than 20Gy to the chest she is going to qualify for an annual screening MRI – at age 25 or 8 year post exposure** *(whichever is later).*

Relatives with Cancer: A first degree relative with breast cancer increases your lifetime risk from 8% to 13%. Two first degree relatives increases your risk to 21%.

Actual Mutations:

BRCA 1	Chromosome 17. More common than type 2. Increased risk for breast, ovary, and various GI cancers.
BRCA 2	Chromosome 13. Male carriers have a higher risk with 2. Increased risk for breast, ovary, and various GI cancers.
Li Fraumeni	Their p53 does NOT work, and they are high risk for all kinds of rare cancers.
Cowden Syndrome	Risk for breast cancer, follicular thyroid cancer, endometrial cancer, and **Lhermitte-Duclos** (a brain hamartoma).
Bannayan-Riley Ruvalcaba	Associated with developmental disorders at a young age.
NF-1	"Moderate Risk" of breast cancer

High Yield Take Home Points Regarding Risk:

- Anything that gets you more estrogen increases your risk
- BRCA 1 is more common than BRCA 2 (in women).
- Men with BRCA 2 get more cancer than men with BRCA 1.
- Breast Density is an independent risk factor (denser the breast, the more the risk)
- 20Gy of Radiation to your chest as a kid buys you a screening MRI – at 25 or 8 years after exposure *(*whichever is longer)*
- Cowden Syndrome – Bowel Hamartoma, Follicular Thyroid Cancer, Lhermitte-Duclos, and Breast Cancer
- All current risk models underestimate life time risk.
- Tyrer Cuzick is the most comprehensive risk model, but does not include breast density.
- Exercise *(probably more like not being fat)* reduces the risk of breast cancer
- Tamoxifen and Raloxifene (SERMs) reduce breast cancer incidence of ER/PR

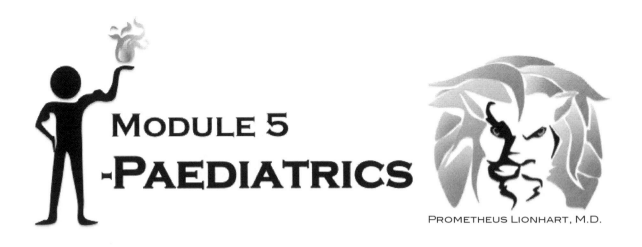

Module 5
-Paediatrics

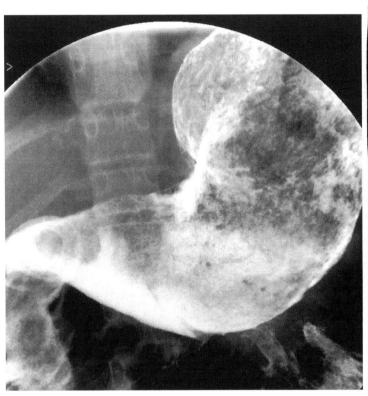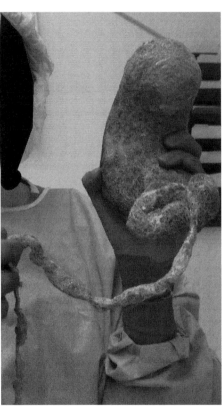

Airway

Croup

This is the most common cause of acute upper airway obstruction in young children. The peak incidence is between 6 months and 3 years (average 1 year). They have a **barky "croupy" cough**. It's viral. The thing to realize is that the lateral and frontal neck x-ray is done not to diagnosis croup, but to exclude something else. Having said that, the so called *"steeple sign"* – with loss of the normal lateral convexities of the subglotic trachea is your buzzword, and if it's shown, that will be the finding. Questions are still more likely to center around facts (age and etiology). **The culprit is often parainfluenza virus.**

Epiglottitis

In contrast to the self limited croup, this one can kill you. It's mediated by H. Influenza and the classic age is 3.5 years old (there is a recent increase in teenagers - so don't be fooled by that age). The lateral x-ray will show marked swelling of the epiglottis *(thumb sign)*. A fake out is the "omega epiglottis" which is caused by oblique imaging. You can look for thickening of the aryepiglottic folds to distinguish.

Trivia: Death by asphyxiation is from the aryepiglotic folds (not the epiglottis)

Exudative Tracheitis

This is an uncommon but serious (possibly deadly) situation that is found in slightly older kids. It's caused by an exudative infection of the trachea (sorta like diptheria). It's usually from Staph A. and affects kids between 6-10. The buzzword is *linear soft tissue filling defect within the airway*.

Croup	Epiglottitis	Exudative Tracheitis
6 months – 3 years (peak 1 year)	Classic = 3.5 years, but now seen with teenagers too	6-10 years
Steeple Sign: loss of the normal shoulders (lateral convexities) of the subglottic trachea	**Thumb Sign:** marked enlargement of epiglottis	Linear soft tissue filling defect (a membrane) seen within the airway
Viral (*Most Common - parainfluenza*)	H-Flu	Staph. A

Retropharyngeal Cellulitis and Abscess

This most commonly affects young kids (age 6 months -12 months). They will most likely show this with a lateral x-ray demonstrating **massive retropharyngeal soft tissue thickening**. For the real world, you can get pseudothickening when the neck is not truly lateral. To tell the difference between positioning and the real thing, a repeat with an extended neck is the next step.

On CT it will be very obvious (the fake out would be a more lateral low density suppurative node).

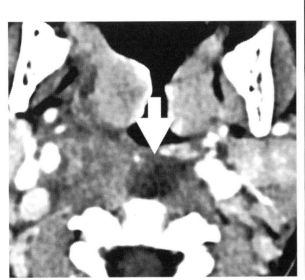

Retropharyngeal Abscess
-Midline -

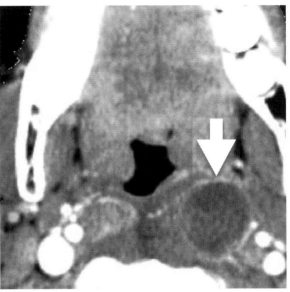

Suppurative Node
- Just Medial to the Carotid

Subglottic Hemangioma

The hemangioma is the most common soft tissue mass in the trachea, and they are most commonly located in the subglottic region. In croup there is symmetric narrowing with loss of shoulders on both sides (Steeple Sign). In contradistinction, subglottic hemangiomas have loss of just one of the sides.

Trivia
- *Tends to favor the left side,*
- *50% are associated with cutaneous hemangiomas,*
- *7% have the PHACES syndrome.*

PHACES
P- Posterior fossa *(Dandy Walker)*
H- Hemangiomas
A- Arterial anomalies
C- Coarctation of aorta, cardiac defects
E- Eye abnormalities
S- Subglottic hemangiomas

Gamesmanship -
Frontal and Lateral Neck Radiographs

For the frontal, there are two main things to think about.

(1) Croup and
(2) Subglottic Hemangioma

You can tell them apart by the shouldering.

If you can't tell…. try and let the history bias you. Cough? Fever? Think Croup.

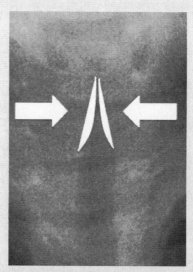 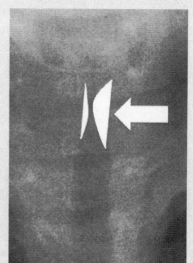

For the lateral, there are 4 main things to think about:

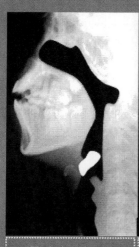 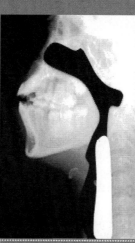 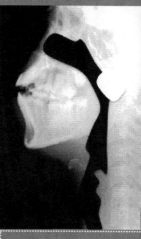 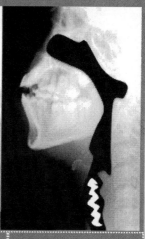

Epiglottitis	Retropharyngeal Abscess	Tonsils (adenoids)	Exudative Tracheitis
Looks like a thumb If the ordering suspects the diagnosis, do NOT bring this kid to x-ray. Have them do a portable.	Too wide (>6mm at C2, or >22mm at C6) **Next Step = CT** *don't forget to look in the mediastinum for "Danger Zone" extension.*	Not seen till about 3-6 months, and not big till around 1-2 years. Too big when they encroach the airway	Linear Filling Defect It's usually staph

Newborn Chest

Meconium Aspiration

This typically occurs secondary to stress (hypoxia), and is *more common in term or post-mature babies (the question stem could say "post term" delivery)*. The pathophysiology is all secondary to chemical aspiration.

Things to know are:
- *The buzzword "ropy appearance" of asymmetric lung densities*
- *Hyperinflation with alternative areas of atelectasis*
- *Pneumothorax in 20-40% of cases*

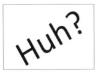 *How can it have hyperinflation?? Aren't the lungs full of sticky shit (literally) ???* The poop in the lungs act like miniature ball-valves ("floaters" I call them), causing air trapping - hence the increased lung volumes.

Transient Tachypnea of the Newborn (TTN)

The classic clinical scenario is a history of c-section (vagina squeezes the fluid out of lungs normally). Other classic scenario histories include "diabetic mother" and/or "maternal sedation." Findings are going to start at 6 hours, peak at one day, and be done by 3 days. You are going to see coarse interstitial marking and fluid in the fissures.

Things to know are:
- *Classic histories: C-Section, Maternal Sedation, Maternal Diabetes*
- *Onset: Peaks at day 1, Resolved by Day 3*
- *Lung Volumes – Normal to Increased*

Surfactant-Deficient Disease (SDD)

This is also called hyaline membrane disease, or RDS. It's a disease of pre-mature kids. The idea is that they are born without surfactant (the stuff that makes your lungs stretchy and keeps aveolar surfaces open). It's serious business and is the most common cause of death in premature newborns. You get **low lung volumes and bilateral granular opacities** (just like B-hemolyic pneumonia). But, unlike B-hemolytic pneumonia you **do NOT get pleural effusions**. As a piece of useful clinical knowledge, a normal plain film at 6 hours excludes SDD.

Surfactant Replacement Therapy

They can spray this crap in the kids lungs, and it makes a huge difference (decreased death rate etc…). Lung volumes get better, and granular opacities will clear centrally after treatment. The post treatment look of bleb-like lucencies can mimic PIE.

Things to know:
- *Increased Risk of Pulmonary Hemorrhage*
- *Increased Risk of PDA*

Neonatal Pneumonia (not Beta-Hemolytic Strep)

Lots of causes. Typical look is patchy, asymmetric perihilar densities, and hyperinflation. Will look similar to surfactant deficient disease but will be full term.

Neonatal Pneumonia (Beta-Hemolytic Strep)

This is the most common type of pneumonia in newborns. It's acquired during exit of the dirty birth canal. It affects premature infants more than term infants. It has some different looks when compared to other pneumonias (why I discuss it separately).

Things to know:
- *It often has low lung volumes (other pneumonias have high)*
- *Granular Opacities is a buzzword (for this and SDD)*
- *Often has pleural effusion (SDD will not)*

Persistent Pulmonary HTN

Also called, persistent fetal circulation. Normally the high pulmonary pressures seen in utero (that cause blood to shunt around the lungs), decrease as soon as the baby takes his/her first breath. When high pressures persist in the lungs it can be primary (the work of Satan), or secondary from hypoxia (meconium aspiration, pneumonia, etc…). The CXR is going to show the cause of the pulmonary HTN (pneumonia), rather than the HTN itself.

Solving Cases Using Buzzwords

When I say *"Post Term Baby,"*
You Say *Meconium Aspiration*

When I say *"C-Section,"*
You say *Transient Tachypnea*

When I say *"Maternal Sedation"*
You say *Transient Tachypnea*

When I say *"Premature"*
You say *RDS*

> How this works:
>
> Blah Blah Blah , **Post Term Delivery** of a beautiful baby girl. What is the diagnosis?
>
> (A) RDS
> (B) Transient Tachypnea
> **(C) Meconium Aspiration**

Solving Cases Using Lung Volumes:

High:

- Meconium Aspiration
- Transient Tachypnea
- Neonatal Pneumonia

Low:

- Surfactant Deficiency (no pleural effusion)
- Beta-Hemolytic Pneumonia (gets pleural effusions)

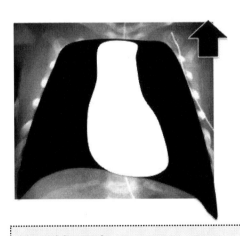
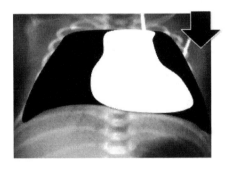

> How this works:
>
> Blah Blah Blah , **This Picture** of a beautiful baby girl. What is the diagnosis?
>
> **(A) RDS**
> (B) Transient Tachypnea
> (C) Meconium Aspiration

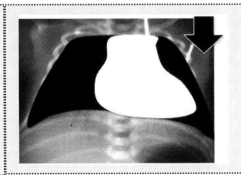

Complications of Life in the NICU

Pulmonary Interstitial Emphysema (PIE)

When you have surfactant deficiency and they put you on a ventilator (which pulverizes your lungs with PEEP), you can end up with air escaping the aveoli and ending up in the interstitium and lymphatics. On CXR it looks like **linear lucencies (buzzword)**. It's a warning sign for impending Pneumothorax. Most cases of PIE occur in the first week of time (bronchopulmonary dysplasia – which looks similar – occurs in patients older than 2 weeks). **Surfactant therapy can also mimic PIE.** The treatment is to switch ventilation methods and or place them affected side down.

A total zebra is the progression of PIE to a large cystic mass. The thing can even cause mediastinal mass effect.

Things to know:
- *Consequence of ventilation*
- *Usually occurs in the first week of life*
- *Buzzword = Linear Lucencies*
- *Warning Sign for Impending Pneumothorax*
- *Treatment is to put them affected side down*

Chronic Lung Disease (Bronchopulmonary Dysplasia - BPD)

This is the kid born premature (with resulting surfactant deficiency), who ended up on a ventilator. Prolonged ventilation in a tiny (<1000 grams), premature kid (<32 weeks) is your classic scenario. So, after week two you start to get hazy lungs, which over the next few months coarsen and give you some bubble like lucencies. **"Band like opacities" is a buzzword.**

Congenital Chest

Pulmonary Hypoplasia

This can be primary or secondary. Secondary causes seem to lend themselves more readily to multiple choice questions. Secondary causes can be from decreased hemi-thoracic volume, decreased vascular supply, or decreased fluid. The most common is the decreased thoracic volume, typically from a space occupying mass such as a **congenital diaphragmatic hernia** (with bowel in the chest), but sometimes from a neuroblastoma or sequestration. Decreased fluid, refers to the **Potter Sequence** (no kidneys -> no pee -> no fluid -> hypoplastic lungs).

Bronchopulmonary Sequestration

These are grouped into intralobar and extralobar with the distinction being which has a pleural covering. The venous drainage is different (intra to pulmonary veins, extra to systemic veins). **You can NOT tell the difference radiographically.** The *practical difference is age of presentation*; intralobar presents in adolescence or adulthood with recurrent pneumonias, extralobar presents in infancy with respiratory compromise.

- **Intralobar:** Much more common (75%). Presents in adolescence or adulthood as recurrent pneumonias (bacteria migrates in from pores of Kohn). **Most commonly in the left lower lobe** posterior segment (2/3s). Uncommon in the upper lobes. In contradistinction from extralobar sequestration, it is rarely associated with other developmental abnormalities. *Pathology books love to say "NO pleural cover" - but you can't see that shit on CT or MR.*

- **Extralobar:** Less common of the two (25%). Presents in infancy with respiratory compromise (primarily because of the associated anomalies - Congenital cystic adenomatoid malformation (CCAM), congenital diaphragmatic hernia, vertebral anomalies, congenital heart disease, pulmonary hypoplasia). It rarely gets infected since it has its own pleural covering. These are sometimes described as part of a bronchopulmonary foregut malformation, and may actually have (rarely) a patent channel to the stomach, or distal esophagus. *Pathology books love to say "has a pleural cover" - but you can't see that shit on CT or MR.*

Gamesmanship: I say recurrent pneumonia in same area, you say intralobar sequestration.

Bronchogenic Cysts

Typically an incidental finding. They are generally solitary and unilocular. They typically do NOT communicate with the airway, so if they have gas in them you should worry about infection.

Congenital Cystic Adenomatoid Malformation (CCAM) - *(Also Know As - CPAM)*

As the name suggests it's a malformation of adenomatoid stuff that replaces normal lung. Most of the time it only affects one lobe. There is no lobar preference (unlike CLE which favors the left upper lobe). There are cystic and solid types (type 1 cystic, type 3 solid, type 2 in the middle). There is a crop of knuckle heads who want to call these things CPAMs and have 5 types, which I'm sure is evidence based and will really make an impact in the way these things are treated. CCAMs communicate with the airway, and therefore fill with air. Most of these things (like 90%) will spontaneously decrease in size in the third trimester. The treatment (at least in the USA) is to cut these things out, because of the iddy bitty theoretical risk of malignant transformation (pleuropulmonary blastoma, rhabdomyosarcoma).

Q: *What if you see a systemic arterial feeder (one coming off the aorta) going to the CCAM ?*
A: Then it's not a CCAM, it's a Sequestration. — sneaky

Congenital Lobar Emphysema (CLE)

The idea behind this one is that you have bronchial pathology (maybe atresia depending on what you read), that leads to a ball-valve anomaly and progressive air trapping. On CXR, it looks like a lucent, hyperexpanded lobe.

Things to know:
- *It's not actually emphysema – just air trapping secondary to bronchial anomaly*
- *It prefers the left upper lobe (40%)*
- *Treatment is lobectomy*

Gamesmanship
- *They can show you a series of CXRs. The first one has an opacity in the lung (the affected lung clears fluid slower than normal lung). The next x-ray will show the opacity resolved. The following x-ray will show it getting more and more lucent. Until it's actually pushing the heart over. This is the classic way to show it in case conference, or case books.*

Congenital Diaphragmatic Hernia (CDHs)

Most commonly they are **B**ochdalek type. **B** is in the **B**ack – they are typically posterior and to the left. The appearance on CXR is usually pretty obvious.

Things to know:
- *Usually in the Back, and on the left (Bochdalek)*
- *If it's on the right - there is an association with GBS Pneumonia*
- *Mortality Rate is related to the degree of pulmonary Hypoplasia*
- *Most have Congenital Heart Disease*
- *Essentially all are malrotated*

Gamesmanship
- *One trick is to show the NG tube curving into the chest.*

Locational Strategy

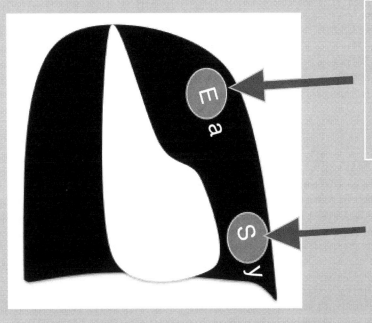

Left Upper Lobe:

Think **Congenital Lobar Emphysema (CLE)** first

But, remember CCAM has no lobar prevalence, so it can be anywhere

Left Lower Lobe:

Think **Sequestration** First

Congenital Diaphragmatic Hernia (CDHs) favors this side too

Case 1. Newborn with congenital heart disease

A. Intralobar Sequestration
B. Extralobar Sequestration
C. Congenital Lobar Emphysema

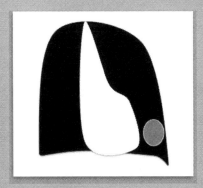

Case 2. 10 year old with recurrent pneumonia

A. Intralobar Sequestration
B. Extralobar Sequestration
C. Congenital Lobar Emphysema

**Intralobar is seen older kids,
**Extralobar is seen in infants with co-morbids
** CLE is in the upper lobe

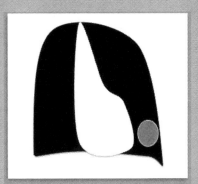

Special Situations in Peds Chests

Viral – In all ages this is way more common than bacterial infection. Peribronchial edema is the buzzword for the CXR finding. "Dirty" or "Busy" Hilum. You also end up with debris and mucus in the airway which causes two things (1) hyperinflation and (2) subsegmental atelectasis.

Round Pneumonia – Kids get round pneumonia. They love to show this, and try to trick you into thinking it's a mass. Younger than 8 you are thinking round pneumonia, round pneumonia, round pneumonia – with S. Pneumonia being the culprit. The PhD trivia is that these occur because you don't have good collateral ventilation pathways. Round pneumonia is usually solitary, and likes the posterior lower lobes. Take home message: *No CT to exclude cancer, just get a follow up x-ray.*

Swyer James – This is the classic unilateral lucent lung. It typically occurs after a viral lung infection in childhood resulting in post infectious obliterative bronchiolitis. The size of the affected lobe is smaller than a normal lobe (it's not hyperexpanded).

Papillomatosis - Perinatal HPV can cause these soft tissue masses within the airway and lungs. It's also seen in adults who smoke. *"Multiple lung nodules which demonstrate cavitation"* is the classic scenario. Some testable trivia includes the 2% risk of squamous cell cancer, and that manipulation can lead to dissemination. The appearance of cysts and nodules can look like LCH (discussed more in the thoracic chapter), although the trachea is also involved.

Sickle Cell / Acute Chest – Kids with sickle cell can get "Acute chest." Acute chest actually occurs more in kids than adults (usually between age 2-4). This is the leading cause of death in sickle cell patients. Some people think the pathology is as such: you infarct a rib -> that hurts a lot, so you don't breath deep -> atelectasis and infection. Others think you get pulmonary microvascular occlusion and infarction. Regardless, if you see opacities in the CXR of a kid with sickle cell, you should think of this.

Gamesmanship (how do you know it's sickle cell?)
- *Kid with Big Heart*
- *Kid with bone infarcts (look at the humeral heads)*
- *Kid with H shaped vertebra (look on lateral)*

Bronchial Foreign Body: The key concept is that it causes **air trapping**. The lung may look more lucent (from air trapping) of the affected side. You **put the affected side down and it will remain lucent** (from air trapping). Another random piece of trivia, is that under fluoro the mediastinum will shift AWAY from the affected side on expiration.

Cystic Fibrosis- So the sodium pump doesn't work and they end up with thick secretions and poor pulmonary clearance. The real damage is done by recurrent infections.

Things to know:
- *Bronchiectasis (begins cylindrical and progresses to varicoid)*
- *It has an **apical predominance** (lower lobes are less affected)*
- *Hyperinflation*
- *They get Pulmonary Arterial Hypertension*
- *Mucus plugging (finger in glove sign)*
- *Men are infertile (vas deferens is missing)*

CF Related Trickery

- *Fatty Replaced Pancreas on CT*
- *Abdominal Films with Constipation*
- *Biliary Cirrhosis (from blockage of intrahepatic bile ducts), and resulting portal HTN*

Primary Ciliary Dyskinesia – The motile part of the cilia doesn't work. They can't clear their lungs and get recurrent infections. These guys have lots of bronchiectasis just like CF. BUT, this time its lower lobe predominant (CF was upper lobe).

Things to know:
- *Bronchiectasis (**lower lobes**)*
- *50% will have Kartageners (situs inversus). So, 50% will not*
- *Men are infertile (sperm tails don't work)*
- *Women are subfertile (cilia needed to push eggs around)*

This vs That:

Cystic Fibrosis	Primary Ciliary Dyskinesia
Upper Lobe Predominant - Brochiectasis	Lower Lobe Predominant - Bronchiectasis
Infertile - Men are Missing the Vas Deferens	Infertile - Men's Sperm Don't Swim For Shit

Mediastinal Masses

Anterior:

- **Normal Thymus:** This is the most common mediastinal "mass." It's terribly embarrassing to call a normal thymus a mass, but can actually be tricky sometimes. It can be pretty big in kids less than 5 (especially in infants). Triangular shape of the thymus is sometimes called the "sail sign." Not to be confused with the other 20 sail signs in various parts of the body, or the spinnaker sail sign, which is when pneumomediastinum lifts up the thymus.

> **That Asshole is Guilty!**
>
> Things that make you think the thymus is a cancer!
>
> - *Abnormal Size for patients Age (really big in a 15 year old)*
> - *Heterogenous appearance*
> - *Calcification*
> - *Compression of airway or vascular structure*

- **Thymic Rebound:** In times of acute stress (pneumonia, radiation, chemotherapy, burns), the thymus will shrink. In the recovery phase it will rebound back to normal, and sometimes larger than before. During this rebound it **can be PET avid**.

- **Lymphoma:** This is the **most common abnormal mediastinal mass in children** (older children and teenagers). Lymphoma vs Thymus can be tricky. Thymus is more in kids under 10, Lymphoma is seen more in kids over 10. When you get around age 10, you need to look for cervical lymph nodes to make you think lymphoma. If you see calcification, and the lesion has NOT been treated you may be dealing with a teratoma. Calcification is uncommon in an untreated lymphoma.

- *Complications: Compression of SVC, Compression of Pulmonary Veins, Pericardial Effusion, Airway Compression.*

- **Germ Cell Tumor (GCT):** On imaging, this is a large anterior mediastinal mass arising from or at least next to the thymus. It comes in three main flavors, each of which has a few pieces of trivia worth knowing:

    - **Teratoma** - Mostly Cystic, with **fat** and calcium
    - **Seminoma** - Bulky and Lobulated. ***"Straddles the midline"***
    - **NSGCT** - Big and Ugly - Hemorrhage and Necrosis. Can get crazy and invade the lung.

> ***The only risk factor for extra gonadal germ cell tumors is Klinefelter's Syndrome***
>
> **Klinefelter patients** have the worst syndrome ever. They have small penises, they get male breast cancer, and as if things couldn't possibly get worse… they get germ cell tumors in their chest. In fact, **they are at 300x the risk of getting a GCT**. Pineal gland Germ Cells have also been reported in Klinefelter patients, giving them vertical gaze palsy. In that case, they can't even look up to the sky and say "Why God** ?! Why Me!? Why Klinefelter's!?"
>
> ***God, Allah, Mother Earth, Celestial Deity NOS*

Middle:

- **Lymphadenopathy** – Middle mediastinal lymphadenopathy is most often from granulomatous disease (TB or Fungal), or from lymphoma.

- **Duplication Cysts** – These fall into three categories (a) bronchogenic, (b) enteric, (c) neuroenteric. The neuroenterics are posterior mediastinal, the other two are middle mediastinal.

- **Bronchogenic** – water attenuation – close to the trachea or bronchus. Bronchogenic cysts tend to be middle mediastinal (esophageal cysts tend to be posterior mediastinal).

- **Enteric** – water attenuation close to the esophagus (lower in the mediastinum)

Posterior:

- **Neuroblastoma** – This is the most common posterior mediastinal mass in a child under 2. This is discussed in complete detail in the GU PEDs section. I'll just mention that compared to abdominal neuroblastoma, thoracic neuroblastoma has a better outcome. They may involve the ribs and vertebral bodies. Also, remember that Wilms usually mets (more than neuroblastoma) to the lungs, so if it's in the lungs don't forget about Wilms.

- **Ewing Sarcoma** – *This is discussed in complete detail in the MSK PEDs section - in book 1 - module 2.*

- **Askin Tumor (Primitive Neuroectodermal tumor of the chest wall):** This is now considered part of the Ewing Sarcoma spectrum, and is sometimes called an Ewing sarcoma of the chest wall. They tend to displace adjacent structure rather than invade early on (when they get big they can invade). They look heterogenous, and the solid parts will enhance.

- **Neuroenteric Cyst** – By convention these are associated with vertebral anomalies (think scoliosis). The cyst does NOT communicate with CSF, is well demarcated, and is water density.

- **Extramedullary Hematopoiesis** - This occurs in patients with myeloproliferative disorders or bone marrow infiltration (including sickle cell). Usually, this manifests as a big liver and big spleen. However, in a minority of cases you can get soft tissue density around the spine (paraspinal masses), which are bilateral, smooth, and sharply delineated.

Strategy - The Anterior Mediastinal Mass

Lymphoma - In a kid just assume it's Hodgkins (which means it's gonna involve the thymus). *Why assume Hodgkins ?* Hodgkins is 4x more common than NHL. Hodgkins involves the thymus 90% of the time.

Q: *How the hell do you tell a big ass normal thymus in a little baby vs a lymphoma?*
A: My main move is to go age. **Under 10 = Thymus, Over 10 = Lymphoma.**

Thymic Rebound - If the test writer is headed in this direction they MUST either (a) <u>bias you with a history</u> saying stuff like **"got off chemo"** or **"got off corticosteroids"** or (b) show you a series of axial CTs with the thing growing and maintaining normal morphology. I think "a" is much more likely.

My Other Funk: In general just think morphology / density:

- **Soft Tissue - Kinda Homogenous** = Think **Lymphoma or Hyperplasia**

- **Fat** = **Germ Cell Tumor** (*Why God!? Why Klinefelters!?*)

- **Water** = Congenital Shit - Think **Lymphangiomas**

Strategy - The Posterior Mediastinal Mass

First Rule of Peds Multiple Choice Test Taking - **TIMING! AGE!**

Under 10 - Think **malignant**, Think **neuroblastoma.**

2nd Decade - Think **benign.**

If it's a round mass- Think about **Ganglioneuromas & Neurofibromas**

If it's cystic (and there is scoliosis) think **Neuroenteric Cyst**

If they show you coarse bone trabeculation - with an adjacent mass (or a **history of anemia**) - Think **Extramedullary Hematopoiesis**

Strategy - The B.F.M.
"Big Fucking Mass"

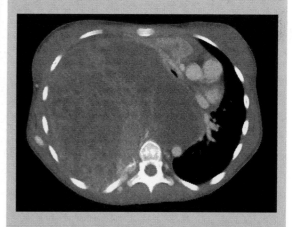

If you see a B.F.M. in the chest of a kid, you basically have two choices:

(1) **Askin Tumor (PNET / Ewings) -**
   *AGE 10+, look for an eaten up rib.
(2) **Pleuropulmonary Blastoma**
   *AGE is typically less than 2.

Primary Lung Tumors:

Pleuropulmonary Blastoma (PPB) – This is a primary intrathroacic malignancy. They can look a lot like CCAMs and even have different types (cystic, mixed, solid). These things are usually right sided, pleural based, and without chest wall invasion or calcifications. **No rib invasion** *(helps distinguish it from the Askin - if they won't tell you the age)*, No calcification. The more solid types can have mets to the brain and bones. The cystic type seem to occur more in kids less than a year old, and be more benign.

Things to know about PPBs:
- Big Fucking Mass (B.F.M.) in the chest of a 1-2 year old
- Shouldn't have an eaten up rib (Askin tumors often do)
- 10% of the time they have a multilocular cystic nephroma.

Catheters / Lines

Umbilical Venous Catheter (UVC) – A UVC passes from the umbilical vein to the left portal vein to the ductus venosus to a hepatic vein to the IVC. You don't want the thing to lodge in the portal vein because you can infarct the liver. The ideal spot is at the IVC – Right Atrium junction.

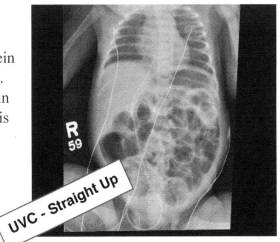

Umbilical Artery Catheter (UAC) – A UAC passes from the umbilicus, down to the umbilical artery, into an iliac artery then to the aorta. Positioning counts, as the major risk factor is renal arterial thrombosis. You want to avoid the renal arteries by going high (T8-T10), or low (L3-L5)

Things to know about UACs:
- *It goes down first*
- *It should be placed either high (T8-T10) or low (L3-L5)*

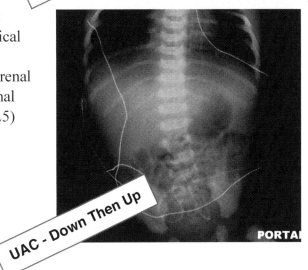

GI

Esophageal Atresia / TE fistula: This can occur in multiple subtypes, with the classic ways of showing it being a **frontal CXR with an NG tube stopped in the upper neck**, or a fluoro study (shown lateral) with a blind ending sac or communication with the tracheal tree.

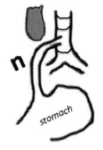
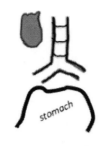
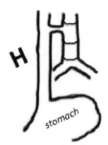

N-Type Fistula (85%)   Esophageal Atresia NO Fistula (10%)   H-Type Atresia (1%)

There are 5 main subtypes, only 3 of which are worth knowing (being familiar with) for the purpose of the exam.

Things to Know About Esophageal Atresia / TE Fistula:
- *Most Important Thing To Know are the VACTERL associations (more on this later)*
- *The most common subtype is the N-Type (blind ended esophagus, with distal esophagus hooked up to trachea*
- *Excessive Air in the Stomach = H type (can also be with N type)*
- *No Air in the Stomach = Esophageal Atresia*
- *The presence of a right arch (4%) must be described prior to surgery (changes the approach).*

VACTERL: This is extremely high yield. VACTERL is a way of remembering that certain associations are seen more commonly when together (when you see one, look for the others).

They occur with different frequency:

V – Vertebral Anomalies (37%)
A – Anal (imperforate anus) (63%)
C – Cardiac (77%)
TE – Tracheoesophageal Fistula or Esophageal Atresia (40%)
R – Renal (72%)
L – Limb (radial ray) – 58%

VACTERL association is diagnosed when 3 or more of the defined anomalies affect a patient.

Therefore, keep investigating when 1-2 of these anomalies are found.

The **heart** and **kidneys** are the **most commonly affected** organs in this association.

Trivia: If both limbs are involved, then both kidneys tend to be involved. If one limb is involved, then one kidney tends to be involved.

Esophageal Foreign Bodies: Kids love to stick things in their mouths (noses and ears). This can cause a lot of problems including direct compression of the airway, perforation, or even fistula to the trachea. Stuff stuck in the esophagus needs to be removed.

One trick to be aware of is that on a frontal CXR, a coin that is seen totally in the coronal plane is more likely in the esophagus. A coin seen turned 90 degrees is more likely in the trachea (because in the rigid trachea it must turn long ways against the elastic posterior membrane).

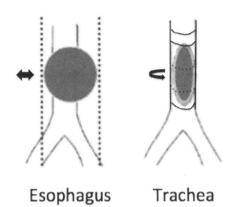

Additional trivia relates to swallowed batteries, magnets, and pennies

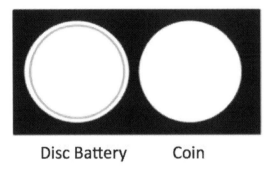

- **Swallowed Magnets** – One magnet is ok. Two or more magnets is a problem. The reason is that they can attract each other across intestinal walls leading to obstruction, necrosis, perforation, and a law suit. They need a surgical consult. Also... MRI is contraindicated.

- **Disc Batteries** – They look like coins, except they have two rings. The literature is not clear, but it appears that modern batteries rarely leak (leaking is bad – caustic chemicals, heavy metals etc..). So most people will watch the transit with serial x-rays. If it gets stuck, they go and get it. If you leave it in longer than a week or so, the risk of it leaking increases.

- **Pennies** - Those minted prior to 1982 (copper pennies) are safe. Those **minted after 1982 contain mostly Zinc** which when combined with stomach acid **can cause gastric ulcerations**, and if absorbed in great enough quantity can cause zinc toxicosis (which is mainly pancreatic dysfunction / pancreatitis). The ulcers are the more likely thing to happen, so just remember that.

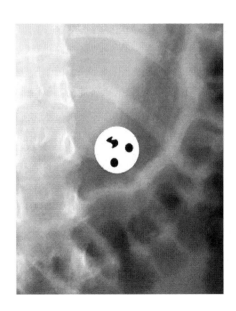

   So how the hell can you tell the date of a penny that is swallowed? Either (a) the question stem will have to say something like - "2 year old child playing with father's collection of 1984 pennies", or the more likely (b) **showing you the penny with characteristic radiolucent holes** - from erosion.

Vascular Impressions

This is a very high yield topic for the purpose of multiple choice exams.

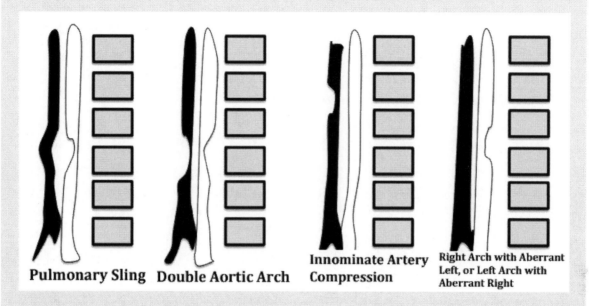

Pulmonary Sling   Double Aortic Arch   Innominate Artery Compression   Right Arch with Aberrant Left, or Left Arch with Aberrant Right

Trivia to Know:

Pulmonary Sling:
- The **only variant that goes between the esophagus and the trachea**.
- Classic question, is that this is **associated with trachea stenosis.**
- High association with other cardiopulmonary and systemic anomalies: hypoplastic right lung, horseshoe lung, TE-fistula, imperforate anus, and complete tracheal rings.

Double Aortic Arch:
- Most Common **SYMPTOMATIC** vascular ring anomaly

Left Arch with Aberrant Right Subclavian Artery
- Most Common Aortic Arch Anomaly — not necessarily symptomatic.
- **"Dysphagia Lusoria"** - fancy Latin speak (therefore high yield) for trouble swallowing in the setting of this variant anatomy
- **"Diverticulum of Kommerell"** pouch like aneurysmal dilatation of the proximal portion of an aberrant right subclavian artery

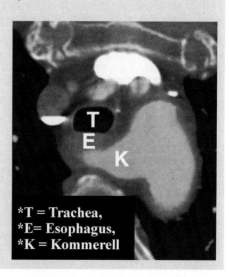

*T = Trachea,
*E = Esophagus,
*K = Kommerell

Bowel Obstruction (in the neonate)

Bowel obstruction in the neonate can be thought of as either high or low. Here are causes you should keep in your mind when you think the question stem is leading toward obstruction.

Neonatal Obstruction	
High	**Low**
Midgut Volvulus / Malrotation	Hirschsprung Disease
Duodenal Atresia	Meconium Plug Syndrome
Duodenal Web	Ileal Atresia
Annular Pancreas	Meconium Ileus
Jejunal Atresia	Anal Atresia / Colonic Atresia

Why might you think the question is leading you toward obstruction? Anytime you are dealing with a neonate, and the history mentions **"vomiting," "belly pain,"** or **"hasn't passed a stool yet."**

The following sections will walk through an algorithm, starting with plain films for diagnosis (and sometimes management).

Section 1: "Bubbles"

People who do peds radiology are obsessed with bubbles on baby grams. The idea is to develop a pattern based approach to bowel obstruction in the newborn.

At the institution I trained at, this was taught as 8 classic patterns:

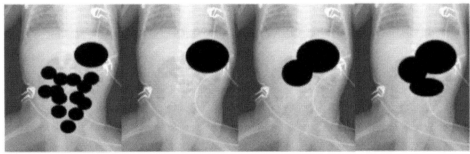

Normal   Single Bubble   Double Bubble   Triple Bubble

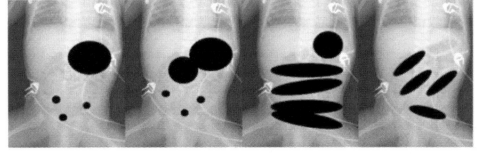

Single Bubble -plus distal gas   Double Bubble -plus distal gas   Diffusely Dilated   Diffusely Mildly Dilated

 **Single Bubble = Gastric (antral or pyloric) atresia.**

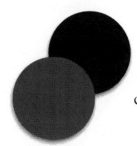 **Double Bubble** = *Duodenal Atresia (highly specific)*. Some authors will say that UGI is not necessary because of how highly specific this is. The degree of distention will be more pronounced than with midgut volvulus (which is a more acute process). Thought to be secondary to failure to canalize during development (often an isolated atresia)

Trivia Regarding Duodenal Atresia:
- *30% have Downs*
- *40% have polyhydramnios and are premature*
- *The "single atresia" - cannulation error*
- *On multiple choice test the "double bubble" can be shown on 3rd trimester OB ultrasound, plain film, or on MRI.*

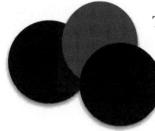 **Triple Bubble = Jejunal Atresia**. When you call jejunal atresia, you often prompt search for additional atresias (colonic). Just remember that jejunal atresia is secondary to a vascular insult during development.

- *The "multiple atresia" - vascular error.*

Single Bubble with Distal Gas = Can mean nothing (lotta air swallowing). If the clinical history is bilious vomiting, this is ominous and can be midgut volvulus (surgical emergency). Next test would be emergent Upper GI.

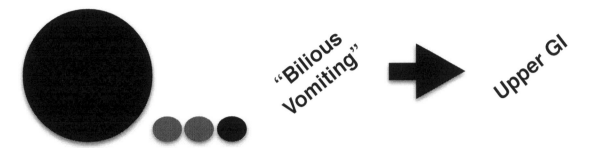

Double Bubble with Distal Gas = Seeing distal gas excludes duodenal atresia. The DDx is a duodenal web, duodenal stenosis, or midgut volvulus. Next step would be upper GI.

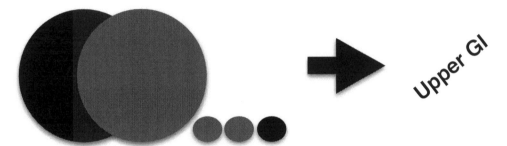

Multiple Diffusely Dilated Loops = Suggestive of a low obstruction (ileum or colon). Next step is contrast enema. If the contrast enema is normal you need to follow with upper GI (to exclude an atypical look for midgut volvulus).

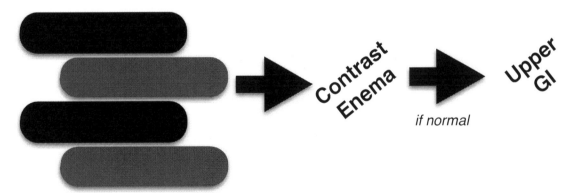

Mildly Dilated, Scattered Loops = "Sick Belly" – Can be seen with proximal or distal obstruction. Will need Upper GI and contrast enema.

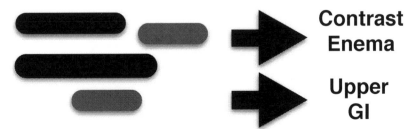

Section 2 : Upper GI Patterns

Upper GI on kids is fair game in multiple choice tests, and real life. Often the answer of this test can equal a trip to the OR for kids, so it's no trivial endeavor.

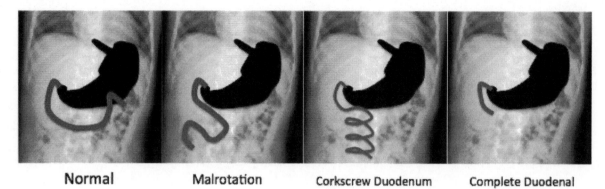

Normal   Malrotation   Corkscrew Duodenum   Complete Duodenal Obstruction

Malrotation – Normally, the developmental rotation of the gut places the ligament of Trietz to the left of the spine (at the level of the duodenal bulb). If mother nature fucks up and this doesn't happen, you end up with <u>the duodenum to the right of the midline</u> (spine). These patients are at increased risk for mid gut volvulus, and internal hernias. If you see the appearance of malrotation and the clinical history is bilious vomiting, then you must suspect midgut volvulus.

Trivia regarding Malrotation
- *Associated with Heterotaxy Syndromes. Associated with Omphaloceles.*
- *Classically shown as the SMA to the right of the SMV (on US or CT).*
- *False Positive on UGI – Distal Bowel Obstruction, displacing the duodenum (because of ligamentous laxity).*

Corkscrew Duodenum - This is diagnostic of midgut volvulus (surgical emergency). The appearance is an Aunt Minnie.

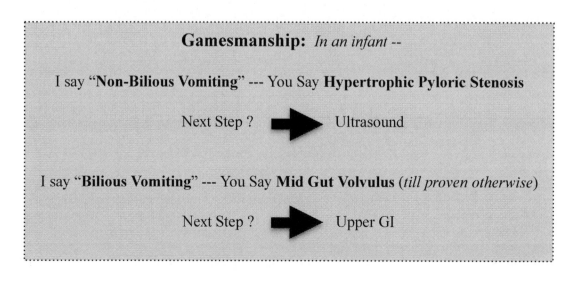

Ladd's Bands – In older children (or even adults) obstruction in the setting of malrotation will present as intermittent episodes of spontaneous duodenal obstruction. The cause is not midgut volvulus (a surgical emergency) but rather kinking from Ladd's Bands.

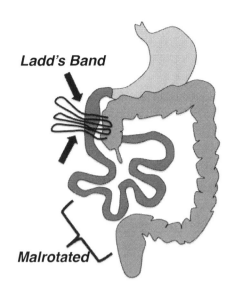

So what the hell is a "Ladd's Band"? We are talking about a fibrous stalk of peritoneal tissues that fixes the cecum to the abdominal wall, and can obstruct the duodenum.

Ladd's Procedure –

Procedure to prevent mid gut volvulus. Traditionally, the Ladd's Bands are divided, and the appendix is taken out. The small bowel ends up on the right, and the large bowel ends up on the left. They are fixed in place by adhesions (just by opening the abdomen).

It is still possible to develop volvulus post Ladd's (but it's rare – 2-5%).

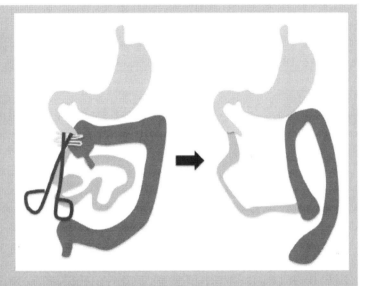

Ladds Procedure:
- Divide the Adhesive Ladds Bands
- Widen the Mesentery to a safe distance
- Take out the appendix (bill extra for that)

Complete Duodenal Obstruction – Strongly associated with midgut volvulus. If you were thinking duodenal atresia, look for distal air (any will do) to exclude that thought. Plus, as discussed above, you want to see a dilated duodenum (double bubble) for duodenal atresia. **Partial Duodenal Obstruction** – If the kid is vomiting this might be from extrinsic narrowing (ladd band, annular pancreas), or intrinsic (duodenal web, duodenal stenosis). You can't tell.

Hypertrophic Pyloric Stenosis – Thickening of the gastric pyloric musculature, which results in progressive obstruction. Step 1 buzzword is "non-bilious vomiting." Here is the most likely multiple choice trick; **this does NOT occur at birth or after 3 months.**

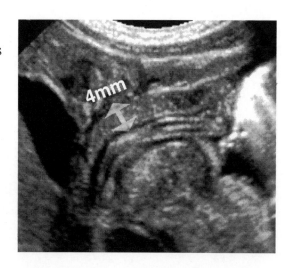

There is a specific age range 2-12 weeks (peak at 3-6 weeks).

Criteria is 4mm and 14mm (4mm single wall, 14mm length).

The primary differential is pylorospasm (which will relax during exam). The most common pitfall during the exam is gastric over distention, which can lead to displacement of the antrum and pylorus – leading to false negative.

False positive can result from off axis measurement.

The phenomenon of *"paradoxial aciduria"* has been described, and is a common buzzword.

Gastric Volvulus- This comes in two flavors; organoaxial and mesenteroaxial.

- *Organoaxial* – The <u>greater curvature flips over the lesser curvature</u> (rotation along the long axis). This is seen in old ladies with paraesophageal hernias.

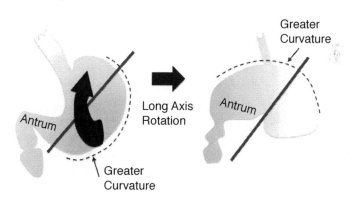

- *Mesenteroaxial* – Twisting over the mesentery (rotation along short axis). The *antrum flips near the GE junction.* **Can cause ischemia** and needs to be fixed. Additionally this type causes obstruction. *This type is* **more common in kids.**

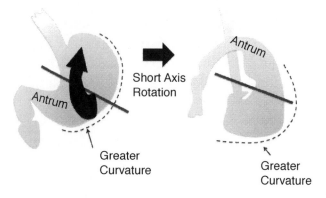

Duodenal Web: This is best thought of as *"almost duodenal atresia."* The reason I say that is just like duodenal atresia this occurs from a failure to canalize, but instead of a total failure of canalization (like duodenal atresia) this bowel is only partially canalized, leaving behind a potentially obstructive web.

Trivia to know:
- Because the web is distal to ampulla of Vater - you get **bile stained emesis**
- **Associated with** malrotation and **Downs syndrome**
- The **"wind sock"** deformity is seen more in older kids - where the web like diaphragm has gotten stretched.

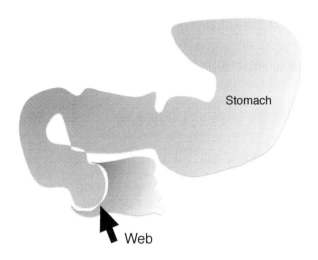

Annular Pancreas: Essentially an embryologic screw up (failure of ventral bud to rotate with the duodenum), that results in encasement of the duodenum.

In Kids = Think Duodenal Obstruction

In Adults = Think Pancreatitis

How it's shown:

- On CT: Look for pancreatic tissue (same enhancement as the nearby normal pancreas) encircling the descending duodenum.

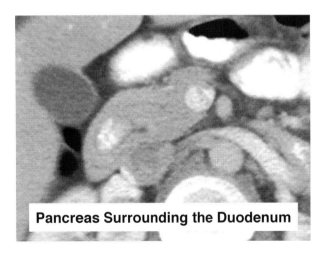

- On Fluoro: Look for an extrinsic narrowing the duodenum. Obviously this is non-specific (typical barium - voodoo), use the location and clinical history to bias yourself.

Section 3: "Low Obstructions" in a Neonate

Just like the upper GI and "bubble" plain film in sections 1 & 2, the lower obstruction can be approached with a pattern based method. You basically have 4 choices: Normal, Short Microcolon, Long Microcolon, and a Caliber Change from micro to normal.

Normal:
- This is what normal looks like:

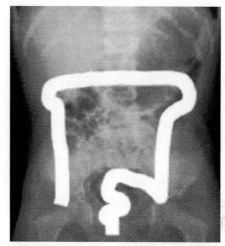

Short Microcolon -
- Think about <u>Colonic Atresia</u>

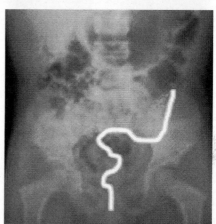

Long Microcolon - This can be seen with meconium ileus or distal ileal atresia.

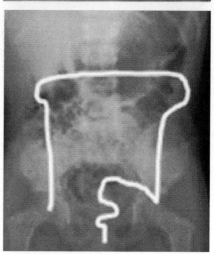

•**Meconium Ileus – ONLY in patients with CF**. The pathology is the result of thick sticky meconium causing obstruction of the distal ileum. Contrast will reach ileal loops, and demonstrate multiple filling defects (meconium). This can be addressed with an enema.

•**Distal Ileal Atresia -** This is the result of intrauterine vascular insult. **Contrast will NOT reach ileal loops**. This needs surgery.

Caliber Change – This can be seen with small left colon syndrome or Hirschsprungs

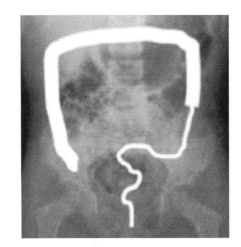

- **Small Left Colon Syndrome** – This is a transient functional colonic obstruction, that is self limited and relieved by contrast enema.

    *Most Testable Fact: It is **NOT associated with CF**.

    *2nd Most Testable Fact: It is seen in **infants of diabetic mothers** or mothers who have received magnesium sulfate for eclampsia.

- **Hirschsprung Disease** – Failure of the ganglion cells to migrate and innervate the distal colon. Affected portions of the colon are small in caliber, whereas the normally innervated colon appears dilated.

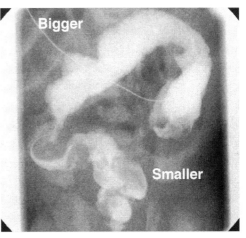

Trivia:
- It's 4:1 more common in boys.
- 10% association with downs.
- Diagnosis is made by rectal biopsy.

How its Shown:
- Enema - **Rectum smaller than the Sigmoid** "Recto-sigmoid ratio < 1"
- Enema - **Rectum with "sawtooth pattern"** Represents bowel spasm

Presentation:
(1) Newborn who fails to have BM,
(2) One month old who shows up "sick as stink" with NEC bowel

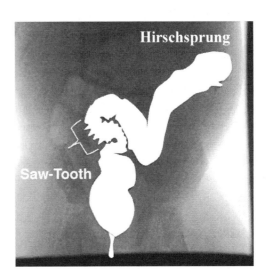

- **Total Colonic Aganglionosis** - This is super rare variant of Hirschsprungs, and **can mimic microcolon**. The piece of commonly asked trivia is that it can also affect the terminal ileus.

Meconium Peritonitis: This is a somewhat random GI topic, with a very characteristic look. It's a **calcified mass in the mid abdomen**, traditionally shown on plain film. It is the result of a sterile peritoneal reaction to an intra utero bowel perforation. The bowel perforation could be the result of atresia or meconium ileus. Usually, the perforation seals off prior to birth and there is no leak.

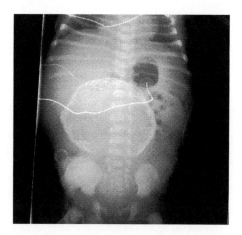

Imperforate or Ectopic Anus: This can range from simple membranous anal atresia to an arrest of the colon as it descends through puborectalis sling. The thing to known is fistula to genitourinary tract. Imperforate anus is also associated with a tethered cord (probably need a screening ultrasound).

- *I say "Baby with no asshole", you say "VACTERL"*
- *I say "Baby with no asshole", you say "Screening US for tethered cord"*

Obstruction in an Older Child:

"My belly hurts" questions in an older child, should make you think of 6 main things - the classic AA-II-MM or "AIM" differential.

> *The classic DDx in "AIM" –*
>
> - Appendicitis, Adhesions
> - Inguinal Hernia, Intussusception
> - Midgut Volvulus, Meckels Diverticulum

Appendicitis – In children older than 4 this is the most common cause for bowel obstruction. If they show this in the PEDs section it's most likely to be on ultrasound. In that case you can expect a blind ending tube, non compressible, and bigger than 6mm.

Inguinal Hernia: This is covered in more depth in the GI chapter. Big points are that **indirect hernias are more common in kids,** they are lateral to the inferior epigastric, and incarceration is the most common complication. Umbilical hernias are common in kids, but rarely incarcerate.

Trivia to know: This is the most common cause of obstruction in boy 1 month - 1 year.

Intussusception – The age range is 3 months – 3 years, before or after that you should think of lead points (90% between 3 months and 3 years don't have lead points). The normal mechanism is forward peristalsis resulting in invagination of proximal bowel (the intussusceptum) into lumen of the distal bowel (the intussuscipiens). They have to be bigger than 2.5cm to matter (in most cases- these are enterocolic), those that are less than 2.0 cm are usually small bowel-small bowel and may reduce spontaneously within minutes. Just like an appendix, in the peds section, I would anticipate this shown on ultrasound as either the target sign, or pseudo-kidney.

There are 3 main ways to ask questions about this: (1) *what is it ?*- these should be straight forward as targets or pseudo kidneys, (2) *leads points* - stuff like HSP (vasculitis), meckle diverticulum, enteric duplication cysts, and (3) *reduction trivia.*

Reducing Intussusception Trivia:
- *Contraindications: Free Air (check plain film). Peritonitis (based on exam)*
- *Recurrence: Usually within 72 hours*
- *Success Rates – 80-90% with air*
- *Risk of Perforation – 0.5%*
- *Air causes less peritonitis (spillage of fecal material) than barium*
- *Pressure should NOT exceed 120mmHg*

Target Signs of Intussusception

Not all targets are created equal.

Target > 2.5cm = Illeocolic - getting air enema

Target < 2.5cm = Small Bowel - Small Bowel, not getting air enema.

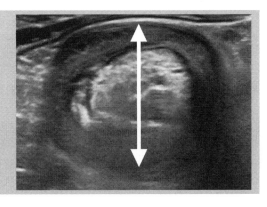

Meckels Diverticulum: This is a congenital diverticulum of the distal ileum. A piece of total trivia is that it is a persistent piece of the omphalomesenteric duct. Step 1 style, "rule of 2s" occurs in 2% of the population, has 2 types of heterotopic mucosa (gastric and pancreatic), located 2 feet from the IC valve, it's usually 2 inches long (and 2cm in diameter), and usually has symptoms before the child is 2. If it has gastric mucosa (the ones that bleed typically do) it will take up Tc-Pertechnetate just like the stomach (hence the Meckel's scan).

High Yield Trivia (Regarding Complications)
- *Can get diverticulitis in the Meckels (mimic appendix)*
- *GI Bleed from Gastric Mucosa (causes 30% of symptomatic cases)*
- *Can be a lead point for intussusception (seen with inverted diverticulum)*
- *Can Cause Obstruction*

Special Topics:

Enteric Duplication Cysts – These are developmental anomalies (failure to canalize). They don't have to communicate with the GI lumen but can. They are most commonly in the ileal region (40%). They have been known to cause in utero bowel obstruction / perforation.

Strategy: A common way to show this is a cyst in the abdomen (on ultrasound). If you have a random cyst in the abdomen you need to ask yourself - *"does this have gut signature?"*

- Cyst with Gut Signature = Enteric Duplication Cyst
- Cyst without Gut Signature = Omental Cyst
- WTF is "Gut Signature ?" - It's alternating bands of hyper and hypo echoic signal - supposedly representing different layers of bowel.

Trivia to know: 30% of the time they are **associated with vertebral anomalies**.

Distal Intestinal Obstruction Syndrome – This is a cause of bowel obstruction in an older kid (20 year old) with cystic fibrosis. This is sometimes called the *"meconium ileus equivalent,"* because you end up with a distal obstruction (as the name implies) secondary to dried up thick stool. It more commonly involves the ileum / right colon. Kids who get this, are the ones who aren't compliant with their pancreatic enzymes.

Necrotising Enterocolitis (NEC)- This is bad news. The general thinking is that you have an immature bowel mucosa (from being premature or having a heart problem), and you get translocated bugs through this immature bowel. It's best thought of as a combination of ischemic and infective pathology.

Who gets it?
- **Premature Kids** (90% within the first 10 days of life)
- Low Birth Weight Kids (< 1500 grams)
- **Cardiac Patients** (sometimes occult) – they can be full term
- Kids who had perinatal asphyxia
- **Hirschsprung Kids** that go home and come back – they **present around month 1**.

What does it look like?
- Pneumatosis – most definitive finding ; Look for Portal Venous Gas Next
- Focal Dilated Bowel (especially in the right lower quadrant) – the terminal ileum / right colon is the region most affected by NEC
- Featureless small bowel , with separation (suggesting edema).
- Unchanging bowel gas pattern – this would be a dirty trick – showing several plain films from progressing days, with the bowel gas pattern remaining the same.

Pneumatosis vs Poop - The age old question.
- First question - has the kid been feed? No food = No poop.
- Second question - is it staying still? Poop will move, Pneumatosis will stay still.

Useless Trivia:
- Use of maternal breast milk is the only parameter associated with decreased incidence of NEC.

Gastroschisis – Extraabominal evisceration of neonatal bowel (sometimes stomach and liver) through a paraumbilical wall defect.

Trivia to know:
- It does NOT have a surrounding membrane (omphalocele does)
- It's **always on the RIGHT side.**
- Associated anomalies are rare (unlike omphalocele).
- Maternal Serum AFP will be elevated (higher than that of omphalocele)
- Outcome is usually good
- For some reason they get bad reflux after repair.

Omphalocele – This is a congenital midline defect, with herniation of gut at the base of the umbilical cord.

Trivia to know:
- It DOES have a surrounding membrane (gastroschisis does not)
- **Associated anomalies are common** (unlike gastroschisis)
- Trisomy 18 is the most common associated chromosomal anomaly
- Other associations: Cardiac (50%), Other GI, CNS, GU, Turners, Klinefelters, Beckwith-Wiedemann.
- Outcomes are not that good, because of associated syndromes.
- Umbilical Cord Cysts (Allantoic Cysts) are associated.

Physiologic Gut Herniation – This is a normal phenomenon that occurs around 6-8 weeks. The idea is that the bowel grows faster than the abdominal cavity, and to accommodate this growth it herniates out of the abdominal cavity into the base of the cord. The midgut then rotates and everything comes back to normal.

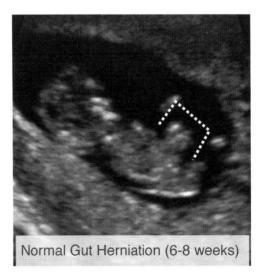
Normal Gut Herniation (6-8 weeks)

Trivia to know
- **It's normal**
- Should NOT contain herniated liver
- Should only be seen in early pregnancy (6-8 weeks)

Mesenteric Adenitis - Self-limiting, usually viral inflammatory condition of mesenteric lymph nodes. It is a **classic clinical mimic of appendicitis**. The finding is a <u>cluster of large right lower quadrant lymph nodes.</u>

GI Organs

Spleen

Polysplenia and Asplenia – Heterotaxia syndromes are clutch for multiple choice tests. This is discussed in the GI section, but because it's such a high yield topic I'll repeat myself. The major game played on written tests is "left side vs right side."

So what the hell does that mean? I like to start in the lungs. The right side has two fissures (major and minor). The left side has just one fissure. So if I show you a CXR with two fissures on each side, (a left sided minor fissure), then the patient has two right sides. Thus the term "bilateral right sidedness."

What else is a right sided structure? The liver. So, these patients won't have a spleen (the spleen is a left sided structure).

The opposite is true. Bilateral left sided patients have polysplenia.

Heterotaxia Syndromes	
Right Sided	**Left Sided**
Two Fissures in Left Lung	One Fissure in Right Lung
Asplenia	Polysplenia
Increased Cardiac Malforations	Less Cardiac Malformations
Reversed Aorta/IVC	Azygous Continuation of the IVC

Infarcted Spleen – Just say sickle cell.

Liver

Tumors: With regard to the liver tumors I like to use an age-based system to figure it out. Mass in the liver, first think – what is the age. Then use the narrow DDx to figure it out.

Age 0-3: With kids that are newborns you should think about 3 tumors:

Hemangioendothelioma: Often < 1. Associated with high output CHF, this is classically shown as a large heart on CXR plus a mass in the liver. The Aorta above the hepatic branches of the celiac is often enlarged relative to the aorta below the celiac because of differential flow. Skin hemangiomas present 50%. **Endothelial growth factor is elevated**. These can be associated with Kasabach-Merritt Syndrome (the platelet eater).

How do they do? - Actually well. They tend to spontaneously involute without therapy over months-years - as they progressively calcify.

Hepatoblastoma: Most common primary liver tumor of childhood (< 5). The big thing to know is that it's associated with a bunch of syndromes – mainly hemi-hypertrophy, Wilms, Beckwith-Weidemann crowd. *Prematurity is a risk factor.* This is usually a well circumscribed solitary right sided mass, that may extend into the portal veins, hepatic veins, and IVC. Calcifications are present 50% of the time. **AFP is elevated.** Another piece of trivia is the hepatoblastoma **may cause a precocious puberty** from making bHCG.

I would know 3 things: (1) Associated with Wilms, (2) AFP, (3) Precocious Puberty

Mesenchymal Hamartoma: This is the predominately **cystic mass** (or multiple cysts), sometimes called a "developmental anomaly." Because it's a "developmental anomaly" it shouldn't surprise you that the **AFP is negative**. Calcifications are UNCOMMON. What is common is a large portal vein branch feeding the tumor.

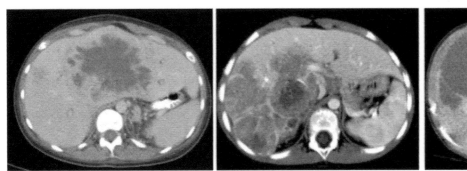
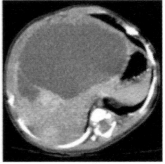
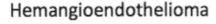

Hemangioendothelioma   Hepatoblastoma   Mesenchymal Hamartoma

Age >5

HCC: This is actually the second most common liver cancer in kids. You'll see them in kids with cirrhosis (biliary atresia, fanconi syndrome, glycogen storage disease). **AFP will be elevated.**

Fibrolamellar Subtype: This is typically seen in a younger patients (<35) without cirrhosis and a normal AFP. The **buzzword is central scar**. The scar is similar to the one seen in FNH with a few differences. This scar does NOT enhance, and is T2 Bright. As a point of trivia, this tumor is Gallium avid. This tumor **calcifies more often than conventional HCC.**

Undifferentiated Embryonal Sarcoma: This is the pissed off cousin of the mesenchymal hamartoma. It's also cystic, but the mass is much more aggressive. It will be a hypodense mass with septations and fibrous pseudocapsule. This mass has been known to rupture.

Any Age:

Mets: Think about Wilms tumor or Neuroblastoma

Now, there are several other entities that can occur in the liver of young children / teenagers including; Hepatic Adenoma, Hemangiomas, Focal Nodular Hyperplasia, and Angio Sarcoma. The bulk of these are discussed in greater detail in the adult GI chapter.

Congenital:

Choledochal cysts are congenital dilations of the bile ducts –classified into 5 types by some dude named Todani. The high yield trivia is type 1 is focal dilation of the CBD and is by far the most common. Type 2 and 3 are super rare. Type 2 is basically a diverticulum of the bile duct. Type 3 is a "choledochocele." Type 4 is both intra and extra hepatic. Type 5 is Caroli's, and is intrahepatic only. I'll hit this again in the GI chapter.

Caroli's is an AR disease associated with polycystic kidney disease and medullary sponge kidney. The hallmark is intrahepatic duct dilation, that is large and secular. Buzzword is **"central dot sign"** which corresponds to the portal vein surrounded by dilated bile ducts.

AR Polycystic Kidney Disease: This will be discussed in greater detail in the renal section, but kids with AR polycystic kidney disease will have cysts in the kidneys, and variable degrees of fibrosis in the liver. The degree of fibrosis is actually the opposite of cystic formation in the kidneys (bad kidneys ok liver, ok kidneys bad liver).

Hereditary Hemorrhagic Telangiectasia (Osler-Weber-Rendu): Autosomal dominant disorder characterized by multiple AVMs in the liver and lungs. It leads to cirrhosis, and a massively dilated hepatic artery. The *lung AVMs set you up for brain abscess.*

Biliary Atresia: If you have prolonged newborn jaundice (> 2 weeks) you should think about two things (1) neonatal hepatitis, and (2) Biliary Atresia. It's critical to get this diagnosis right because they need corrective surgery (Kasai Procedure) prior to 3 months. Patients with biliary atresia really only have **atresia of the ducts outside the liver** (absence of extrahepatic ducts), in fact *they have proliferation of the intrahepatic ducts.* They will develop cirrhosis without treatment and not do well.

Trivia to Know about Biliary Atresia:
- Associations with Polysplenia, and Trisomy 18
- **Gallbladder may be absent** *(normal gallbladder – supports neonatal hepatitis)*
- Triangle Cord Sign – triangular echogenic structure by the portal vein – possibly remnant of the CBD.
- Hepatobiliary Scintigraphy with 99m Tc-IDA is the test of choice to distinguish (discussed in the Nukes Chapter).
- Alagille Syndrome: This is a total zebra. All you need to know is hereditary cholestasis, from paucity of intrahepatic bile ducts, and peripheral pulmonary stenosis. *The purpose of a liver biopsy in biliary atresia is to exclude this diagnosis.*
- Gallstones: If you see a pediatric patient with gallstones you should immediately think sickle cell.

If You Remember 4 Things for Peds GI:

Absent Gallbladder =	Biliary Atresia
SMA / SMV Reversal =	Malrotation
Absent Spleen / Poly Spleen =	Heterotaxias
VACTERL	

Pancreas

CF - The pancreas is nearly always (90%) with CF patients. Inspissated secretions cause proximal duct obstruction leading to the two main changes in CF: (1) Fibrosis (decreased T1 and T2 signal) and the more common one (2) fatty replacement (increased T1).

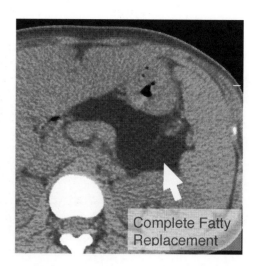

Patient's with CF diagnosed as adults tend to have more pancreas problems than those diagnosed as children. Those with residual pancreatic exocrine function can have bouts of recurrent acute pancreatitis. Small (1-3mm) pancreatic cysts are common.

High Yield Trivia:
- **Complete fatty replacement** is the most common imaging finding in adult CF
- Markedly enlarged with fatty replacement has been termed **lipomatous pseudohypertrophy of the pancreas.** *This is a buzzword.*
- Fibrosing Colonopathy: Wall thickening of the proximal colon as a complication of enzyme replacement therapy.

 Shwachman-Diamond Syndrome - The 2nd most common cause of pancreatic insufficiency in kids (CF #1). Basically, it's a kid with diarrhea, short stature, and eczema. Will also cause lipomatous pseudohypertrophy of the pancreas.

 Dorsal Pancreatic Agenesis - You only have a ventral bud (the dorsal bud forgets to form). Since the dorsal buds makes the tail, the appearance is that of a pancreas without a tail. All you need to know is that (1) this sets you up for diabetes *(most of your beta cells are in the tail)*, and (2) it's associated with polysplenia.

Pancreatitis – The most common cause of pancreatitis in the pediatric setting is trauma (seat belt).

NAT: Another critical point to make is that non-accidental trauma can present as pancreatitis. If the kid isn't old enough to ride a bike (handle bar injury) or didn't have a car wreck (seat belt injury) you need to think NAT is the trick.

Pediatric Pancreatic Mass - Rapid Fire:
— Age 1 = Pancreatoblastoma
— Age 6 = Adenocarcinoma
— Age 15: Solid Pseudopapillary Tumor of the Pancreas

Congenital - Kidneys

Renal Agenesis – This comes in one of two flavors; (1) Both Kidneys Absent - this one is gonna be potter sequence related, (2) One Kidney Absent - this one is gonna have reproductive associations.

Most likely way to test this: Show unilateral agenesis on prenatal US - as an absent renal artery (in view of the aorta) or oligohydramnios - with followup questions on associations. Or make it super obvious with a CT / MRI and ask association questions.

Unilateral Absence Association
- 70% of women with unilateral renal agenesis have associated genital anomalies (usually **unicornuate uterus, or a rudimentary horn**).
- 20% of men are missing the epididymis, and vas deferens on the same side they are missing the kidney. PLUS they have a seminal vesicle cyst on that side.

> **Mayer-Rokitansky-Kuster-Hauser.** – Mullerian duct anomalies including absence or atresia of the uterus / unicornuate uterus. Associated with unilateral renal agenesis.

Potter Sequence: Insult (maybe ACE inhibitors) = kidneys don't form, if kidneys don't form you can't make piss, if you can't make piss you can't develop lungs (pulmonary hypoplasia).

Lying Down Adrenal or "Pancake Adrenal" Sign – describes the elongated appearance of the adrenal not normally molded by the adjacent kidney. It can be used to differentiate surgical absent vs congenital absent.

Horseshoe Kidney – This is the most common fusion anomaly. The kidney gets hung up on the IMA. Questions are most likely to revolve around the complications / risks:

- *Complications from Position* - Easy to get smashed against vertebral body - kid shouldn't play football or wrestle.
- *Complications from Drainage Problems:* Stones, Infection, and Increased risk of Cancer (from chronic inflammation) - big ones are Wilms, TCC, and the Zebra **Renal Carcinoid.**
- *Association Syndrome Trivia* - Turner's Syndrome is the classic testable association.

Crossed Fused Renal Ectopia – One kidney comes across the midline and fuses with the other. Each kidney has it's own orthotropic ureteral office to drain through. It's critically important to the patient to know that ***"the Ectopic Kidney is Inferior."*** The left kidney more commonly crosses over to the right. Complications include stones, infection, and hyponephrosis (50%).

Prune Belly (Eagle Barrett Syndrome) – This malformation complex occurs in males and includes the following triad:

- *Crappy Abdominal Musculature*
- *Hydroureteronephrosis*
- *Cryptorchidism (bladder distention interferes with descent of testes)*

Congenital UPJ Obstruction – This is the most common congenital anomaly of the GU tract in neonates. About 20% of the time, these are bilateral. Most (80%) of these are thought to be caused by intrinsic defects in the circular muscle bundle of the renal pelvis. Treatment is a pyeloplasty. A Radiologist can actually add value by **looking for vessels crossing the UPJ** prior to pyeloplasty, as this changes the management.

Q: 1970 called and they want to know how to tell the difference between a prominent extrarenal pelvis vs a congenital UPJ obstruction.
A: "Whitaker Test", which is a urodynamics study combined with an antegrade pyelogram.

Classic History: Teenager with flank pain after drinking "lots of fluids."

Classic Trivia: These do NOT have dilated ureters (NO HYDROURETER).

Autosomal Recessive Polycystic Kidney Disease (ARPKD) – These guys get HTN, and renal failure. The liver involvement is different than the adult form (ADPKD). Instead of cysts they have abnormal bile ducts and fibrosis. This congenital hepatic fibrosis is ALWAYS present in ARPKD. The **ratio of liver and kidney disease is inverse**. The worse the liver is the better the kidneys do. The better the liver is the worse the kidneys are. Death is often from portal hypertension.

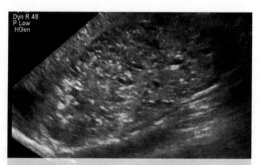

ARPKD: Big Bright, with Lost Corticomedullary Differentiation.

On ultrasound the kidneys are smoothly enlarged and diffusely echogenic, with a loss of corticomedullary differentiation. In utero you sometimes will not see urine in the bladder.

Neonatal Renal Vein Thrombosis – This is an associated condition of **maternal diabetes**. It is typically unilateral (usually left). The theory is that it starts peripherally and progresses toward the hilum. When acute, will cause renal enlargement and chronically, will result in renal atrophy.

Neonatal Renal Artery Thrombosis – This occurs secondary to **umbilical artery catheters**. Unlike renal vein thrombosis it does NOT present with renal enlargement but instead severe hypertension.

Congenital Ureter and Urethra

Congenital (primary) MEGAureter – This is a "wastebasket" term, for an enlarged ureter which is intrinsic to the ureter (NOT the result of a distal obstruction). Causes include (1) Distal adynamic segment (analogous to achalasia, or colonic Hirschsprungs), (2) reflux at the UVJ, (3) it just wants to be big (totally idiopathic). The distal adynamic type "obstructing primary megaureter" can have some hydro, but generally speaking an *absence of dilation of the collecting system* helps distinguish this from an actual obstruction.

Retrocaval Ureter (circumcaval)- This is actually a problem with the development of the IVC, which grows in a manner that pins the ureter. Most of the time it's asymptomatic, but can cause partial obstruction and recurrent UTI. IVP will show a "reverse J" or "fishhook" appearance of the ureter.

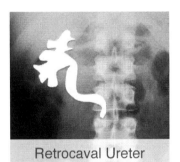

Retrocaval Ureter

Duplicated System – The main thing to know about duplicated systems is the so called "**Weigert-Meyer Rule**" where the upper pole inserts inferior and medially. The upper pole is prone to ureterocele formation and obstruction. The lower pole is prone to reflux. Kidneys with duplicated systems tend to be larger than normal kidneys. In girls a duplicated system can lead to incontinence (ureter may insert below the sphincter - sometimes into the vagina).

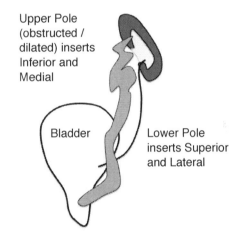

- *Upper Pole Obstructs*
- *Lower Pole Refluxes*

Ureterocele – A cystic dilation of the intravesicular ureter, secondary to obstruction at the ureteral orifice. IVP (or US) will show the *"cobra head" sign*, with contrast surrounded by a lucent rim, protruding from the contrast filled bladder. This is associated with a duplicated system (specifically the upper pole).

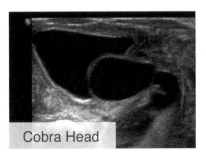

Cobra Head

Ectopic Ureter – The ureter inserts distal to the external spincter in the vestibule. More common in females and associated with incontinence (not associated with incontinence in men). Ureteroceles are best demonstrated during the early filling phase of the VCUG

Posterior Urethral Valves: This is a fold in the posterior urethra, that leads to outflow obstruction, and eventual renal failure (if it's not fixed). It is the most common cause of urethral obstruction in male infants.

Now, this can be shown a variety of ways; it could be shown in the classic VCUG. The key finding on VCUG is an *abrupt caliber change between the dilated posterior urethra and normal caliber anterior urethra.*

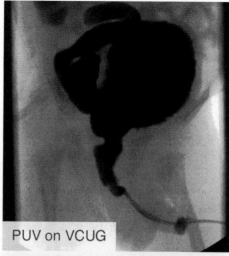

Another, much sneakier way to show this is with a fetal MRI. The MRI would have to show hydro in the kidney and a "key hole" bladder appearance.

"Peri-renal fluid collection" is a buzzword, and it's the result of forniceal rupture. Obviously that is non-specific and can be seen with any obstructive pathology.

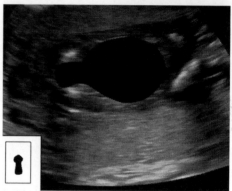

Vesicoureteral Reflux (VUR) – Normally the ureter enters the bladder at an oblique angle so that a "valve" is developed. If the angle of insertion is abnormal (horizontal) reflux can develop. This can occur in the asymptomatic child, but is seen in 50% of children with UTIs. The recommendations for when the boy/girl with a UTI should get a VCUG to evaluate for VUR is in flux (not likely to be tested). Most of the time VUR resolves by age 5-6.

There is a grading system for VUR which goes 1-5.
- *One is reflux half way up the ureter,*
- *Two is reflux into a non-dilated collecting system, (calyces still pointy),*
- *Three you have dilation of the collecting system, and calyces get blunted*
- *Four the system gets mildly tortuous,*
- *Five the system is very tortuous.*

A sneaky trick would be to show the echogenic mound near the UVJ, that results from injection of "deflux", which is a treatment urologist try. Essentially, they make a bubble with this proprietary compound in the soft tissues near the UVJ and it creates a valve (sorta). Anyway, they show it in a lot of case books and text books so just keep your eyes peeled.

Additional Pearl is that chronic reflux can lead to scarring. This **scarring can result in hypertension** and/or chronic renal failure.

Congenital Bladder

The Urachus: The umbilical attachment to the bladder (started out being called the allantois, then called the Urachus). This usually atrophies into the umbilical ligament. Persistent canalization can occur along a spectrum (patent, sinus, diverticulum, cyst).

- *Trivia:* Most common complication of urachal remnant = infection
- *Trivia:* Urachal anomalies are twice as common in boys (relative to girls)
- *Trivia:* **The most important piece of trivia is that when these guys get cancer, it's adenocarcinoma** (90% of cases). To hint at this multiple choice test writers will often use the phrase "midline bladder structure"

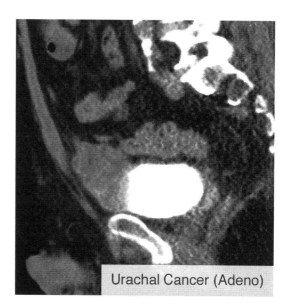
Urachal Cancer (Adeno)

Renal Masses

When it comes to solid renal masses – an age based strategy is the ticket.

Neonate	Around Age 4	Teenager
Nephroblastomatosis	Wilms	RCC
Mesoblastic Nephroma	Wilms Variants	Lymphoma
	Lymphoma	
	Multilocular Cystic Nephroma	

Solids Age 0-3

Nephroblastomatosis – These are persistent nephrogenic rests beyond 36 weeks. It's sorta normal (found in 1% of infants). But, can be a precursor to Wilms so you follow it. When Wilms is bilateral, 99% of the time it had nephroblastomatosis first. It goes away on its own (normally). *It should NOT have necrosis – this makes you think Wilms.* It has a variable appearance, and is often described as "homogeneous." Also more commonly a focal homogeneous ball, the way it's always shown in case conferences and case books is the hypodense rind.

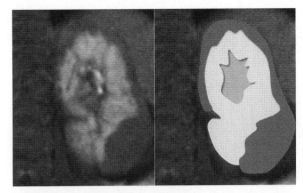

Nephroblastomatosis
-Hypodense Rind -

Ultrasound screening q 3 months till age 7 is the usual routine - to make sure it doesn't go Wilms on you.

Mesoblastic Nephroma - *"Solid renal tumor of infancy."* This is a fetal hamartoma, and generally benign. It is the most common neonatal renal tumor (80% diagnosed in the first month on life). Often involves the renal sinus. Antenatal ultrasound may have shown polyhydramnios.

Pearl: If it really looks like a wilms, but they are just too young (< 1 year) then call it mesoblastic nephroma.

Cystics Age 0-3

Multicystic Dysplastic Kidney You have multiple tiny cysts forming in utereo. What you need to know is (1) that there is "no functioning renal tissue," (2) contralateral renal tract abnormalities occur like 50% of the time (most commonly UPJ obstruction).

MCDK vs Bad Hydro?
- In hydronephrosis the cystic spaces are seen to communicate.
- In difficult cases renal scintigraphy can be useful. MCDK will show no excretory function.

Pearl: MCDK has MACROscopic cysts that do NOT communicate

Solids Around Age 4

Wilms – "Solid renal tumor of childhood." This is the most common solid renal tumor of childhood. This is NOT seen in a newborn. Repeat, you can NOT be born with this tumor. The average age is around 3. It typically spreads via direct invasion.

Associated Syndromes:
- *Overgrowth*
    - *Beckwith-Weidemann* – Macroglossia (most common finding), Omphalocele, Hemihypertrophy, Cardiac, Big Organs.
    - *Sotos* – Macrocephaly, Retarded (CNS stuff), Ugly Face
- *Non-Overgrowth*
    - *WAGR* - Wilms, Aniridia, Genital, Growth Retardation
    - *Drash* – Wilms, Pseudohemaphroditism, Progressive Glomerulonephritis

> *I Say Beckwith-Weidemann*
>
> *You Say,*
> - *Wilms,*
> - *Omphalocele,*
> - *Hepatoblastoma*

Wilms Variants (look just like Wilms)
- **Clear Cell** – likes to go to bones (lytic)
- **Rhabdoid** – "Terrible Prognosis" – Associated with aggressive rhabdoid brain tumors

Wilms Nevers
- **NEVER Biopsy** suspected Wilms (you can seed the tract and up the stage)
- Wilms **NEVER occurs before 2 months of age** (Neuroblastoma can)

> *Wilms in a 1 year old ?*
>
> *Think about associated syndromes. Wilms loves to pal around with Hemihypertrophy, Hyposadias, Cryptorchidism*

Cystics Around Age 4

Multilocular Cystic Nephroma – "Non-communicating, fluid-filled locules, surrounded by thick fibrous capsule." By definition these things are characterized by the absence of a solid component or necrosis. Buzzword is "protrude into the renal pelvis." The question is likely the bimodal occurrence (4 year old boys, and 40 year old women). *I like to think of this as the Michael Jackson lesion – it loves young boys and middle aged women*

Solids in Teenagers

Renal Lymphoma and RCC can occur in teenagers. Renal lymphoma can occur in 5 year old as well. Both of these cancers are discussed in detail in the adult GU chapter (module 4).

Other GU Masses / Cancers

Rhabdomyosarcoma – This is the most common bladder cancer in humans less than 10 years of age. They are often infiltrative, and it's hard to tell where they originate from. **"Paratesticular Mass" is often a buzzword.** They can met to the lungs, bones, and nodes. The Botryoid variant produces a polypoid mass, which looks like a bunch of grapes. *I'll discuss this again in the testicle section on page 206.*

Neuroblastoma - Isn't a Renal Mass, but is frequently contrasted with Wilms so I want to discuss it in the renal section. It is the most common extracranial solid childhood malignancy. They typically occur in very young kids (you can be born with this). 95% of cases occur before age 10. They occur in the abdomen more than the thoracic (adrenal 35%, retroperitoneum 30%, posterior mediastinum 20%, neck 5%).

Staging: Things that up the stage include crossing the midline, and contralateral positive nodes. These things make it Stage 3

Better Prognosis Seen with – Diagnosis in Age < 1, Thoracic Primary, Stage 4S.

Associations:
- NF-1, Hirschsprungs, DiGeorge, Beckwith Wiedemann
- Most are sporadic

> **STAGE 4 S - HIGH YIELD**
>
> - Less than 1 year old
> - Distal Mets are Confined to Skin, Liver, and Bone Marrow
> - Excellent Prognosis.
>
> **A common distractor is to say 4S goes to cortical bone. This is false! It's the marrow.

Random Trivia:
- Opsomyoclonus (dancing eyes, dancing feet) – paraneoplastic syndrome associated with neuroblastoma.
- "Raccoon Eyes" is a common way for orbital neuroblastoma mets to present
- MIBG is superior to Conventional Bone Scan for Neuroblastoma Bone Mets
- Neuroblastoma bone mets are on the "lucent metaphyseal band DDx"
- Sclerotic Bone mets are UNCOMMON
- Urine Catecholamines are always (95%) elevated

Neuroblastoma	Wilms
Age: usually less than 2 (can occur in utero)	Age: Usually around age 4 **(never before 2 months)**
Calcifies 90%	Calcifies Rarely (<10%)
Encases Vessels (doesn't invade)	Invades Vessels (doesn't encase)
Poorly Marginated	Well Circumscribed
Mets to Bones	Doesn't usually met to bones (unless clear cell wilms variant).

Adrenal

Neuroblastoma – *Discussed above in the renal section*

Neonatal Adrenal Hemorrhage – This can occur in the setting of birth trauma or stress.

Hemorrhage vs Neuroblastoma:
- Ultrasound can usually tell the difference (**adrenal hemorrhage is anechoic and avascular,** neuroblastoma is echogenic and hypervascular).
- MRI could also be done to problem solve if necessary (**Adrenal Hemorrhage low T2, Neuroblastoma high T2).**
- The real answer is "what does it do a week later?" Serial ultrasound will show it decrease in size.

GYN / Pelvic

Hydrometrocolpos – Essentially the vagina won't drain the uterus. This condition is characterized on imaging by an expanded fluid filled vaginal cavity with associated distention of the uterus. You can see it presenting in infancy as a mass, or as a teenager with delayed menarche. Causes include imperforate hymen (most common), vaginal stenosis, lower vaginal atresia, and cervical stenosis.

For multiple choice trivia think about this as a "midline pelvic mass", which can cause hydronephrosis (mass effect from distended uterus).

Trivia: Associated with Uterus Didelphys (which often ~75% has a transverse vaginal septum)

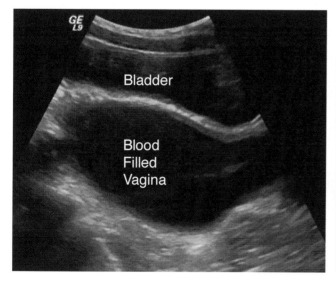
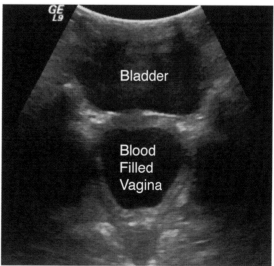

Sacrococcygeal Teratoma – This is the most common tumor of the fetus or infant. These solid and/or cystic masses are typically large and found either on prenatal imaging or birth. Their largeness is a problem and can cause mass effect on the GI system, hip dislocation, and even nerve compression leading to incontinence. They are usually benign (80%), although those presenting in older infants tend to have a higher malignant potential. The location of the mass is either external to the pelvis (47%), internal to the pelvis (9%), or dumbelled both inside and outside (34%).

There is another classification that discusses involvement of the abdomen.

The easiest way to remember it is like this:
-Type 1 - Totally extra pelvic
-Type 2 - Barely pelvic, but not abdominal
-Type 3 - Some abdominal
-Type 4 - Totally inside abdomen ** *this one has the highest rate of malignancy.*

Trivia: They have to cut the coccyx off during resection. Incomplete resection of the coccyx is associated with a high recurrence rate.

—

Ovary – A complete discussion of ovarian masses is found in the GYN chapter. I'll briefly cover some PEDs specific ovarian issues.

Torsion: In an adult, ovarian torsion is almost always due to a mass. In a child, torsion can occur with a normal ovary, secondary to excessive mobility of the ovary. As described in the GYN chapter you are going to see an enlarged (swollen) ovary, with peripheral follicles, with or without arterial flow.

Masses: About two thirds of ovarian neoplasms are benign dermoids/teratomas (discussed in detail in the GYN chapter). The other one third cancer. The cancers are usually germ cells (75%). Again, mural nodules and thick septations should clue you in that these might be cancer. Peritoneal implants, ascites, lymphadenopathy, are all bad signs and would over-ride characteristics of the mass.

Scrotum

Random Scrotum Trivia

Hydrocele: Collection of serous fluid and is the most common cause of painless scrotal swelling. Congenital hydroceles result from a patent processus vaginalis that permits entry of peritoneal fluid into the scrotal sac.

Complicated Hydrocele (one with septations): This is either a hematocele vs pyocele. The distinction is clinical.

Varicocele: Most of these are idiopathic and found in adolescents and young adults. They are more frequent on the left. They are uncommon on the right, and if isolated (not bilateral) should stir suspicion for abdominal pathology (nutcracker syndrome, RCC, retroperitoneal fibrosis).

"Next Step" - Isolated right sided varicocele = Abdomen CT.

HSP: This vasculitis is the most common cause of idiopathic scrotal edema (more on this in the vascular chapter).

Acute Pain in or around the Scrotum

The top three considerations in a child with acute scrotal pain are (1) torsion of the testicular appendage, (2) testicular torsion, and (3) epididymo-orchitis.

Epididymitis – The epidymal head is the most common part involved. Increased size and hyperemia are your ultrasound findings. This <u>occurs in two peaks</u>: under 2 and over 6. You can have infection of the epididymis alone or infection of the epididymis and testicle (isolated orchitis is rare).

Orchitis – Nearly always occurs as a progressed epididymitis. When *isolated the answer is mumps*.

Torsion of the Testicular Appendages – This is the <u>most common cause of acute scrotal pain in age 7-14.</u> The testicular appendage is some vestigial remnant of a mesonephric duct. Typical history is a sudden onset of pain, with a **Blue Dot Sign** on physical exam (looks like a blue dot). Enlargement of the testicular appendage to greater than 5 mm is considered by some as the best indicator of torsion

Torsion of the Testicle – Results from the testis and spermatic cord twisting within the serosal space leading to ischemia. The testable trivia is that it is caused by a *failure of the tunica vaginalis and testis to connect* or a **"Bell Clapper Deformity"**. This deformity is usually bilateral, so if you twist one they will often orchiopexy the other one. If it was 1950 you'd call in your nuclear medicine tech for scintigraphy. Now you just get a Doppler ultrasound. Findings will be absent or asymmetrically decreased flow, asymmetric enlargement, and slightly decreased echogenicity of the involved ball.

Extra-Testicular Mass:

Paratesticular Rhabdomyosarcoma: By far the most common extra-testicular mass in young men and the only one really worth mentioning. If you see a mass in the scrotum that is not for sure in the testicle this is it (unless the history is kick to the balls from a spiteful young lady - and you are dealing with a big fucking hematoma). If it's truly a mass - this is the answer.

Trivia:
- The most common location is actually the head/neck - specifically the orbit and nasopharynx.
- There is a bimodal peak (2-4, then 15-17).

Testicular Masses

Testicular Masses can be thought of as intratesticular or extratesticular. With regard to intratesticular masses, ultrasound can show you that there is indeed a mass but there are no imaging features that really help you tell which one is which. **If the mass is extratesticular, the most likely diagnosis is an embryonal rhabdomyosarcoma** from the spermatic cord or epididymis

Testicular Mircolithiasis – This appears as multiple small echogenic foci within the testes. Testicular microlithiasis is usually an incidental finding in scrotal US examinations performed for unrelated reasons. It might have a relationship with Germ Cell Tumors (controversial). Follow-up in 6 months, then yearly is probably the recommendation (maybe - it's very controversial, and therefore unlikely to be asked).

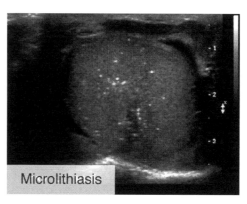
Microlithiasis

Testicular Cancer: The histologic breakdown is as follows:

- Germ Cell (90%)
    - Seminoma (40%) – seen more in the 4th decade
    - Non Seminoma (60%)
        - Teratoma, Yolk Sacs, Mixed Germ Cells, Etc…
- Non Germ Cell (10%)
    - Sertoli
    - Leydig

Testicular Calcifications

Tiny (micro) = Seminoma

BIG = Germ Cell Tumor

The two Germ Cell Tumors seen in the first decade of life are the yolk sac tumor, and the teratoma.

Yolk Sac Tumor: Heterogeneous Testicular Mass in < 2 year old = Yolk Sac Tumor. **AFP** is usually super elevated.

Teratoma – Pure testicular teratomas are only seen in young kids < 2. Mixed teratomas are seen in 25 year olds. Unlike ovarian teratoma, these guys often have aggressive biological behavior.

Choriocarcinoma: This is a aggressive highly vascular tumor, seen more in the 2nd decade.

Sertoli Cell Tumors – These testicular tumors are usually bilateral and are visualized on US as "burned-out" tumors (dense echogenic foci that represent calcified scars). A subtype of Sertoli cell tumor associated with Peutz-Jeghers syndrome typically occurs in children. If they show you the Peurtz-Jegher lips and bilateral scrotal masses, this is the answer.

Testicular Lymphoma – Just be aware that lymphoma can "hide" in the testes because of the blood testes barrier. Immunosuppressed patients are at increased risk for developing extranodal/ testicular lymphoma. On US, the normal homogeneous echogenic testicular tissue is replaced focally or diffusely with hypoechoic vascular lymphomatous tissue **Buzzword = multiple hypoechoic masses of the testicle.**

Peds MSK

Fracture: In general, little kids bend they don't break. You end up with lots of buckles and greensticks. For problem solving you can get a repeat in 7-10 days as periosteal reaction is expected in 7-10 days. Kids tend to heal completely, often with no sign of prior fracture.

Involvement of the Physis: The major concern is growth arrest, probably best asked by showing a **physeal bar** ("early" bony bridge crossing the growth plate). You can get bars from prior infection, but a history of trauma is gonna be the more classic way to ask it.

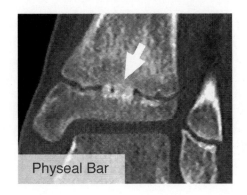

Salter-Harris Classification lends itself well to multiple choice:

Type 1 : S – Slipped

Complete physeal fracture, with or without displacement.

Type 2: A – Above (or "Away from the Joint")

Fracture involves the metaphysis. This is the most common type (75%).

Type 3: L – Lower (3 is the backwards "E" for Epiphysis)

Fracture involves the epiphysis. These guys have a chance of growth arrest, and will often require surgery to maintain alignment

Type 4: T – Through

Fracture involves the metaphysis and epiphysis. These guys don't do as well, often end up with growth arrest, or focal fusion. They require anatomic reduction and often surgery.

Type 5: R – Ruined

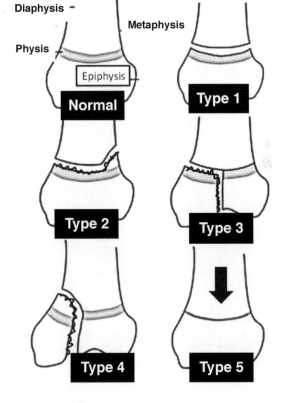

Compression of the growth plate. It occurs from axial loading injuries, and has a very poor prognosis. These are easy to miss, and often found when looking back at comparisons (hopefully ones your partner read). The buzzword is **"bony bridge across physis"**.

Toddler's Fracture: Oblique fracture of the midshaft of the tibia seen in a child just starting to walk (new stress on bone). If it's a spiral type you probably should query non-accidental trauma. The typical age is 9 months – 3 years.

Stress Fracture in Children: This is an injury which occurs after repetitive trauma, usually after new activity (walking). The most common site of fracture is the tibia – proximal posterior cortex. The tibial fracture is the so called "toddler fracture" described above. Other classic stress fractures include the **calcaneal fracture – seen after the child has had a cast removed and returns to normal activity.**

The Elbow:
My God... these peds elbows.

Every first year resident knows that elevation of the fat pad (sail sign) should make you think joint effusion and possible occult fracture. Don't forget that sometimes you can see a thin anterior pad, but you should never see the posterior pad (posterior is positive). I like to bias myself with statistics, when I'm hunting for the peds elbow fracture. The most common fracture is going to be a supracondylar fracture (>60%), followed by lateral condyle (20%), and medial epicondyle (10%).

Radiocapitellar Line: This is a line through the center of the radius, which should intersect the middle of the capitellum on every view (regardless of position). If the radius is dislocated it will NOT pass through the center of the capitellum

Anterior Humeral Line: This time you need a true lateral. A line along the anterior surface of humerus, which should pass through the middle third of the capitellum. With a supracondylar fracture (the most common peds elbow fracture) you'll see this line pass through the anterior third.

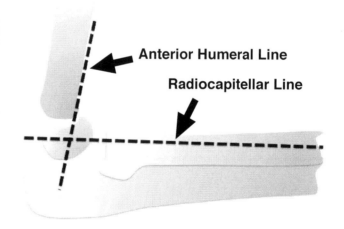

Ossification Centers can be a source of trickery.

Remember they occur in a set order (CRITOE),
- *Capitellum (Age 1),*
- *Radius (Age 3),*
- *Internal (medial epicondyle – Age 5),*
- *Trochlea (Age 7),*
- *Olecranon (Age 9), and*
- *External (lateral epicondyle – Age 11).*

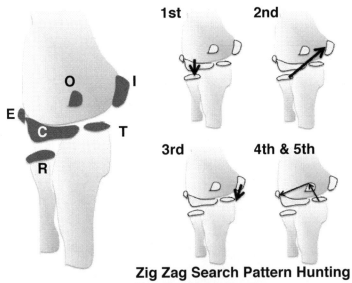

Zig Zag Search Pattern Hunting For the Next Center

Elbow Tricks:

Lateral Condyle Fx: This is the **second most common distal humerus fracture** in kids. Some dude named Milch classified them. The thing to know is a fracture that passes through the capitello-trochlear groove is unstable (Milch II). Since it's really hard to tell this, **treatment is based on the displacement of the fracture fragment (> or < 2mm).**

Trochlea – it can have multiple ossification centers, so it **can have a fragmented appearance.**

Medial Epicondyle Avulsion (Little League Elbow) – There are two major tricks with this one. (1) Because it's an extra articular structure, its avulsions **will not necessarily result in a joint effusion.** (2) It **can get interposed** between the articular surface of the humerus and olecranon. Avulsed fragments can get stuck in the joint, even when there is no dislocation.

   Anytime you see a dislocation – ask yourself
- *Is the patient 5 years old? And if so*
- *Where is the medial epicondyle.*

   The importance of IT (crIToe) –
- *You should never see the trochlea, and not see the internal (medial epicondyle), if you do it's probably a displaced fragment*

Common vs Uncommon: *Don't get it twisted.*

Common Elbow Fractures	Uncommon Elbow Fractures
Lateral Condylar Fx	Lateral Epicondyle Fx
Medial Epicondyle Fx	Medial Condyle

Nursemaids Elbow: When a child's arm is pulled on, the radial head may sublux into the annular ligament. X-rays typically don't help, unless you supinate the arm during lateral position (which often relocates the arm).

Avulsion Injuries:

Kids tendons tend to be stronger than their bones, so avulsion injuries are more common (when compared to adults). The pelvis is the classic location to test this.

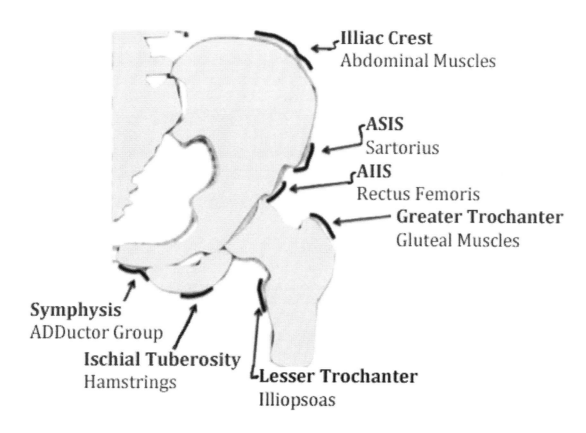

Chronic Fatigue Injuries:

Sinding-Larsen-Johansson – This is a chronic traction injury at the **insertion of the patellar tendon on the patella**. It's seen in active adolescents between age 10-14. **Kids with cerebral palsy** are prone to it.

Osgood-Schlatter – This is due to repeated micro trauma to the patellar tendon on its insertion at the tibial tuberosity. It's bilateral 25% of the time, and more common in boys.

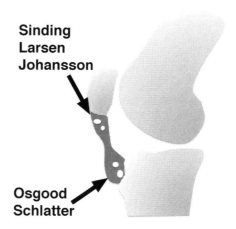

Distal Femoral Metaphyseal Irregularity (Cortical Desmoid): This is a lucency seen along the back of the posteriomedial aspect of the distal femoral metaphysis. If they show you a lateral knee x-ray, and there is an irregularity or lucency on the back of the femur this is it. It's often bilateral. Buzzwords include <u>"Scoop like defect"</u> with an "irregular but intact cortex."

This is a total incidental finding and is a don't touch lesion. **Don't biopsy it, Don't MRI it.**

Just leave it alone. If you really want to know, it's probably a chronic tug lesion from the adductor magnus.

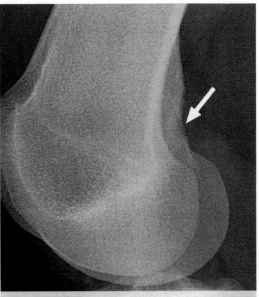

Cortical Desmoid - Scoop Like Defect

Blounts *(tibia vara).* Varus angulation occurring at the medial aspect of the proximal tibia *(varus bowing occurs at the metaphysis not the knee).* This is often bilateral, and NOT often seen before age 2 *(two sides, not before two).* Later in the disease progression the medial metaphysis will be depressed and an osseous outgrowth classically develops. You can see it in two different age groups; (a) early – which is around age 2 and (b) late – which is around age 12.

- Two Sides - Not Before Two
- Two Different Ages (2-3, 12)

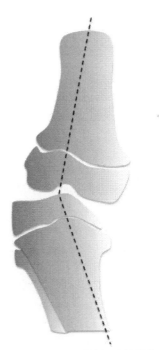

Blount's -Tibia VARA

Periosteal Reaction in the Newborn:

Congenital Rubella: Bony changes are seen in 50% of cases, with the classic buzzword being **"celery stalk"** appearance, from generalized lucency of the metaphysis. This is usually seen in the first few weeks of life.

Syphilis: Bony changes are seen in 95% of cases. Bony changes do NOT occur until 6-8 weeks of life (Rubella changes are earlier). Metaphyseal lucent bands and periosteal reaction along long bones can be seen. The classic buzzword is **"Wimberger Sign"** or **destruction of the medial portion of the proximal metaphysis of the tibia.**

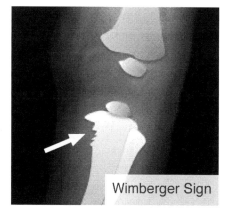

Caffey Disease – Have you ever seen that giant multiple volume set of peds radiology books? Yeah, same guy. This thing is a self limiting disorder of soft tissue swelling, periosteal reaction, and irritability **seen within the first 6 months of life**. The **classic picture is the really hot mandible on bone scan**. The mandible is the most common location (clavicle, and ulna are the other classic sites). It's rare as hell, and probably not even real. There have been more sightings of Chupacabra in the last 50 years.

Prostaglandin Therapy – Prostaglandin E1 and E2 (often used to keep a PDA open) can cause a periosteal reaction. The classic trick is to show a chest x-ray with sternotomy wires (or other hints of congenital heart), and then periosteal reaction in the arm bones.

Neuroblastoma Mets – This is really the only childhood malignancy that occurs in newborns and mets to bones.

Physiologic Growth: So this is often called "Physiologic Periostitis of the Newborn", which is totally false and wrong. It **does NOT happen in newborns**. *You see this around 3 months* of age, and it should resolve by six months. **Proximal involvement (femur) comes before distal involvement (tibia).** It **always involves the diaphysis**.

*It is **NOT** physiologic periostitis if:*
- *You see it before 1 month*
- *You see it in the tibia before the femur*
- *It does not involve the diaphysis.*

Abuse – Some people abuse drugs, some just can't stand screaming kids, some suffer both shortcomings. More on this later.

Other "Aggressive Processes" in Kids

Langerhans Cell Histiocytosis (LCH) – Also known as EG (eosinophilic granuloma). It's twice as common in boys. Skeletal manifestations are highly variable, but lets just talk about the classic ones:

- *Skull* – **Most common site.** Has "**beveled edge**" from uneven destruction of the inner and outer tables. If you see a round lucent lesion in the skull of a child think this (and neuroblastoma mets).

- *Ribs* – Multiple lucent lesions, with an expanded appearance

- *Spine* – **Vertebra plana**

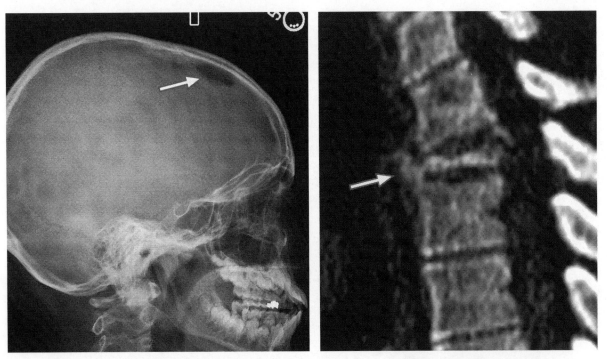

LGH - *Beveled Edge Skull Lesion*   **LGH** - *Vertebra Plana*

Ewing Sarcoma, and ***Osteosarcoma*** are covered in depth in the MSK chapter

Osteomyelitis – It usually occurs in babies (30% of cases less than 2 years old). It's usually hematogenous (adults it directly spreads - typically from a diabetic ulcer).

There are some changes that occur over time, which are potentially testable.

Newborns - They have open growth plates and perforating vessels which travel from the metaphysis to the epiphysis. Infection typically starts in the metaphysis (it has the most blood supply because it is growing the fastest), and then can spread via these perforators to the epiphysis.

Kids - Later in childhood, the perforators regress and the avascular epiphyseal plate stops infection from crossing over. This creates a "septic tank" scenario, where infection tends to smolder. In fact, 75% of cases involve the metaphyses of long bones (femur most common).

Adults - When the growth plates fuse, the barrier of an avascular plate is no longer present, and infection can again cross over to the epiphysis to cause mayhem.

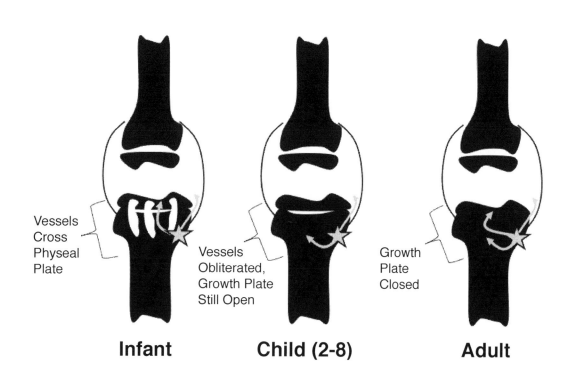

Trivia to know:
- Hematogenous spread more common in kids (direct spread in adult)
- Metaphysis most common location, with target changes as explained above
- Bony changes don't occur on x-ray for around 10 days.
- It's serious business and can rapidly destroy the cartilage if it spreads into the joint

Skeletal Dysplasia

There is a bunch of vocabulary to learn regarding dysplasias:

English	Fancy Doctor Speak
Short Fingers	Brachydactyly
Too Many Fingers	Polydactyly
Two or More Fused Fingers ("Sock Hand" – I call it)	Syndactyly
Contractures of Fingers	Camptodactyly
Inclinded Fingers (Usually 5th)	Clinodactyly
Long, Spider-Like Fingers	Arachnodactyly
Limb is Absent	Amelia
Limb is mostly Absent	Meromelia
Hands / Feet (distal limbs) are Short	Acromelic
Forearm or Lower Leg are short (middle limbs)	Mesomelic
Femur or Humerus (proximal limbs) are short	Rhizomelic
Short All Over	Micromelic

How I remember the lengths: Meso is in the middle, Acro sounds like acromegaly (they get big hands), and the other one is the other one (Rhizo).

There are tons of skeletal dsyplasias and extensive knowledge of them is way way way way beyond the scope of the exam. Instead I'm going to mention 3 dwarfs, and a few other miscellaneous conditions.

Dwarfs:

Achondroplasia – This is the most common skeletal dysplasia, and are the mostly likely to be seen at the mall (or on television). It results from a fibroblast growth factor receptor problem (most dwarfisms do). It is a **rhizomelic** (short femur, short humerus) dwarf. They often have weird big heads, trident hands (3rd and 4th fingers are long), narrowing of the interpedicular distance, and the tombstone pelvis. Advanced paternal age is a risk factor. They make good actors, excellent rodeo clowns, and various parts of their bodies (if cooked properly) have magical powers.

Thanatophoric – This is the **most common lethal dwarfism**. The have **rhizomelic shortening** (humerus, femur). The femurs are sometimes called **telephone receivers**. They have short ribs and a long thorax, and small iliac bones. The **vertebral bones are flat** (platyspondyly), and the **skull can be cloverleaf shaped**.

Asphyxiating Thoracic Dystrophy (Jeune) – This is usually fatal as well. The big finding is the "Bell shaped thorax" with **short ribs**. 15% will have too many fingers (polydactyly). If they live, they have kidney problems (chronic nephritis). You can differentiate a dead Thanatophoric dwarf, from a dead Jeune dwarf by looking at their vertebral bodies. The Jeune bodies are normal (the thanatophorics are flat).

Additional Dwarf pearls;
- *Ellis-Van Crevald is the dwarf with multiple fingers.*
- *Pseudoachondroplasia is this weird thing not present at birth, and spares the skull.*
- *Pyknodysostosis is osteopetrosis, in a dwarf, with a wide angled jaw, and osteoarcolysis.*

The Dwarf Blitz - 5 Things I Would Remember About Dwarfs

1. **The Vocab**: Rhizo (humerus, femur) vs Acro (hands, feet) vs Meso (forearm, tib/fib)
2. **Most dwarfs are Rhizomelic** - if forced to choose, always guess this
3. The pedicles are supposed to widen slightly as you descend the spinal column, **Achondroplasia** has the opposite - they narrow. If you see a live dwarf, with short femurs / humerus, and **narrowing of the pedicles** then this is the answer. *(technically thantophorics can get this too - but it's more classic for achondroplasia)*
4. Thanatophoric is your main dead dwarf. Usually the standout feature is the **telephone receiver femur** (and a crazy cloverleaf head)
5. **Jeune** is another dead dwarf - but the **short ribs** really stand out.

Misc Conditions:

Osteogenesis Imperfecta – They have a collagen defect and make brittle bones. Depending on the severity it can be totally lethal or more mild. It's classically shown with a **totally lucent skull**, or **multiple fractures with hyperplastic callus**. Another classic trick is to show the legs with the **fibula longer than the tibia**. They have **wormian bones**, and often flat or beaked vertebral bodies. Other trivia is the blue sclera, hearing impairment (**otosclerosis**), and that they tend to suck at football.

Osteopetrosis – They have a defect in the way osteoclasts work, so you end up with disorganized bone that is sclerotic and weak (prone to fracture). There are a bunch of different types, with variable severity. The infantile type is lethal because it takes out your bone marrow. With less severe forms, you can have abnormal diminished osteoclastic activity that varies during skeletal growth, and results in alternating bands of sclerosis parallel to the growth plate. Most likely the way this will be shown is the "bone-in-bone" appearance in the vertebral body or carpals. Picture frame vertebrae is another buzzword. Alternatively, they can show you a diffusely sclerotic skeleton, with diffuse loss of the corticomedullary junction in the long tubular bones.

Pycnodysostosis - Osteopetrosis + Wormian Bones + Acro-Osteolysis. They also have "wide (or obtuse) angled mandible", which apparently is a buzzword.

Klippel Feil – You get **congenital fusion of the cervical spine** (sorta like JRA). The cervical vertebral bodies will be tall and skinny. There is often a sprengel deformity (high riding scapula). Another common piece of trivia is to show the omovertebral bone – which is just some big stupid looking vertebral body.

Hunters / Hurlers / Morquio: All three of these are mucopolysaccharidoses. Findings include **oval shaped vertebral bodies with anterior beak**. The beak is actually mid in Morquio, and inferior in Hurlers. **Clavicles and ribs are often thick (narrow more medially) – like a canoe-paddle**. The pelvis shape is described as the opposite of achondroplasia – the iliac wings are tall and flaired. The hand x-ray is the most commonly shown in case books and gives you **wide metacarpal bones with proximal tapering**.

Few More Trivia points on Morquio:
- *They are dwarfs*
- *The most common cause of death is cervical myelopathy at C2*
- *The bony changes actually progress during the first few years of life*

Gauchers – This is the most common lysosomal storage disease. It gives you a big spleen, and big liver among a few bone signs.

- *AVN of the Femoral Heads*
- *H Shaped Vertebra*
- *Bone Infarcts (lots of them)*
- *Erlenmeyer Flask Shaped Femurs*

Caudal Regression Syndrome – This is a spectrum that includes sacral and or coccyx agenesis. You see it with VACTERL and Currarino Triads Syndromes.

Scoliosis – Lateral curvature of the spine, which is usually idiopathic in girls. It can also be from vertebral segmentation problems. NF can cause it as well (that's a piece of trivia).

Radial Dysplasia- Absence or hypoplasia of the radius (usually with a missing thumb) is a differential case (VACTER, Holt-Oram, Fanconi Anemia, Throbocytopenia Absent Radius). As a point of trivia TAR kids will have a thumb.

Neurofibromatosis – Just briefly remember that type 1 can cause **anterior tibial bowing**, and **pseudo-athrosis at the distal fibula**. This is an Aunt Minnie. You can also get scoliosis.

Hand Foot Syndrome - The classic history is hand or foot pain / swelling in an infant with sickle cell. This is a dactylitis, and felt to be related to ischemia. It will resolve on its own, after a few weeks. <u>Radiographs can show a periostitis two weeks after the pain goes away.</u>

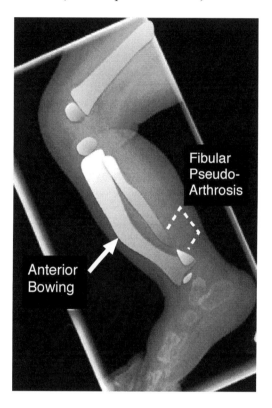

219

Feet

Congenital foot is a complicated and confusing topic, about which I will avoid great detail because it is well beyond the scope of the exam. I am going to at least try and drop some knowledge on how I learned to work these problems out.

Step 1: Vocabulary. Just knowing the lingo is very helpful for getting the diagnosis on multiple choice foot questions.

- *Talipes = Congenital ,*
- *Pes = Foot or Acquired*
- *Equines = "Plantar Flexed Ankle", Heel Cord is often tight, and the heel won't touch the floor*
- *Calcaneus = Opposite of Equinus. The Calcaneus is actually angled up*
- *Varus = Forefoot in*
- *Valgus = Forefoot out*
- *Cavus = High Arch*
- *Planus = Counter part of Cavus – flat foot*
- *Supination – Inward rotation – "Sole of foot in"*
- *Pronation – Outward rotation – "Sole of foot out"*

Step 2: Hindfoot Valgus vs Varus

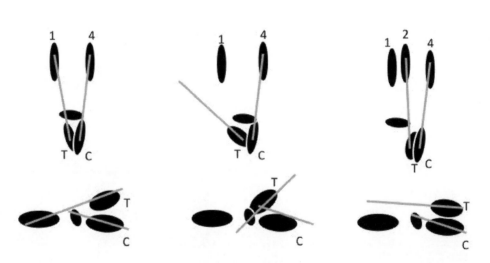

Normal

First look at the normal acute angle the talus and calcaneus make on a lateral view.

Hindfoot Valgus

Think about this as the talus sliding nose down off the calcaneus. This make the angle wider.

If the talus slides off you lose your longitudinal arch - which essentially characterizes hindfoot valgus.

Also, note that the nose down (nearly **vertical**) appearance of the talus .

Hindfoot Varus

This is the opposite situation, in which you have a narrowing of the angle between the talus and calcaneus.

Notice the two bones lay nearly parallel - like two **"clubs"** laying on top of each other.

Step 3 - Knowing the two main disorders. The flat foot (valgus), and the club foot (varus).

Flat Foot (Pes Planus)- This can be congenital or acquired. The peds section will cover congenital and the adult MSK section will cover acquired. The congenital types can be grouped into flexible or rigid (the flexible types are more common in kids). The distinction can be made with plantar flexion views (flexible improves with stress). The ridged subtypes can be further subdivided into tarsal coalition and vertical talus. In any case you have a **hindfoot <u>valgus.</u>**

> ***Tarsal Coalition*** – There are two main types (talus to the calcaneus, and talus to the navicular). They are pretty equal in incidence, and about 50% of the time are bilateral. You can have bony or fibrous/cartilaginous subtypes. The fibrous/cartilaginous types are more common than the bony types.
>
>> **Talocalcaneal**– Occurs at the middle facet. Has the "continuous C-sign" produced from an "absent middle facet" on the lateral view. Talar beaking (spur on the anterior talus) is also seen in about 25% of cases.
>>
>> **Calcaneonavicular**– Occurs at the anterior facet. Has the "anteater sign"
>
> ***Vertical Talus*** (equinus hindfoot valgus) – This is sometimes called the "rocker-bottom foot" because the talus is in extreme plantar flexion with dorsal dislocation of the Navicular – resulting in a locked talus in plantar flexion. As a point of trivia this is often associated with myelomeningocele.

Club Foot (Talipes Equino <u>Varus</u>)- Translation – Congenital Plantar Flexed Ankle Forefoot. This is sorta why I lead with the vocab, all the congenital feet can be figured out based on the translated language. This thing is more common in boys, and bilateral about half the time. The toes are pointed down (equines), and the talocalcaneal angle is acute (varus).

Key features:
- Hindfoot varus (decreased talocalcaneal angle)
- Medial deviation and inversion of the forefoot
- Elevated Plantar Arch

Trivia: The most common surgical complication is over correction resulting in a "rocker bottom" flat foot deformity.

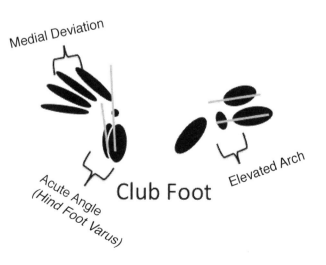

Hip Dysplasia

Developmental Dysplasia of the Hip - This is seen more commonly in females, children born breech, and oligohydramnios. The physical exam buzzwords are asymmetric skin or gluteal folds, leg length discrepancy, palpable clunk, or delayed ambulation. It's bilateral about 1/3 of the time. Ultrasound is done to evaluate (after physical exam), and is excellent until the bones ossify (then you need x-rays). A common trick is to be careful making a measurement in the first week of life - the laxity immediately after birth (related to maternal estrogen,) can screw up the measurements.

Angles:

On ultrasound the **alpha angle, should be more than 60 degrees**. Anything less than that and your cup is not deep enough to hold your ball. The plain film equivalent in the **acetabular angle, which is the complimentary angle (and therefore should be less than 30).**

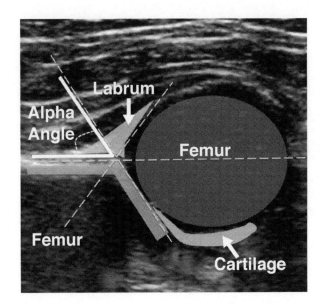

Getting them confused? Remember that the *"Alpha Angle is the Alpha Male"* - and therefore the bigger of the two angles. **But don't forget the DDH is more common in women (not alpha males).

The acetabular angle should decrease from 30 degrees at birth to 22 degrees at age 1. DDH is the classic cause of an increased angle, but neuromuscular disorder can also increase it.

The position of the femoral epiphysis (or where it will be) should be below Hilgenreiner's line "**H**", and medial to Perkin's Line "**P**". Shenton's Line "**S**" should be continuous.

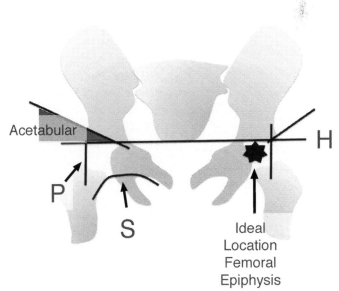

222

Proximal Focal Femoral Deficiency – This is a congenital zebra, which ranges from absent proximal femur to hypoplastic proximal femur. You get a varus deformity. This is a mimic of DDH, but DDH will have normal femur leg length.

Septic Arthritis- This is serious business, and considered the most urgent cause of painful hip in a child. Wide joint space (lateral displacement of femoral head), should prompt an ultrasound, and that should prompt a joint tap. If you have low suspicion and don't want to tap the hip, You could pull on the leg under fluoro and try and get gas in the joint. This air arthrogram sign supposedly excludes a joint effusion (and therefore a septic joint) – depending on who you ask.

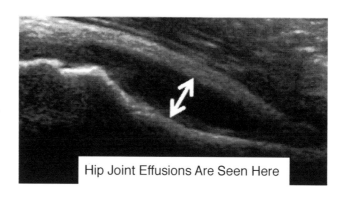

Hip Joint Effusions Are Seen Here

Slipped Capital Femoral Epiphysis (SCFE) – This is **a type 1 salter harris**, through the proximal femoral physis. What makes this unique is that unlike most SH 1s, this guy has a bad prognosis if not fixed. The classic history is **fat African American adolescent (age 12-15)** with hip pain. It's bilateral in 1/3 of cases (both hips don't usually present at same time). The **frog leg view is the money – this is always the answer on next step questions**.

Legg-Calve-Perthes – This is AVN of the proximal femoral epiphysis. It's seen more in boys than girls (4:1), and favors **white people around age 5-8**. This is **bilateral about 10% of the time (less than SCFE)**. The subchondral lucency (crescent sign) is best seen on a frog leg. Other early signs include an asymmetric small ossified femoral epiphysis. MRI has more sensitivity. The flat collapsed femoral head makes it obvious.

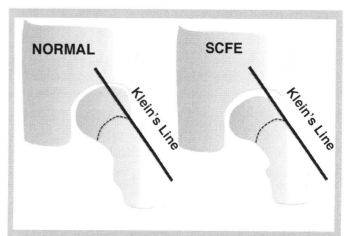

"Klein's Line" - Drawn along the edge of the femur and should normally intersect with lateral superior femoral epiphysis. This line is used to evaluate for SCFE. When the line doesn't cross the lateral epiphysis think SCFE.

***Testable Trivia -** <u>Frog Leg View</u> is more sensitive for this measurement

Perthes	SCFE
White Kids	Overweight Black Kids
Age 5-8	Age 12-15
Bilateral 10%	Bilateral 30%

223

Metabolic

Rickets – Not enough vitamin D. Affects the most rapidly growing bones (mostly knees and wrists). Buzzwords **"fraying, cupping, and irregularity along the physeal margin."** They are at increased risk for SCFE. "Rachitic rosary" appearance from expansion of the anterior rib ends at the costochondral junctions. As a pearl, **rickets is never seen in a newborn** (Mom's vitamin D is still doing its thing).

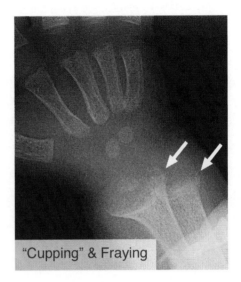
"Cupping" & Fraying

Hypophosphatasia - This looks like **Rickets in a newborn**. They will have frayed metaphyses and bowed long bones. The underlying pathology is a deficient serum alkaline phosphatase. There is variability in severity with lethal perinatal / natal forms, and more mild adult forms.

Scurvy – Not enough vitamin C. This is rare as hell outside of a pirate ship in the 1400s. For the purpose of trivia (which multiple choice tests love) the following stuff is high yield:

- Does NOT occur before 6 months of age (maternal stores buffer)
    - Bleeding Disorders Common
    - Subperiosteal hemorrhage (lifts up the periosteum)
- Hemarthrosis
- "Scorbutic rosary" appearance from expansion of the costochondral junctions (very similar to rickets).

Lead Poisoning – This is most commonly seen in kids less than two who eat paint chips. The classic finding is a **wide sclerotic metaphyseal line (lead line),** in an area of rapid growth (knee). It will not spare the fibula (as a normal variant line might).

Lucent Metaphyseal Bands – This is a classic peds DDx.

- *Leukemia*
- *Infection (TORCH)*
- *Neuroblastoma Mets*
- *Endocrine (rickets, Scurvy)*

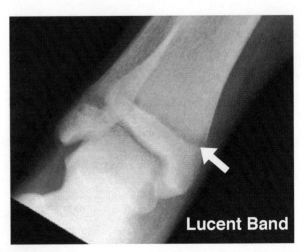
Lucent Band

Non-Accidental Trauma (NAT)

"Some People Just Can't Take Screaming Kids." Any suspicious fracture should prompt a skeletal survey ("baby gram" does NOT count). Suspicious fractures would include highly specific fractures (metaphyseal corner fracture, posterior rib fractures), or fractures that don't make sense - toddler fracture in a non-ambulatory child.

Posterior Medial Rib Fracture: In a child under the age of 3, this is pretty reliable. Supposedly this type of fracture can only be made from squeezing a child.

Metaphyseal Corner Fractures: When this is present in a non-ambulatory patient (infant) it is HIGHLY specific. The only exception is obstetric trauma. After age 1, this becomes less specific.

Skull Fracture: The general idea is anything other than a parietal bone fracture (which is supposedly seen more with an actual accident) is concerning.

Solid Organ and Lumen Injury - Don't forget about this as a presentation for NAT. Duodenal hematoma and pancreatitis (from trauma) in an infant - should get you to say NAT. Just think *"belly trauma in a kid that is too young to fall on the handle bars of their bike"*.

Dating the Fracture:

- *Periosteal Reaction:* This means the fracture is less than a week old.
- *Complete healing:* This occurs in around 12 weeks.
- *Exceptions:* Metaphyseal, skull, and costochondral junction fractures will often heal without any periosteal reaction.

Child Abuse Mimics

Rickets and OI , can have multiple fractures at different sites and are the two most commonly described mimics.

Wormian bones and bone mineral density issues are clues that you are dealing with a mimic. They will have to show you one or the other (or both) if they are gonna get sneaky.

Peds Neuro

Brain tumors and developmental anomalies are discussed in detail in the Neuro Chapter. This section of the pediatric chapter will focus briefly on head ultrasound, and some random head and neck conditions. I'll hit a lot of this stuff again in the near chapter.

Peds Head and Neck:

Choanal Atresia – This results from a oronasal membrane that separates the nasal cavity from the oral cavity. It can be unilateral or bilateral (symptomatic immediately if bilateral). Classic story is *"can't pass NG tube."* The most important imaging finding is thickening of the vomer. It's associated with CHARGE syndrome

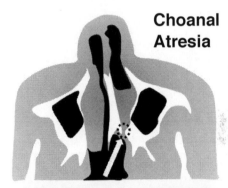

Congenital Piriform Aperture Stenosis – This results from abnormal development of the medial nasal eminences, and subsequent **failure of formation of the primary palate**. The piriform aperture of the nasal cavity is stenotic (as the name suggests), and the palate is narrow. The classic picture is the associated **central maxillary "MEGA-incisor."** Midline defects of the brain (corpus callosal agenesis, and holoprosencephaly) are associated.

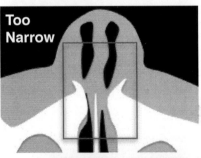

Next Step - You have to image the brain

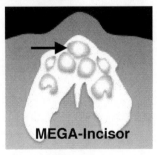

Branchial Cleft Cyst – There are several types but by far the **most common is a 2nd Branchial Cleft Cyst** (95%). The **angle of the mandible** is a classic location. They can get infection, but are often asymptomatic. Extension of the cyst between the ICA and ECA (**notch sign**) just above the carotid bifurcation is pathognomonic.

- I say lateral cyst in the neck, you say branchial cleft cyst

- I say midline cyst in the neck, you say thyroglossal duct cyst

Fibromatosis Coli – This is a **benign mass in the sternocleidomastoid** in neonates who present with torticollis (chin points towards the opposite side). Ultrasound can look scary, until you realize it's just the enlarged SCM. Sometimes <u>it looks like there are two</u> of them, but that's because the SCM has two heads. It goes away on its own, sometimes they do passive physical therapy.

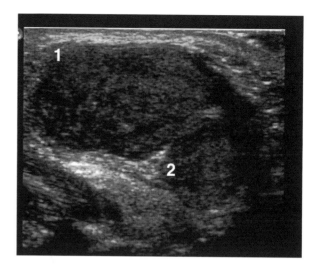

Orbital Calcifications:

Retinoblastoma: Discussed in detail in the neuro chapter. Calcifications are present in like 90% of cases. You can have bilateral disease, (and trilateral - involving the pineal gland with a pineoblastoma). The common thinking is the unilateral ones are sporadic, and the bilateral (and trilateral) ones are autosomal dominant related to chromosome 13. The RB suppressor on 13 links up with lots of other tumors (melanoma, fibrosarcoma, osteosarcoma, etc..).

Less than 3	Older than 3
Retinoblastoma	Toxo
CMV	Retinal Astrocytoma
Colobomatous	

Bad JuJu Chromosome 13

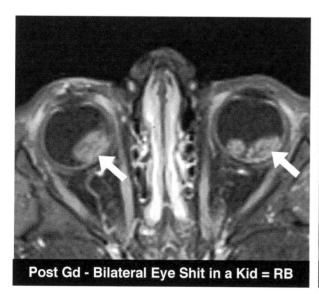

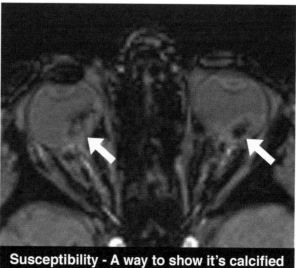

Peds Spine

Low lying cord / Tethered cord: Because the canal grows faster than the cord, a fixed attachment ("tethering") results in cord stretching and subsequent ischemia. This can be primary (isolated), or secondary (associated with myelomeningocele, filum terminale lipoma, or trauma). *The secondary types are more likely shown on MR (to showcase the associated mass - fluid collection), the primary types are more likely shown on US - as a straight counting game.*

Imaging Features: Low conus (**below L2**), and thickened filum terminale (> 2mm).

A common piece of trivia used as a distractor is that meningomyelocele is associated with Chiari malformations, lipomyelomeningocele is NOT.

High Yield Trivia

- <u>Anal Atresia</u> = High Risk For Occult Cord Problems (including tethering) – should get screened
- Low lying / tethered cords are closely linked with <u>Spina Bifida</u> (tufts of hair)
- Low Dimples (below the gluteal crease) **Do NOT** need screening,
- High Dimples (above the gluteal crease) **DO** need screening.

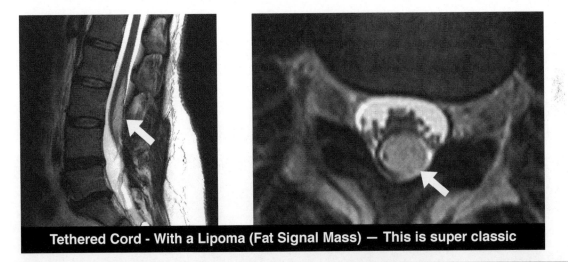

Tethered Cord - With a Lipoma (Fat Signal Mass) — This is super classic

For Screening Purposes:

Just remember low dimples (below the butt crease) don't get screened, but basically everyone else does.

Most Likely Question Style: "Which of the following does NOT get screened ?"
(Answer = low dimple).

Brain:

Periventricular Leukomalacia: This is the result of an ischemic / hemorrhagic injury, typically from a hypoxic insult during birthing. The kids who are at risk for this are premature, and little (less than 1500g). It favors the watershed areas (characteristically the white matter dorsal and lateral to the lateral ventricles). This will eventually cavitate into periventricular cystic changes, which occurs around 1-3 weeks post injury. Honestly, until they start to cavitate, you can't see it well, ultrasound just isn't sensitive early on. About 50% of kids with this will develop cerebral palsy.

Germinal Matrix Hemorrhage: This is seen in premature infants. By 32 weeks germinal matrix is only present at the caudothalamic groove. By 36 weeks, you basically can't have it *(if no GM then no GM hemorrhage)*. The earlier they are born the more common they are. Up to 40% occur in the first 5 hours, and most have occurred by day 4 (90%). There is a grading system (1-4).

Take home point - **No GM Hemorrhage in a full term infant.** The scenario will always call the kid a premature infant (probably earlier than 30 weeks).

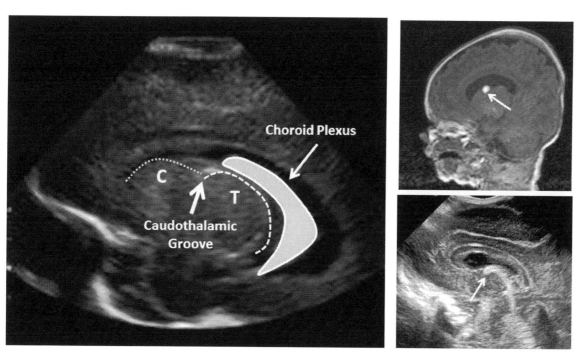

Grade 1 GM Hemorrhage
- Blood in the CT Groove

Premature Suture Closure Buzzwords:	
Sagittal	Dolichocephaly (long and skinny)
Metopic	Trigonocephaly (pointed forehead)
Coronal	Brachycephaly (also gets orbit issues "harlequin-eye)
Unilateral Lambdoid	Plagiocephaly
Bilateral Lambdoid	Turricephaly

For additional details of Congenial Brain Disorders please refer to the detailed discussion in the Neuro chapter *(found in the next module).*

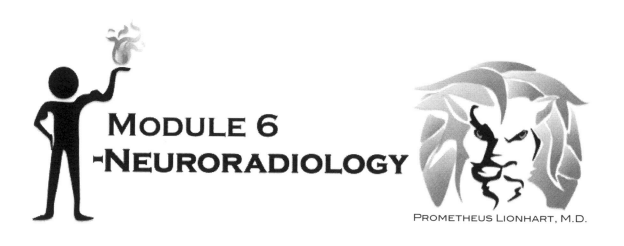

MODULE 6
-NEURORADIOLOGY

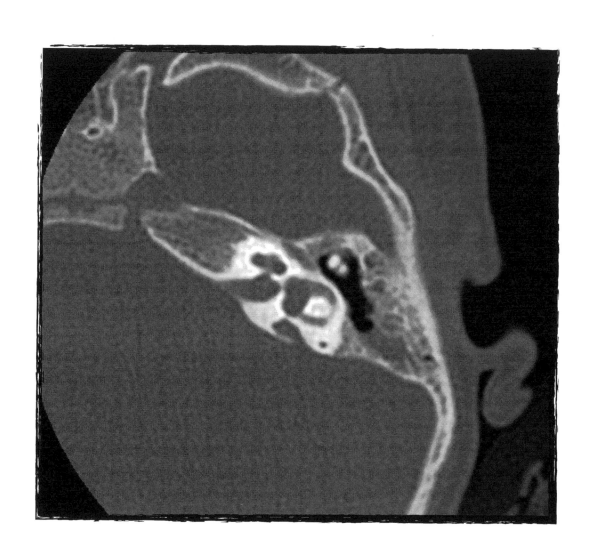

Section 1: Brain

Anatomy

There is a ton of anatomy that can be asked on a multiple choice test. My idea is to break it down into three categories: (1) soft tissue – brain parenchyma (*including normal development*), (2) bony anatomy – which is basically foramina, and (3) vascular anatomy.

Soft Tissue Brain Anatomy:

Central Sulcus - This anatomic landmark separates the frontal lobe from the parietal lobe. Old school grey bearded Radiologists (likely the ones who are important enough to write test questions) love to ask how you find this important structure. There are about 10 ways to do this, which brings me to the main reason this is a great pimping question. Even if you can name 9 ways to do it, they can still correct you by naming the 10th way. I noticed during my time as a "trainee" that Attendings tend to be excellent at knowing the answers to the questions they are asking.

Practically speaking this is the strategy I use for findings the central sulcus:

Pretty high up on the brain, maybe the 3rd or 4th cut, I find the cingulate sulcus. This is called the **"pars bracket sign"** - because the bi-hemispheric symmetric pars marginalis form an anteriorly open bracket. The bracket is immediately behind the central sulcus. This is *present about 95% of the time* - it's actually pretty reliable.

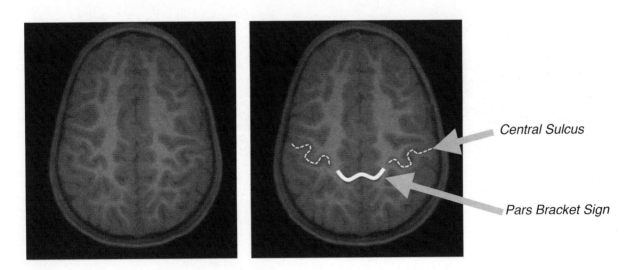

232

Central Sulcus Trivia - Here are the other less practical ways to do it.

- Superior frontal sulcus / Pre-central sulcus sign: The posterior end of the superior frontal sulcus, joins the pre-central sulcus
- Inverted omega (sigmoid hook) corresponds to the motor hand
- Bifid posterior central sulcus: Posterior CS has a bifid appearance about 85%
- *Thin post-central gyrus sign* – The precentral gyrus is thicker than the post central gyrus (ratio 1 : 1.5).
- *Intersection* – The intraparietal sulcus intersects the post central sulcus (works almost always)
- *Midline sulcus sign* – The most prominent sulcus that reaches the midline is the central sulcus (works about 70%).

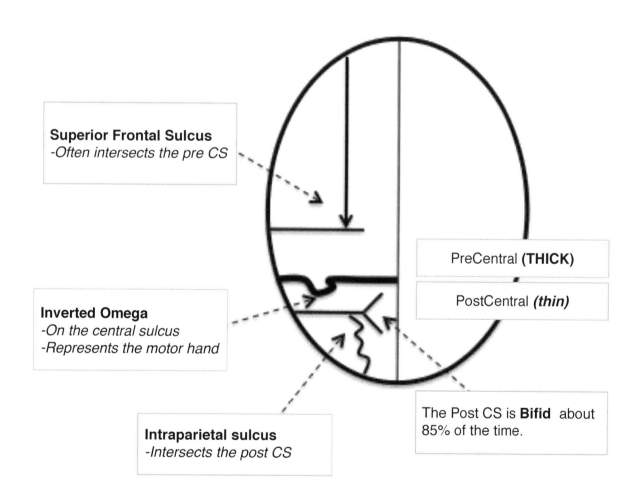

Homoculous Trivia:

- The inverted omega (posteriorly directed knob) on the central sulcus / gyrus designates the motor cortex controlling hand function.

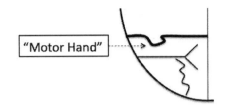

- ACA territory gets legs, MCA territory hits the rest.

Normal Cerebral Cortex: As a point of trivia, the cortex is normally 6 layers thick, and the hippocampus is normally 3 layers thick. I only mention this because the hippocampus can look slightly brighter on FLAIR compared to other cortical areas, and this is the reason why (supposedly).

Dilated Perivascular Spaces (Virchow-Robins): These are fluid filled spaces that accompany perforating vessels. They are a normal variant and very common. They can be enlarged and associated with multiple pathologies; mucopolysaccharidoses (Hurlers and Hunters), "gelatinous pseudocysts" in cryptococcal meningitis, and atrophy with advancing age. They don't contain CSF, but instead have interstitial fluid. The common locations for these are: around the lenticulostriate arteries in the lower third of the basal ganglia, in the centrum semiovale, and in the midbrain.

Ventricular Anatomy: Just a quick refresher on this. You have two lateral ventricles that communicate with the third ventricle via the interventricular foramen (of Monroe), which in turn communicates with the fourth ventricle via the cerebral aqueduct. The fluid in the fourth ventricle escapes via the median aperture (foramen of Magendie), and the lateral apertures (foramen of Luschka). A small amount of fluid will pass downward into the spinal subarachnoid spaces, but most will rise through the tentorial notch and over the surface of the brain where it is reabsorbed by the arachnoid vili and granulations into the venous sinus system. Blockage at any site will cause a noncommunicating hydrocephalus. Blockage of reabsorption at the vili / granulation will also cause a noncommunicating hydrocephalus.

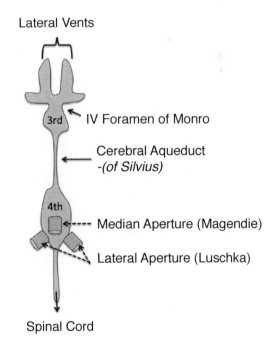

Arachnoid Granulations: These are regions where the arachnoid projects into the venous system allowing for CSF to be reabsorbed. There are hypodense on CT (similar to CSF), and usually round or oval. This round shape helps distinguish them from clot in a venous sinus (which is going to be linear). On MR they are typically T2 bright (iso to CSF), but can be bright on FLAIR (although this varies a lot an therefore probably won't be tested). These things can scallop the inner table (probably from CSF pulsation)

Cavum Variants:

- *Cavum Septum Pellucidum* - Seen in 100% of preterm infants, 80% of term infants, and 15% of adults. Rarely, can dilate and cause obstructive hydrocephalus
- *Cavum Vergae* – A posterior continuation of the cavum septum pellucidum (*never exists without a cavum septum pellucidum*)
- *Cavum Velum Interpositum* - Extension of the quadrigeminal plate cistern to foramen of Monro. Seen on sagittal as above the 3rd ventricle and below the fornices.

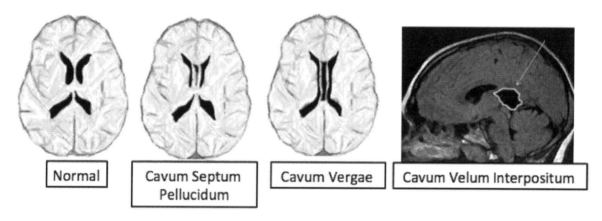

Basal cisterns: The basal cisterns are good for two things (1) looking for mass effect and (2) anatomy questions. Some people say the suprasellar cisterns look like a pentagon. The five corners of the star lend themselves easily to multiple choice questions: the top of the star is the interhemispheric fissure, the anterior points are the sylvian cisterns, and the posterior points are the ambient cisterns. The quadrigeminal plate looks like a smile.

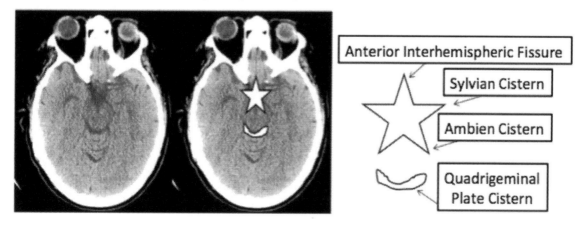

Brain Development:

Brain Myelination: The baby brain has essentially the opposite signal characteristics as the adult brain. **The T1 pattern of a baby, is similar to the T2 pattern of an adult.** The T2 pattern of a baby, is similar to the T1 pattern of an adult. This appearance is the result of myelination changes. The process of myelination occurs in a predetermined order, and therefore lends itself easily to multiple choice testing. The basic concept to understand first is that immature myelin has a higher water content relative to mature myelin and therefore is brighter on T2 and darker on T1. During the maturation process water will decrease, and fat (brain cholesterol and glycolipids) will increase. Therefore mature white matter will be brighter on T1 and darker on T2.

Immature Myelin	*Mature Myelin*
High Water, Low Fat	Low Water, High Fat
Relatively T1 dark, T2 bright	Relatively T1 bright, T2 dark

As a point of highly testable trivia: the T1 changes precede the T2 changes (adult T1 pattern seen around age 1, adult T2 pattern seen around age 2). Should be easy to remember *(1 for T1, 2 for T2)*.

Take Home Point: T1 is most useful for assessing myelination in the first year (especially 0-6 months), T2 is most useful for assessing myelination in the second year (especially 6 months to 18 months).

Order of progression: Just remember, inferior to superior, posterior to anterior, central to peripheral, and sensory fibers prior to motor fibers. The testable trivia, is that **the subcortical white matter is the last part of the brain to myelinate**, with the occipital white matter around 12 months, and the frontal regions finishing around 18 months. The "terminal zones" of myelination occur in the subcortical frontotemporoparietal regions – finishing around 40 months. Another high yield piece of testable trivia is that the **brainstem, and posterior limb of the internal capsule are normally myelinated at birth.**

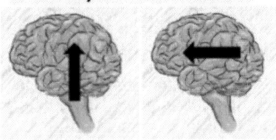

Inferior to Superior, Posterior to Anterior

Corpus Callosum: I'll touch on this again in the developmental/congenital section but it's high yield enough to repeat. **The corpus callosum forms front to back (then rostrum last).** Therefore hypoplasia of the corpus callosum is usually absence of the splenium (with the genu intact).

High Yield Points Regarding Brain Development

Myelination Occurs Inferior to Superior, and Posterior to Anterior

The Corpus Callosum Forms Front to Back (with the rostrum last)

Both the Anterior and Posterior Pituitary are Bright at Birth (posterior only bright around 2 months – 2 years)

Calverial Bone Marrow will be active (T1 hypointense) in young kids and fatty (T1 hyperintense) in older kids

The sinuses form in the following order: Maxillary, Ethmoid, Sphenoid, and Frontal Last

Brain Iron increases with age (globus pallidus darkens up).

Bony Anatomy:

Skull Base: The most likely multiple choice questions regarding the skull base are anatomy questions. Specifically, the *"what goes where?"* question is very easy to write.

Foramen	Contents
Foramen Ovale	CN V3, and Accessory Meningeal Artery
Foramen Rotundum	CN V2 ("**R2V2**"),
Superior Orbital Fissure	CN 3, CN 4, CN V1, CN6
Inferior Orbital Fissure	CN V2
Foramen Spinosum	Middle Meningeal Artery
Jugular Foramen	*Pars Nervosa:* Jugular Vein, CN 9, *Pars Vascularis:* CN 10, CN 11
Hypoglossal Canal	CN12
Optic Canal	CN 2, and Opthalmic Artery

The Jugular Foramen

The jugular foramen has two parts which are separated by a bony "jugular spine"

Pars Nervosa - The nervous guy in the front. This contains the Glossopharyngeal nerve (CN9), along with it's tympanic brach - the "Jacobson's Nerve"

Pars Vascularis - This is the "vascular part" which actually contains the jugular bulb, along with the Vagus nerve (CN 10), along with it's auricular branch "Arnold's Nerve," and the Spinal Accessory Nerve (CN 11)

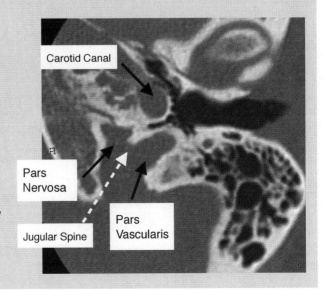

Remember, that they don't have to show you the hole in the axial plane. They can be sneaky and show it in the coronal or sagittal planes. In fact, showing foramen rotundum in the coronal and sagittal planes is a very common sneaky trick.

With regard to the relationship between **spinosum and ovale**, I like to think of this as the foot print a woman's high heeled shoe might make in the snow, with the oval part being ovale, and the pointy heel as spinosum.

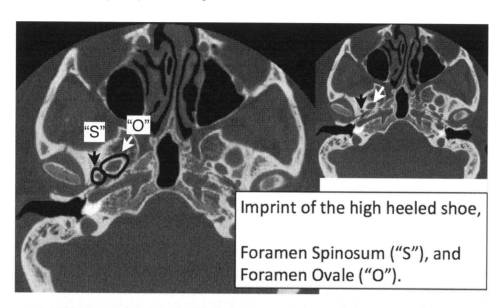

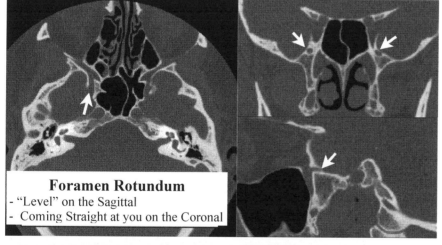

With regard to **Rotundum**, think about it as being totally level or horizontal on the sagittal view.

On the coronal view, it looks like you are staring into a gun

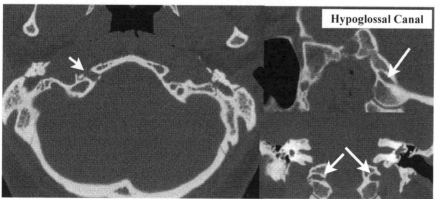

The **hypoglossal canal** is very posterior and inferior.

This makes it unique as a skull base foramen.

The relationship between the superior orbital fissure (SOF), the inferior orbital fissure (IOF), foramen rotundum (FR), and the pterygopalatine fossa (PPF) is an important one, that can really lead to some sneaky multiple choice questions (mainly what goes through what). I've attempted to outline this relationship on both sagittal and coronal views.

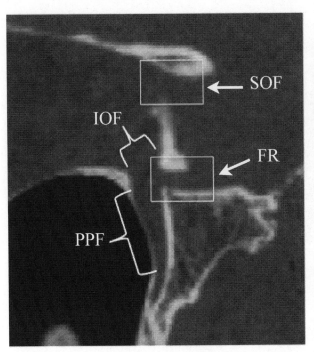

Sagittal

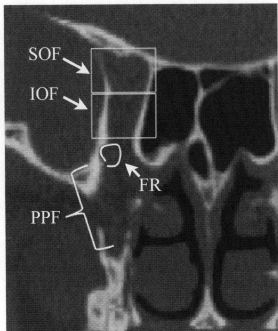

Coronal

Cavernous Sinus: - The question is going to be, what's in it (probably asked as what is NOT in it). CN3, 4, CN V1, CNV2, CN6, and the carotid. **CN2 and CN V3 do NOT run through it**.

The only other anatomy trivia I can think of is that CN6 runs next to the carotid, the rest of the nerves are along the wall. This is why you can get lateral rectus palsy earlier with cavernous sinus pathologies.

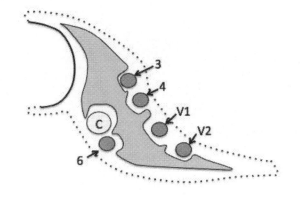

240

Skull fusion (Craniosynostosis): The craniosynostoses are discussed in more detail in the congenital section. I'll briefly touch on what is normal. The sutures exist to allow for rapid brain growth over the first few years of life. The brain will double in size within the first 6 months, and double again by the second year of life. The majority of skull growth occurs by age 3, at which time most of the sutures will fuse. Some, like the petro-occipital, will remain open into adulthood. When they fuse too early that causes a problem. The long Latin / French sounding word that goes along with that fusion problem makes for a good multiple choice test question (more on this later).

IAC - Nerve Orientation

The thing to remember is "7UP, and COKE Down" - with the 7th cranial nerve superior to the 8th cranial nerve (the cochlear nerve component). As you might guess, the superior vestibular branch is superior to the inferior one.

If it is shown, it is always shown in this orientation. The ideal sequence to find it is a heavily T2 weighted sequence with super thin cuts through the IAC.

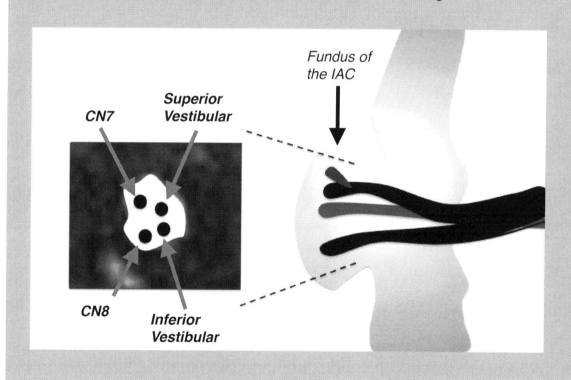

Vascular Anatomy:

Vascular anatomy can be thought of in four sections. (1) The branches of the external carotid (most commonly tested as the order in which the arise from the common carotid). (2) Segments of the internal carotid, with pathology at each level and variants. (3) Vertebral artery, with pathology. (4) Circle of Willis, with pathology and variants.

What are the branches of the external carotid ?

- *Some Administrative assistants Like Fucking Over Poor Medical Students*
    - Superior Thyroid
    - Ascending Pharyngeal
    - Lingual
    - Facial
    - Occipital
    - Posterior Auricular
    - Maxillary
    - Superficial Temporal

Anterior Circulation (Carotids):

Some Trivia about the ICA (Internal Carotid):

- The Bifurcation of the IAC and ECA usually occurs at C3-C4

- Cervical ICA has no branches in the neck - if you see branches either (a) they are anomalous or more likely (b) you are a dumb ass and actually looking at the external carotid. Remember the presence of branches is a way you can tell ICA from ECA on ultrasound.

- Flow reversal in the carotid bulb is common

Segment by Segment Trivia:

C1 (Cervical): 4 main pathologies of interest at this level:

- Atherosclerosis: The origin is a very common location
- Dissection: Can be spontaneous (women), and in Marfans or Ehlers-Danlos, and result in a partial Horner's (ptosis and miosis), followed by MCA territory stroke.
- Can have a retropharyngeal course and get "drained" by ENT accidentally.
- Pharyngeal infection may cause pseudoaneurysm at this level.

C2 (Petrous): - Not much goes on at this level. Sometimes aneurysms (which can be surprisingly big).

C3 (Lacerum): Not much here as far as vascular pathology. The anatomic location is important to neurosurgeons for exposing Meckel's cave via a transfacial approach.

C4 (Cavernous): Aneurysms here are strongly associated with hypertension. This segment is affected by multiple pathologies including the development of cavernous – carotid fistula.

C5 (Clinoid): An aneurysm here could compress the optic nerve and cause blindness.

C6: (Ophthalmic - Supraclinoid): Common site for aneurysm formation. **Origin at the "dural ring" is a buzzword** for this artery.

C7 (Communicating - terminal): An aneurysm here may compress CN III and present with a palsy.

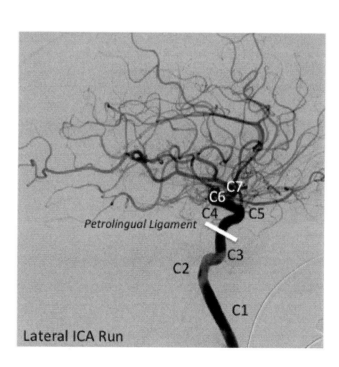

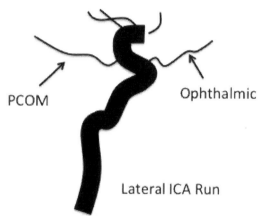

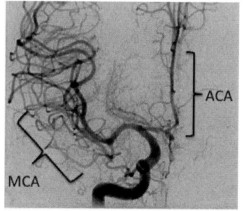

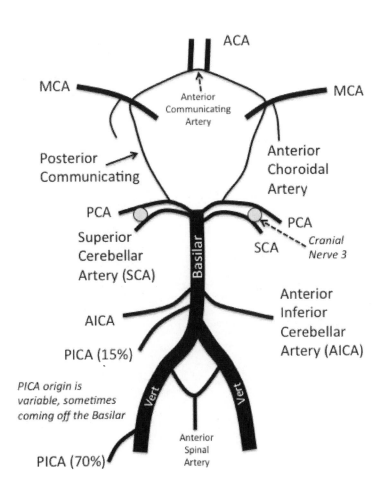
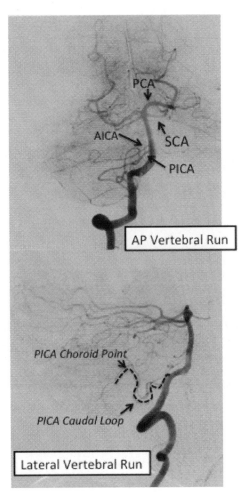

Vascular Variants:

Fetal Origin of PCA: Most common vascular variant (probably) - seen in up to 30% of general population. The term "fetal PCOM" is typically used to refer to a situation where the PCOM is larger (or the same size) as P1. Another piece of trivia is that *anatomy with a fetal PCA has the PCOM superior / lateral to CN3 (instead of superior / medial - in normal anatomy)*.

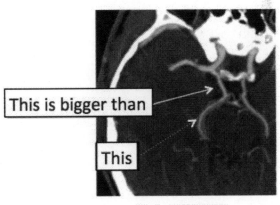

Fetal PCOM

Persistent Trigeminal Artery: Persistent fetal connection between the cavernous ICA to the basilar artery. A characteristic *"tau sign"* on Sagittal MRI has been described. It **increases the risk of aneurysm** (anytime you have branch points).

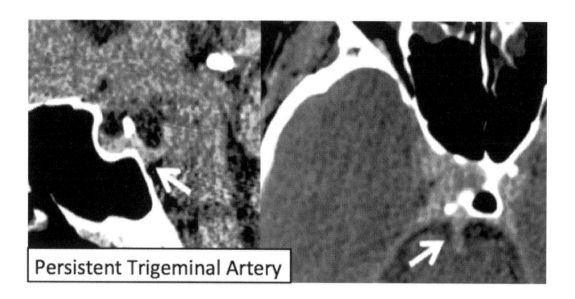

Aberrant Carotid Artery: Typically represents an enlarged inferior tympanic artery anastomosis with an enlarged caroticotympanic artery (with underdevelopment of the cervical ICA). This vessel courses though the tympanic cavity and joins the horizontal carotid canal. It can cause pulsatile tinnitus. The oldest trick in the book is to try and fool you into calling it a paraganglioma.

Don't biopsy it !

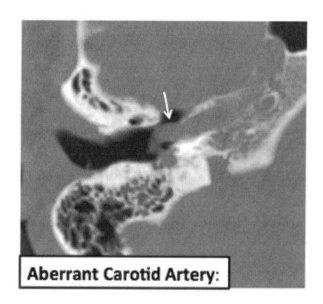

Venous Anatomy:

You can ask questions about the venous anatomy in roughly three ways (1) what is it – on a picture, (2) what is a deep vein vs what is a superficial vein, (3) trivia.

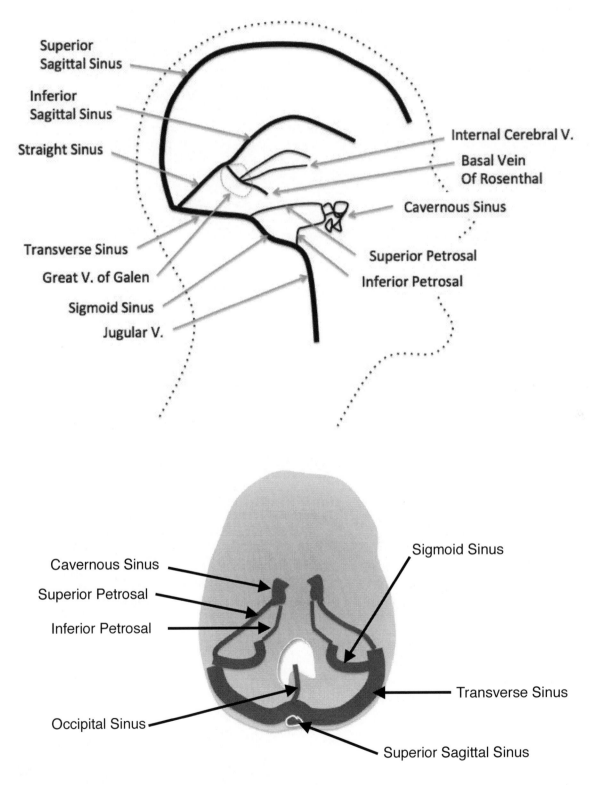

Anastomotic Superficial Veins:

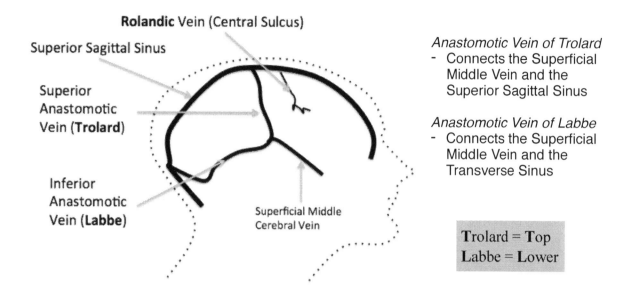

Here is a way to schematically think about the venous drainage -

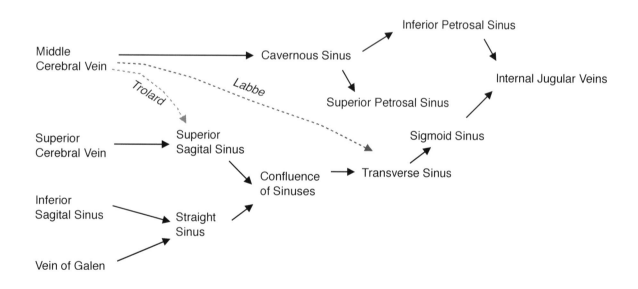

Superficial vs Deep

There is a superficial venous system and a deep venous system. The easiest way to test material like this is your *"which of the following is not?"* or *"which of the following is ?"* type question.

The big ones to remember are in the chart.

Superficial	*Deep*
Superior Cerebral Veins	Basal Vein of Rosenthal
Superior Anastomotic Vein of Trolard	Vein of Galen
Inferior Anastomotic Vein of Labbe	Inferior Petrosal Sinus
Superficial Middle Cerebral Veins	

Venous Trivia:

Collateral Pathways: The dural sinuses have accessory drainage pathways (other than the jugular veins) that allow for connection to extracranial veins. These are good because they can help regulate temperature, and equalize pressure. These are bad because they allow for passage of sinus infection / inflammation, which can result in venous sinus thrombosis.

Inverse Relationship: There is a relationship between the Vein of Labbe, and the Anastomotic Vein of Trolard. Since these dudes share drainage of the same territory, as one gets large the others get small.

Sounds Latin or French: As a general rule, anything that sounds Latin or French has an increased chance of being on the test.

- *Vein of Labbe:* Large draining vein, connecting the superficial middle vein and the transverse sinus
- *Vein of Trolard:* Smaller (usually) vein, connecting the superficial middle vein and sagittal sinus
- *Basal vein of Rosenthal:* Deep vein that passes lateral to the midbrain through the ambient cistern and drains into the vein of Galen. Its course is similar to the PCA.
- *Vein of Galen:* Big vein ("great") formed by the union of two internal cerebral veins.

Sinus Trivial Anatomy Bonus - The Concha Bullosa

This is a common variant where the middle concha is pneumatized. It's pretty much of no consequence clinically unless it's fucking huge - then it can cause obstructive symptoms.

When I was in private practice there was this ENT who told me he wanted it mentioned in all his CT sinus reports.

That way he could justify doing FESS…

He drove a nice car.

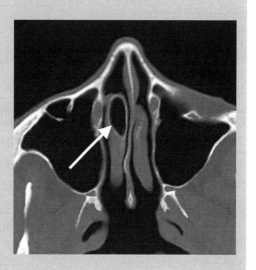

Gamesmanship for Neuro Anatomy

- *First Order Trivia:*
    - *"What is it?"* Style questions are most likely; with possibilities including CTA, MRA, or Angiograms. Considering when the people writing the questions trained, angiograms are probably the most likely.
    - *"What goes through there?"* Neuro foramina
    - *"What doesn't?"* Style questions - CN 2 and CN V3 don't go through the cavernous sinus.

- *Second Order Trivia:*
    - CN 3 Palsy - Think Posterior Communicating Artery Aneurysm
    - CN 6 Palsy - Think increased ICP

Misc Brain Conditions:

Monro-Kellie Doctrine:

The Monro-Kellie doctrine is the idea that the head is a closed shell, and that the three major components: (1) brain, (2) blood – both arterial and venous, and (3) CSF, are in a state of dynamic equilibrium. As the volume of one goes up, the volume of another must go down.

Intracranial Hypotension: If you are leaking CSF, this will decrease the overall fixed volume, the volume of venous blood will increase to maintain the equilibrium. The result is meningeal engorgement (enhancement), distention of the dural venous sinuses, prominence of the intracranial vessels and engorgement of the pituitary. The development of subdural hematoma and hygromas is also a classic look (again, compensating for lost volume).

Idiopathic Intracrainal Hypertension (Pseudotumor Cerebri): Classic scenario of a fat middle aged women with a headache. Etiology is not well understood (making too much CSF, or not absorbing it correctly). It has a lot of associations (hypothyroid, cushings, vitamin A toxicity). The findings follow the equilibrium idea. With increased CSF the ventricles become slit like, the pituitary shrinks (partially empty sella), and the venous sinuses appear compressed. You can also have the appearance of vertical tortuosity of the optic nerves and flattening of the posterior sclera.

Edema:

Cytotoxic: This type of edema can be thought about as intracellular swelling, secondary to malfunction of the Na/K pump. It tends to favor the gray matter, and **looks like loss of the gray-white differentiation**. This is classically **seen with stroke** (or trauma), and is why early signs of stroke involve loss of the GM-WM interface.

Vasogenic: This type of edema is extracellular, secondary to disruption of the blood brain barrier. It looks like **edema tracking through the white matter** (which is less tightly packed than the gray matter). This is classically **seen with tumor and infection**. A response to steroids is characteristic of vasogenic edema.

Communicating: This is an obstruction at the level of villi / granulation, blocking reabsorption. All the ventricles will be dilated (25% of the time the fourth ventricle is normal). There are 4 main causes.

- **Normal Pressure Hydrocephalus:** It's not well understood – and idopathic. The buzz-phrase is "ventricular size out of proportion to atrophy." The frontal and temporal horns of the lateral ventricles are the most affected. "Upward bowing of the corpus callosum" is another catch phrase. On MRI you may see transependymal flow and/or a flow void in the aqueduct and 3rd ventricle. The step 1 trivia is "wet, wacky, and wobbly" – describing the clinical triad of urinary incontinence, confusion, and ataxia. This is treated with surgical shunting.
- **Blood, Pus, and Cancer** – Anything that plugs up the villi – the three most common causes being SAH, Meningitis, and Carcinomatous Meningitis.

Non- Obstructive:

This is sort of a trick question, with the only answer being something that produces CSF. The only answer you need to know is Choroid Plexus Papilloma (discussed in detail in the tumor section).

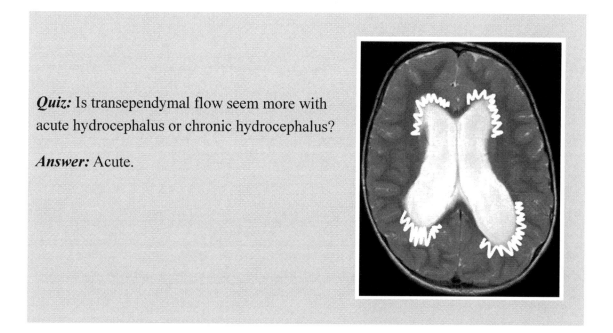

Quiz: Is transependymal flow seem more with acute hydrocephalus or chronic hydrocephalus?

Answer: Acute.

Brain Herniation:

Subfalcine Herniation: This is just a fancy way of saying midline shift (deviation of ipsilateral ventricle and bowing of the falx). The trivia to know is that the ACA may be compressed, and can result in infarct.

Descending Transtentorial Herniation: The uncus and hippocampus herniated through the tentorial incisura. Effacement of the ipsilateral suprasellar cistern occurs first:

Things to know:

- Perforating basilar artery branches get compressed resulting in *"Duret Hemorrhages"* - classically located in the midline at the pontomesencephalic junction (in reality they can also effect cerebellar peduncles).

- CN3 gets compressed between the PCA and Superior Cerebellar Artery causing ipsilateral pupil dilation and ptosis

- "Kernohan's Notch / Phenomenon" – The midbrain on the tentorium forming an indentation (notch) and the physical exam finding of ipsilateral hemiparesis – which Neurologist's call a *"false localizing sign."* Of course, localization on physical exam is stupid in the age of MRI, but it gives Neurologists a reason to carry a reflex hammer and how can one fault them for that.

Ascending Transtentorial Herniation: Think about this in the setting of a posterior fossa mass. The vermis will herniate upward through the tentorial incisura often resulting in severe obstructive hydrocephalus.

Things to know
- The "Smile" of the quadrigeminal cistern will be flattened or reversed
- *"Spinning Top"* is a buzzword, for the appearance of the midbrain from bilateral compression along its posterior aspect
- Severe hydrocephalus (at the level of the aqueduct).

Cerebellar Tonsil Herniation: Can be from severe herniation after downward transtentorial herniation). Alternatively, if in isolation you are thinking more along the lines of Chiari (Chiari I = 1 tonsil 5mm, or both tonsils 3mm).

Neuro-Degenerative / Toxic Metabolic

Multiple Sclerosis:

By far the most common acquired demyelinating disease. Usually affects women 20-40. As a point of trivia in children there is no gender difference. There are multiple types with the relapsing-remitting form being by far the most common (85%). Clinical history of "separated by time and space" is critical. Findings are the classic T2/FLAIR oval and periventricular perpendicularly oriented lesions. Involvement of the calloso-septal interface is 98% specific for MS (and helps differentiate it from vascular lesions and ADEM). In children the posterior fossa is more commonly involved. Acute demyelinating plaques should enhance and restrict diffusion (on multiple choice tests and occasionally in the real world). Brain atrophy is accelerated in MS.

You can sometimes get a big MS plaque that looks like a tumor. **It will ring enhance but classically incomplete (*like a horseshoe*)**, with a leading demyelinating edge. Solitary spinal cord involvement can be seen but it usually is seen in addition to brain lesions. The cervical spine is the most common location in the spine (65%). Spinal cord lesions tend to be peripherally located.

Multiple Sclerosis Variants:

ADEM (Acute Disseminated Encephalomyelitis): Typically presents in childhood or adolescents, after a viral illness or vaccination. Classically has multiple LARGE T2 bright lesions, which enhance in a nodular or ring pattern (open ring). Lesions **do NOT involve the calloso-septal interface**.

Acute Hemorrhagic Leukoencephalitis (Hurst Disease): This a fulminant form of ADEM with massive brain swelling and death. The hemorrhagic part is only seen on autopsy (not imaging).

Devics (neuromyelitis optica): Transverse Myelitis + Optic Neuritis.
Lesions in the Cord and the Optic Nerve

Marburg Variant: Childhood variant that is fulminant and terrible leading to rapid death. It usually has a febrile prodrome. "MARBURG!!!" = DEATH

Toxic / Metabolic

PRES (Posterior Reversible Encephalopathy Syndrome): Seen with hypertension or chemotherapy. Features include asymmetric cortical and subcortical white matter edema (usually in parietal occipital regions). PRES does NOT restrict on diffusion (helps tell you it's not a stroke).

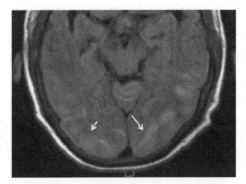

PRES – T2/FLAIR High Signal

Radiation-Induced Demyelination: Seen as T2 bright areas and atrophy corresponding to the radiation portal. Can be seen with hemosiderin deposition, and mineralizing microangiopathy (calcifications involving the basal ganglia and subcortical white matter).

Osmotic Demylination Syndrome (CPM): Seen with rapid correction of sodium (usually in a drunk). Usually T2 bright in the central pons (spares the periphery). Can also have an extra-pontine presentation involving the basal ganglia, external capsule, amygdala, and cerebellum.

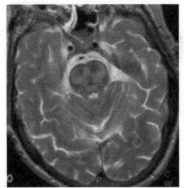

CPM – T2 Bright Central Pons

Wernicke Encephalopathy: Caused by thiamine deficiency. Just think contrast **enhancement of the mammillary bodies** (seen more in alcoholics).

Additionally, think increased T2/FLAIR signal in the bilateral medial thalamus and periaqueductal gray.

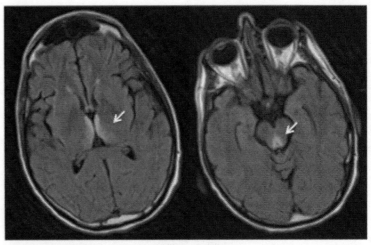

Wernicke
High Signal in Medial Thalamus and Periaqueductal Gray

CNS Findings Secondary to Drugs or Toxins:

- **Carbon Monoxide:** CT Hypodensity / T2 Bright Globus Pallidus (*carbon monoxide causes "globus" warming*).

- **Alcohol:** Brain atrophy, especially the cerebellar vermis.

- **Marchiafava-Bignami**: Seen in drunks. Swelling and T2 bright signal affecting the **corpus callosum** (typically beginning in the body, then genu, and lastly splenium). Will involve the central fibers and spare the dorsal and ventrals fibers (called a **"sandwich sign" on sagittal imaging**).

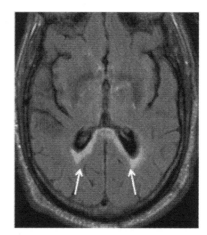

Marchiafava-Bignami
-High T2/FLAIR in the Corpus Callosum

- **Methanol**: Optic nerve atrophy, hemorrhagic **putaminal** and subcortical white matter necrosis

Post-Radiation: There is a latent period, so imaging findings don't typically show up for about two months post therapy.

- *Whole Brain Radiation* changes are typically T2 bright in the periventricular white matter, sparing the subcortical regions early on. Peripheral extension to the subcortical regions occurs later.

- *Localized Radiation:* Usually we are talking about severe focal edema with mass effect and enhancement. Differentiation from residual tumor can be a sneaky sneaky thing, and MR perfusion may be useful in differentiating.

Post Chemotherapy: You will have T2 effects acutely in the white matter, that can progress to atrophy. Enhancement or mass effect is rare unless it is very severe. Children receiving both radiation and chemotherapy can sometimes develop calcifications - "mineralizing microangiopathy."

Disseminated necrotizing leukoencephalopathy: Severe white matter changes, which demonstrate ring enhancement, classically seen with leukemia patients undergoing radiation and chemotherapy. This is bad news and can be fatal.

Neurodegenerative Disorders:

You can do dementia imaging with a variety of imaging modalities, including CT and MRI for structure, and FDG PET and SPECT for function. **Pearl: On FDG PET the motor strip is always preserved in dementia.**

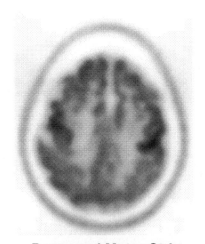

Preserved Motor Strip
—Seen in degenerative dementias

Alzheimer Disease: Most common cause of dementia. Most likely question is **hippocampal atrophy** (which is first), and out of proportion to the rest of the brain atrophy. They could ask temporal horn atrophy > 3mm, which is seen in more than 65% of cases.

Multi-infarct Dementia: This is the second most common cause of dementia. Cortical infarcts and lacunar infarcts are seen on MRI. Most likely to be shown as a PET-FDG case, demonstrating multiple scattered areas of decreased activity

Crossed Cerebellar Diaschisis (CCD): Depressed blood flow and metabolism affecting the cerebellar hemisphere after a contralateral supratentorial insult (infarct, tumor resection, radiation). Creates an Aunt Minnie Appearance:

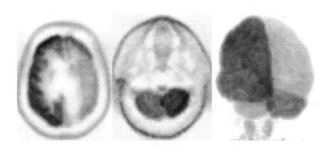

Crossed Cerebellar Diaschisis

Dementia with Lewy Bodies: This is the third most common cause of dementia (second most common neurodegenerative), with a very similar clinical picture to the dementia seen with Parkinsons, with the major difference being that in DLB, the dementia comes first. The hippocampi remain normal in size and you have some decreased FDG uptake in the lateral occipital cortex, with sparing of the mid posterior cingulate gyrus (**Cingulate Island Sign**).

Binswanger Disease: This is a subcortical leukoencephalopathy that affects older people (55 and up), strongly associated with HTN. It's basically a form of *small vessel vascular dementia*. It classically spares the subcortical U fibers *(see page #259 for an explanation on WTF " U Fibers" are)*.

FDG PET - Brain

Alzheimer	Low posterior temporoparietal cortical activity	Identical to Parkinson Dementia
Multi Infarct	Scattered areas of decreased activity	*Lyme, HIV, and Vasculitis are mimics*
Dementia with Lewy Bodies	Low in lateral occipital cortex	Preservation of the mid posterior cingulate gyrus **(Cingulate Island Sign)**
Picks / Frontotemporal / Depression	Low frontal lobe	*Depression is a mimic*
Huntingtons	Low activity in caudate nucleus and putamen	

Infections

My idea for discussing intracranial infections is to think of a few "testable" scenarios. The neonatal infections, the infections related to HIV, the "characteristic" infections, and lastly meningitis and cerebral abscess.

Neonatal Infections:

We are talking about TORCH infections. The first critical thing is that they only really matter in the first two trimesters (doesn't cause as much harm in third trimester). Calcifications and microcephaly are basically present in all of them.

Here are some high yield points regarding the TORCH infections:

CMV: This is the **most common TORCH** (by far!, it's 3x more common than Toxo – which is the second most common). It likes to affect the germinal matrix and causes periventricular tissue necrosis. The result is the most likely test question = **Periventricular calcifications**. Another high yield piece of trivia is that of all the TORCHs **CMV has the highest association with polymircogyria**.

Toxoplasmosis: This is the second most common TORCH. It's seen in women who clean up cat shit. The calcification pattern is more random, and affects the basal ganglia (like most other TORCH infections). The frequency is increased in the 3rd trimester (but only causes a problem in the first two). The most likely test question = **hydrocephalus**.

Rubella: Less common because of vaccines. Calcifications are less common than in other TORCHS. On MR, focal high T2 signal might be seen in white matter (related to vasculopathy and ischemic injury).

HSV: As a point of trivia, it's usually HSV-2 in 90% of cases. Unlike adults, the virus does not primarily affect the limbic system but instead affects the endothelial cells resulting in **thrombus and hemorrhagic infarction** with resulting encephalomalcia and atrophy.

HIV: This is not a TORCH but does occur during pregnancy, at delivery, or through breast feeding. **Brain atrophy predominantly in the frontal lobes** is the main testable piece of trivia. You may also have faint basal ganglia enhancement seen on CT and MRI preceding the appearance of basal ganglia calcification.

CNS TORCH - What you need to remember

- **CMV** = *Most Common, Periventricular Calcifications, Polymicrogyria*
- **Toxo** = *Hydrocephalus, Basal Ganglia Calcifications*
- **Rubella** = *Vasculopathy / Ischemia. High T2 signal - Less Calcifications*
- **HSV** = *Hemorrhagic Infarct, and lead to bad encephalomalcia (hydranencephaly)*
- **HIV** = *Brain Atrophy in frontal lobes*

Infections Immunosuppressed Patients Get (people with AIDS)

The most common opportunistic infection in patients with AIDS is toxo. The most common fungal infection (in people with AIDS) is Cryptococcus. Two other infections worth talking about are JC Virus, and CMV.

HIV Encephalitis: I'll lead with the encephalitis people with AIDS get. This is actually pretty common and affects about 50% of AIDS patients. Usually we are talking about a situation with a CD4 < 200. What you are going to see is **symmetric** increased T2 / FLAIR signal in the deep white matter. **T1 will be normal**. The lesions will not enhance. There may be associated brain atrophy. These tend to **spare the subcortical U-fibers** *(PML will involve them)*.

Progressive Multifocal Leukoencephalopathy (PML): This is caused by the JC virus. We are talking about a situation with a CD4 less than 50. The imaging manifestations are a single or multiple scattered hypodensities, with corresponding **T1 hypointensity** (remember HIV was T1 normal), and **T2/FLAIR hyperintensities out of proportion to mass effect - buzzword**. The lesions have a predilections for the **subcortical U-fibers**. The **asymmetry** of these lesions helps differentiate them from HIV.

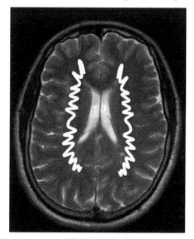
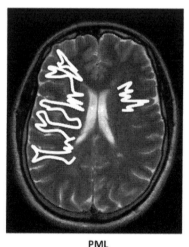
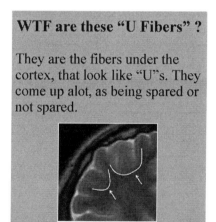

HIV Encephalitis
-Symmetric, and Spare Cortical U Fibers

PML
-Asymmetric, and Involves Cortical U Fibers

WTF are these "U Fibers"?

They are the fibers under the cortex, that look like "U"s. They come up alot, as being spared or not spared.

CMV: Think about brain **atrophy**, periventricular hypodensities (that are T2/FLAIR bright), and **ependymal enhancement**.

Cryptococcus: The most common fungal infection in AIDS. The most common presentation is meningitis that involves the base of the brain (leptomenigneal enhancement). The most likely way this will be shown on a multiple choice exam is **dilated perivascular spaces filled with mucoid gelatinous crap (these will not enhance)**. The second most likely way this will be shown is lesions in the basal ganglia "cryptococcomas" – these are T1 dark, T2 bright, and may ring enhance.

Toxo: Most common opportunistic infection in AIDS. Classically we are talking about T1 dark, T2 bright, ring enhancing (when larger than 1cm) lesions. These guys will NOT show restricted diffusion. Just think **"ring enhancing lesion, with LOTS of edema."** Most likely test question is that Toxo is Thallium Cold, and Lymphoma is thallium hot.

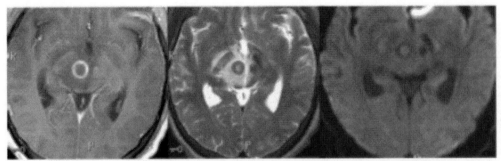

Toxo: Ring Enhancing, Lots of Edema, Not Restricted

Wait - I thought abscess restricted diffusion?
Typical abscess does. However, atypical infections like Toxo or fungal don't always do this, and showing that it does NOT restrict might be a sneaky way to test this.

Toxo	Lymphoma
Ring Enhancing	Ring Enhancing
Hemorrhage more common after treatment	Hemorrhage less common after treatment
Thallium Cold	**Thallium HOT**
PET Cold	Pet Hot
MR Perfusion: Decreased CBV	MR Perfusion: Increased (or Decreased) CBV

Summary:

AIDS Encephalitis	PML	CMV	Toxo	Cryptococcus
Symmetric T2 Bright	Asymmetric T2 Bright	Periventricular T2 Bright	Ring Enhancement	Dilated Perivascular Spaces
	T1 dark	Ependymal Enhancement	Thallium Cold	Basilar Meningitis

MRI Gamesmanship - Enhancement Patterns

In general, to solve MR puzzles you will need to be able to work through some MR sequences. The trick is to have a list of things that are T1 bright, T2 bright, Restrict diffusion, and Enhance. Plus you should know the basic enhancement patterns (homogenous, heterogenous, ring, and incomplete ring).

STROKE vs TUMOR vs ABSCESS vs MS Plaque

T2: For the most part, T2 is not helpful for lesion characterization - as tumors, stroke, MS, infections all have edema.

DWI: This is helpful only if they follow the classic rules. Out of those 4 (Tumor, Abscess, MS, and Stroke) the classical diffusion restrictors are: Abscess, and Stroke. Certain hypercellular tumors (classically lymphoma) can restrict, and demyelinating lesions with acute features can restrict.

Enhancement: In this situation this is probably the most helpful. Out of those 4 (Tumor, Abscess, MS, and Stroke) each should have a different pattern.

- *Tumor* could be heterogeneous or homogenous if high grade (or none if low grade).

- *Abscess* will classically have RING pattern.

- *MS* will classically have an Incomplete RING pattern.

- *Stroke* will have cortical ribbon (gyriform) type enhancement in the sub-acute time period (around 1 week).

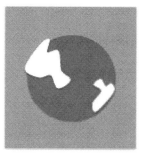  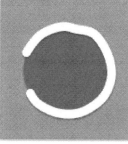 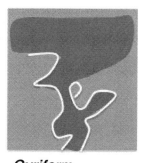

Heterogeneous
-Most likely Tumor (higher grade)

Ring
-Can be lots of stuff: Abscess and Tumor are both prime suspects

Incomplete Ring
-Classic for demyelinating lesion

Gyriform
-Classic for subacute stroke *(can also be seen with PRES or encephalopathy / encephalitis)*

The Characteristic Infections:

TB Meningitis: TB meningitis looks just like regular meningitis, except that it has a predilection for the basal cisterns and may have dystrophic calcifications. There may be **enhancement of the basilar meninges with minimal nodularity.** Complications include vasculitis which may result in infarct (more common in children). Obstructive hydrocephalus is common. *Most likely way to show this is enhancement of the basilar meninges (sarcoid can do that too - so it won't be a distractor unless he/she also has hydrocephalus - in which case pick TB).*

HSV: It's HSV 1 in adults and HSV 2 in neonates. I mention that because (1) it seems like testable trivia and (2) they actually have different imaging appearances (as mentioned above type 2 doesn't love the limbic like type 1). For the purpose of multiple choice test you are going to have a swollen (unilateral or bilateral) **medial temporal lobe**, which will be T2 bright. *Earliest sign is actually restricted diffusion* – related to vasogenic edema. This could be tested by asking "what sequence is more sensitive?", with the answer being the **diffusion is more sensitive than T2**. Blooming on gradient means it's bleeding (common in adults, rare in neonate form). Other trivia is that it **spares the basal ganglia** (distinguishes it from MCA stroke).

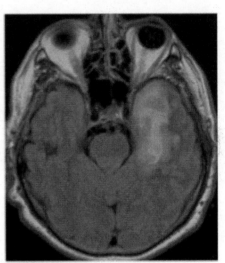

Herpes – Edema in the temporal lobe

Limbic Encephalitis: Not an infection, but a commonly tested mimic. It is a **paraneoplastic syndrome (usually small cell lung cancer)**, that looks very **similar to HSV**. This could be asked by showing a classic HSV image, but then saying HSV titer negative. The second order question would be to ask for lung cancer screening.

West Nile: Several viruses characteristically involve the basal ganglia (Japanese Encephalitis, Murray Valley Fever, West Nile…), the only one realistically testable is West Nile. We are talking about **T2 bright basal ganglia and thalamus, with corresponding restricted diffusion.** Hemorrhage is sometimes seen.

CJD: There are 3 types: sporadic (80-90%), variant (rare), and familial (10%). Random factoid is that it has a characteristic appearance on EEG, and this "14-3-3" protein assay is a CSF test neurologists order. The imaging features are variable and can be unilateral, bilateral, symmetric, or asymmetric. I want to concentrate on the most likely testable appearances of which I think there are 3.

- *(1) DWI Showing Cortical Gyriform restricted signal* – supposedly diffusion is the most sensitive sign, and the cortex is the most common early site of manifestation.
- *(2) "Hockey Stick Sign / Pulvinar Sign"* – Restricted diffusion in the dorsal medial thalamus (which looks like a hockey stick), or in the pulvinar
- *(3) A series of MRs or CTs showing rapidly progressive atrophy*

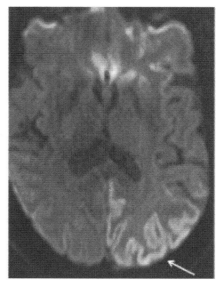

CJD: Gyriform Restricted Diffusion

Neurocysticercosis: Caused by eating pig shit (or undercooked pork). The bug is tinea solium. The most common locations of involvement are the subarachnoid space over the cerebral hemispheres, basal cisterns, brain parenchyma, and ventricles (in that descending order). As a point of trivia, <u>involvement of the basal cisterns carries the worst outcome</u>.

It has 4 stages which could be written in the form of a multiple choice questions (that would be really dirty, and therefore likely):

- Vesicular – thin walled cyst (iso-iso T1/T2 + no edema)
- Colloidal – hyperdense cyst (bright-bright T1/T2 + edema)
- Granular – cyst shrinks, wall thickens (less edema)
- Nodular - small calcified lesion (no edema)

Meningitis and Cerebral Abscess

You can think of meningitis in 4 main categories: bacterial (acute pyogenic), viral (lymphocytic), chronic (TB or Fungal), and non-infectious (sarcoid).

Essentially, we are talking about thick leptomeningeal enhancement, in the appropriate clinical setting. The complications are numerous and include venous thrombosis, vasospasm (leading to the stroke), empyema, ventriculitis, hydrocephalus, abscess etc… and so on and so forth.

Abscess Facts (trivia)
- *DWI - Restricts*
- *MRS – Lactate High*
- *PET FDG – Increased Metabolic*

A very testable piece of trivia is that infants will often get sterile reactive subdurals (much less common than in adults).

Empyema: Can be subdural or epidural (just like blood). Follows the same rules as far as crossing dural attachments (epidurals don't) and crossing the falx (subdurals don't). Subdurals are more common and have more complications relative to epidurals. The vast majority of subdurals are the sequela of frontal sinusitis. The same is true of epidurals with some sources claiming 2/3 of epidurals are secondary to sinusitis. They are often T1 bright and can **restrict on diffusion**.

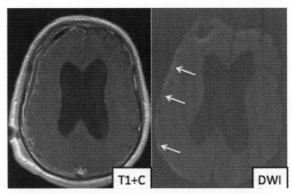

Subdural Empyema: *Dural Enhancement, Restricts*

Intraaxial Infections; We are talking Cerebritis, Abscess, and Ventriculitis:

Again lots of causes via direct spread, or hematogenous spread. The causes worth thinking about include right to left shunts, and pulmonary AVMs. Cerebritis is the early form of intra-axial infection, which can lead to abscess if not treated.

Ventriculits: Usually the result of a shunt placement, or intrathecal chemo. The ventricle will enhance and you can sometimes see ventricular fluid-fluid levels. If septa start to develop you can end up with obstructive patterns of hydrocephalus. The intraventricular extension of abscess is a very serious / ominous "pre-terminal event".

Brain Tumors - The Promethean Method:

I want to introduce my idea for brain tumor diagnosis. The strategy is as follows; (1) decide if it's single or multiple, (2) look at the age of the patient - *adults and kids have different differentials*, (3) look at the location - *different tumors occur in different spots,* (4) now use the characteristics to separate them. The strategy centers around narrowing the differential based off age and location till you are only dealing with 3-4 common things, then using the imaging characteristics to separate them. It's so much easier to do it that way.

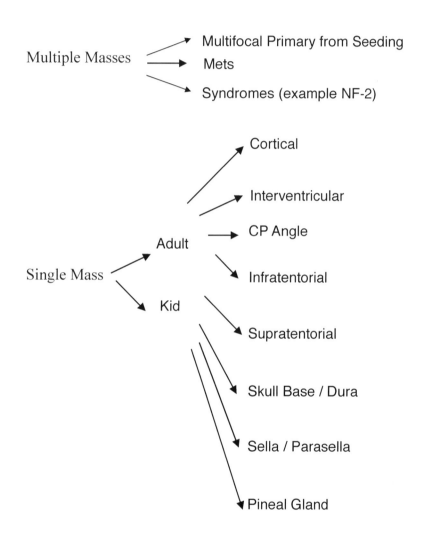

Before we get rolling, the first thing to do is to ask yourself is this a tumor, or is it a mimic? Mimics would be abscess, infarct, or a big MS plaque. This can be tricky. If you see an incomplete ring - you should think giant MS plaque. If they show you diffusion it is either lymphoma or a stroke (or an abscess) - you'll need to use enhancement to straighten that out (remember lymphoma enhances homogeneously).

Two more high yield topics before we start crushing the differentials:

"Intra-axial" vs "Extra-axial"

The Brant and Helms discussion on brain tumors will have you asking "intra-axial" vs "extra-axial" first. This is not always that simple, but it does lend itself very well to multiple choice test questions (therefore it's high yield).

Basically you need to memorize the "signs of extra-axial location"

- CSF Cleft
- Displaced Subarachnoid Vessels
- Cortical Gray matter between the mass and white matter
- Displaced and expanded Subarachnoid spaces
- Broad Dural Base / Tail
- Bony Reaction

Why Do Things Enhance?

Understanding the WHY is very helpful for problem solving. Let me first answer the question "why DON'T things enhance?" They DON'T enhance because of the blood brain barrier. So, when things DO enhance it's because either (a) they are outside the blood brain barrier (they are extra-axial), or (b) because they have melted the blood brain barrier.

In other words, extra axial things (classic example is the meningioma) will enhance. High grade tumors (and infections) enhance. Low grade tumors just aren't nasty enough to take the blood brain barrier down.

Are their exceptions? HA! There always are. And Yes... they are ALWAYS testable.

Gangliogliomas and Pilocytic Astrocytomas are the exceptions - they are low-grade tumors, but they enhance.

Multiple Masses

In adults or kids if you see multiple masses you are dealing with mets (or infection). Differentiating between mets and infection is gonna be done with diffusion (infection will restrict). If they want you to decide between those two they must show you the diffusion otherwise only one or the other will be listed as a choice.

Trivia on Mets

- Most common CNS met in a kid = neuroblastoma (BONES, DURA, ORBIT - not brain)

- Most common location for mets = Supratentorial at the Grey-White Junction (this area has a lot of blood flow + an abrupt vessel caliber change... so you also see hematogenous infection / septic emboli go there first too).

- Most common morphology is "round" or "spherical"

- Remember that mets do NOT have to be multiple. In fact 50% of mets are solitary. In an adult a solitary mass is much more likely to be a met than a primary CNS neoplasm.

- **MRCT** in the mnemonic for bleeding mets (**M**elanoma, **R**enal, **C**arcinoid / **C**horiocarcinoma, **T**hyroid).

- Usually Mets have more surrounding edema than primary neoplasms of similar size.

- *"Next Step Gamesmanship"* - Because the most common intra-axial mass in an adult is a met, if they show you a solitary mass (or multiple masses) and want a next step it's gonna be go hunting for the primary (think lung, breast, colon... the common stuff).

What about a multifocal primary brain tumor, can that happen? Oh yeah there are a few that like to do that (you should still think Met first).

- *Tumors that like to be multifocal:* Lymphoma, Multicentric GBM, Gliomatosis Cerebri
- *Tumors that are multifocal from seeding:* Medulloblastoma, Ependymoma, GBM, Oligodendroglioma
- *Syndromes:* - Tumors with syndromes are more likely to be multifocal.

NF 1	NF 2 "MSME"	Tuberous Sclerosis	VHL
Optic Gliomas	Multiple Schwannomas	Subependymal Tubers	Hemangioblastomas
Astrocytomas	Meningiomas	IV Giant Cell Astrocytomas	
	Ependymomas		

Cortically Based *(P-DOG)*:

Most intra-axial tumors are located in the white matter. So when a tumor spreads to or is primarily located in the gray matter you get a shorter DDx. High yield piece of trivia regarding the cortical tumor / cortical met is that they often have *very little edema* and so a *small cortical met can be occult without IV contrast.*

P-DOG:

- **P**leomorphic Xanthoastrocytoma (PXA)
- **D**ysembryoplastic Neuroepithelial Tumor (DNET)
- **O**ligodendroglioma,
- **G**anglioglioma

Oligodendroglioma: Remember this is the guy that **calcifies 90% of the time**. It's most common in the frontal lobe and the buzzword is **"expands the cortex"**. This takes after its most specific feature of cortical infiltration and marked thickening. It's likely you could get asked about this **1p/19q deletion** which apparently has a better outcome.

Ganglioglioma: This guy can occur at any age, anywhere, and look like anything. However, for the purpose of multiple choice testing the classic scenario would be a 13 year old with seizures, and a temporal lobe mass that is cystic and solid with focal calcifications. There may be overlying bony remodeling.

DNET (Dysembryoplastic Neuroepithelial Tumor): Kid with **drug resistant seizures**. The mass will always be in the **temporal lobe** (on the test – real life 60% temporal). Focal cortical dsyplasia is seen in 80% of the cases. It is hypodense on CT, and on MRI there will be little if any surrounding edema. High T2 signal **"bubbly lesion."**

PXA (Pleomorphic Xanthroastrocytoma): Superficial tumor that is ALWAYS supratentorial and usually involves the **temporal lobe**. They are often in the **cyst with a nodule** category (50%). There is usually no peritumeral T2 signal. The tumor frequently invades the leptomeninges. Looks just like a Desmoplastic Infantile Ganglioglioma - but is not in an infant.

Oligodendroglioma	Ganglioglioma	DNET	PXA
ADULT - (40s-50s)	Any Age	PEDS (< 20)	PEDS (10-20)
Can Enhance	Can Enhance	Does **NOT** Enhance	Will Enhance
Calcification Common	NOT Bubbly	High Signal "Bubbly"	Dural Tail***
"Expands the Cortex"	Can look like Anything		Cyst with Nodule

Interventricular

Tumors can arise from the ventricular wall, septum pellucidum, or choroid plexus.

Ventricular Wall & Septum Pellucidum	Choroid Plexus	Misc
Ependymoma **(PEDS)**	Choroid Plexus Papilloma (**PEDS in Trigone**) (**ADULT in 4th Vent**)	Mets
Medulloblastoma **(PEDS)**	Choroid Plexus Carcinoma (**PEDS**)	Meningioma
SEGA (Subependymal Giant Cell Astrocytoma) = **PEDS** Subependymoma **(ADULT)**	Xanthogranuloma ("Found "in **ADULTS**)	Colloid Cyst
Central Neurocytoma **(YOUNG ADULT)**		

Ventricular Wall / Septum Pellucidum Origin:

Ependymoma: Bimodal distribution on this one (large peak around 6 years of age, tiny peak around 30 years old). I would basically think of this as a **PEDS tumor.**

They come in two flavors:

(a) 4th Ventricle - which is about 70% of the time. with frequent extension into the foramen of Luschka and Magendie. They are the so called "plastic tumor" or *"tooth paste" tumor* because they squeeze out of the 4th ventricle.

(b) Parenchymal Supratentorial - which is about 30% of the time. These are usually big (> 4cm at presentation).

Medulloblastoma: Lets just assume we are talking about the "Classic Medulloblastoma" which is a type of PNET. If you want to understand the genetic spectrum of these things read Osborn's Brain - but that's probably overkill.

This is a **pediatric tumor** - with most occurring before age 10 (technically there is a second peak at 20-40 but for the purpose of multiple choice tests I'm going to ignore it).

These guys are cerebellar (arise from vermis – project into 4th ventricle) tumors that love to met via CSF pathways. The mass is heterogeneous on T1 and T2, and enhances homogeneously. They are much more common than their chief differential consideration the Ependymoma. They are hypercellular and may restrict. They calcify 20% of the time (less than Ependymoma). As mentioned above, they like to "drop met." The buzzword is *"zuckerguss"* which apparently is German for sugar icing, as seen on post contrast imaging of the brain and spinal cord. As a point of absolute trivia, they are *associated with Basal Cell Nevus Syndrome, and Turcots Syndrome.*

Gorlin Syndrome - If you see a **medulloblastoma** next look for **dural calcs**. If you see thick dural calcs you might be dealing with this syndrome. They get **basal cell** skin cancer after radiation, and have odontogenic cysts.

NEXT STEP Trivia: Preoperative imaging of the entire spinal axis should be done in any child with a posterior fossa neoplasm, especially if medulloblastoma or ependymoma is suspected. Evidence of tumor spread is a statically significant predictor of outcome.

Medulloblastoma	Ependymoma
More common	Less Common
Originate from Vermis / FLOOR of the 4th Ventricle	Originate from the ROOF of the 4th ventricle.
Can project into 4th ventricle, do NOT usually extend into basal cisterns	Can extend into basal cisterns like tooth paste pushing though foramina of Luschka and Magendie
Enhance Homogeneously *(more so than Ependymoma anyway)*	Enhance Heterogeneously
Calcify Less (20%)	Calcify More (50%)
Linear "icing-like" enhancement of the brain surface is referred to as "Zuckerguss"	

Subependymal Giant Cell Astrocytoma (SEGA): This is going to be shown in the setting of TS. They will more than likely show you renal AMLs or tell you the kid has seizures / developmental delay.

Because it's syndromic you see it in kids (average age 11).

It will arise from the wall of the lateral wall of the ventricle (near the foramen of Monro), often causing hydrocephalus. It enhances homogeneously.

This vs That: SEGA vs Subependymal Nodule (SEN)- The SEN will stay stable in size, the SEGA will grow. The SEGA is found in the lateral ventricle near the foramen of Monroe, the SEN can occur anywhere along the ventricle. SENs are way more common. Both SEN and SEGA can calcify.

Pearl - Enhancing, partially calcified lesion at the foramen of Monro bigger than 5mm is a SEGA not a SEN.

— (the next 2 IV tumors are in ADULTS) —

Subependymoma: Found in ADULTS. Well circumscribed IV masses **most commonly at the foramen of Monro and the 4th ventricle**. They can cause hydrocephalus. They typically don't enhance. They are T2 bright (like most tumors).

Central Neurocytoma: This is the *most common IV mass in an ADULT aged 20-40*. The buzzword is "**swiss cheese**," because of the numerous cystic spaces on T2. They **calcify** a lot (almost like oligodendrogliomas).

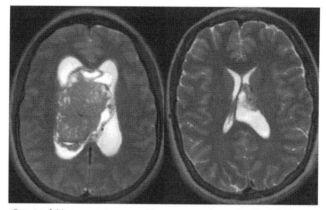

Central Neurocytoma – Two examples, Cystic IV Mass

Choroid Plexus Origin:

Choroid Plexus Papilloma / Carcinoma: Can occur in peds (85% under the age of 5) or adults. They make up about 15% of brain tumors in kids under one. Basically you are dealing with an intraventricular mass, which is often making CSF, so it causes hydrocephalus. *Here is the trick, brain tumors are usually supratentorial in adults and posterior fossa in kids. This tumor is an exception.* Remember exceptions to rules are highly testable.

Trivia -

- **In Adults it's in the 4th Ventricle, in Kids it's in the lateral ventricle (usually trigone).**

- Carcinoma type is ONLY SEE IN KIDS - and are therefore basically ONLY SEEN IN LATERAL VENTRICLE / TRIGONE

- Carcinoma Association with Li-Fraumeni syndrome (bad p53)

- Angiography may show enlarged chorodial arteries which shunt blood to the tumor,

- Carcinoma type of this tumor looks very similar (unless it's invading the parenchyma) and is almost exclusively seen in kids.

- The tumor is typically solitary but rarely you can have CSF dissemination

Xanthogranuloma – This is a benign choroid plexus mass. You see it all the time (7%) and don't even notice it. **The trick is that they restrict on diffusion,** so they are trying to trick you into working them up. They are benign… leave them alone.

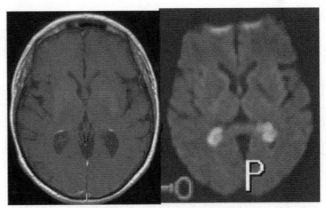

Xanthogranuloma – *Note the Restricted Diffusion*

Misc:

Mets - The most common location of intraventricular metastasis is the trigone of lateral ventricles (because of vascular supply of choroid plexus). The most common primary is controversial - and either lung or renal. If forced to pick I'd go Lung because it's more common overall. I think all things equal renal goes more - but there are less renal cancers. It all depends on how the question is worded.

Colloid Cyst – These are found almost exclusively in the anterior part of the 3rd ventricle behind the foramen of Monro. They **can cause sudden death via acute onset hydrocephalus**. Their appearance is somewhat variable and depends on what they are made of. If they have cholesterol they will be T1 bright, T2 dark. If they don't, they can be T2 bright. The trick is a round well circumscribed mass in the anterior 3rd ventricle. If shown on CT, it will be pretty dense.

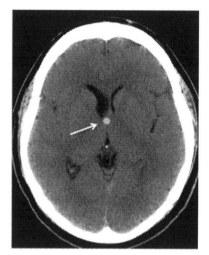

Colloid Cyst –
- *Anterior 3rd Ventricle*
- *Hyperdense on CT*

Meningioma – Can occur in an intraventricular location, most commonly (80%) at the **trigone of the lateral ventricles** (slightly more on the left). Details on meningiomas are discussed below.

Cerebellar Pontine Angle (CPA)

Age is actually less of an issue here because the DDx isn't that big. Most of these are adult tumors, but in the setting of NF-2 you could have earlier onset.

Epidemiology: Vestibular Schwannoma is #1 - making up 75% of the CPA masses, #2 is the meningioma making up 10%, and the Epidermoid is #3 making up about 5%. The rest are uncommon.

Vestibular Schwannoma – These guys account for 75% of CPA masses. When they are bilateral you should immediately think **NF-2** (*one for each side*). Enhances strongly but more heterogeneous than meningomas. May widen the porus acousticus resulting in a "trumpet shaped" IAC.

Meningioma – Second more common CPA mass. One of the few brain tumors that is more common in women. They can calcify, and if you are lucky they will have a dural tail (which is pretty close to pathognomonic – with a few rare exceptions). Because they are extradural they will enhance strongly. Radiation of the head is known to cause meningiomas.

Meningioma	Schwannoma
Enhance Homogeneously	Enhance Less Homogeneously
Don't Usually Invade IAC	Invade IAC
Calcify more often	IAC can have "trumpeted" appearance

Trivia:

- Most common location of a meningioma is over the cerebral convexity.

- They take up octreotide and Tc-MDP on Nuclear Medicine tests (sneaky).

Epidermoid – Can be congenital or **acquired** (after trauma – classically after LP in the spine). Unlike dermoids they are usually off midline. They will follow CSF density and intensity on CT and MRI (*the exception is this zebra called a "white epidermoid" which is T1 bright – just forget I ever mentioned it*). The key points are (1) unlike an arachnoid cyst they are bright on FLAIR (sometimes warm - *they don't completely null)*, and (2) they **will restrict with diffusion**.

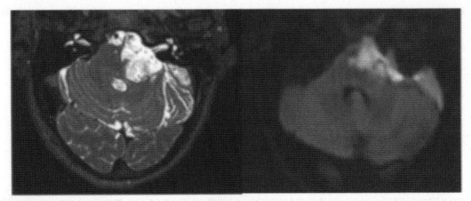

Epidermoid : *Follows CSF Signal – Restricts Diffusion*

Dermoid Cyst – This is about 4x less common than an epidermoid. It's more common in kids / young adults. Usually midline, and usually are found in 3rd decade. They contain lipoid material and are usually hypodense on CT and very bright on T1. They are associated with NF2.

Trivia -

- These are usually midline

- Most common location for a dermoid cyst is the suprasellar cistern (posterior fossa is #2)

This vs That: Dermoid vs Epidermoid — The easy way to think of this is that the Epidermoid behaves like CSF, and the Dermoid behaves like fat.

IAC Lipoma - It can occur, and is basically the only reason you get a T1 when you are working up CPA masses. It will fat sat out - because its a lipoma. There is an association with sensorineural hearing loss, as the vestibulocochlear nerve often courses through it.

Arachnoid Cyst – Common benign lesions that is located within the subarachnoid space and contains CSF. They are increased in frequency in mucopolysaccharidoses (as are perivascular spaces). They are **dark on FLAIR** (like CSF), and **will NOT restrict with diffusion**.

> *How can you tell an epidermoid from an arachnoid cyst?*
>
> The epidermoid restricts, the arachnoid cyst does NOT.

Infratentorial - Most are PEDS (Hemangioblastoma is the exception).

Atypical Teratoma / Rhabdoid – These are highly malignant tumors (WHO IV), and rarely occur in patient's older than 6 years. The average age is actually 2 years, but they certainly occur in the first year of life. They can occur in supra and infratentorial locations (most common in the cerebellum). These are usually **large, pissed off looking tumors with necrosis** and heterogeneous enhancement.

Juvenile Pilocytic Astrocytoma (JPA): Just think cyst with a nodule in a kid. They are WHO grade 1, but the nodule will still enhance. This will be located in the posterior fossa (or optic chiasm).

Diffuse Brain Stem Glioma (DPG): Seen in kids age 3-10. Most common location is the pons, which is usually a high grade fibrillary glioma. It's going to be T2 bright with subtle or no enhancement. The 4th ventricle will be flattened. The imaging features are so classic that no biopsy is needed.

Ganglioglioma: This guy can occur at any age, anywhere, and look like anything… and was discussed under the cortical lesions (page 268)

Medulloblastoma: *Discussed with the IV lesions (page 270)*

Ependymoma: *Discussed with the IV lesions (page 269)*

Hemangioblastoma: First things first – immediately think about this when you see **cyst with a nodule** in an ADULT. Then think **Von Hippel Lindau**, especially if they are multiple. These things are slow growing, indolent vascular tumors, that can cause hydrocephalus from mass effect. About 90% of the time they are found in the cerebellum.

I Say Posterior Fossa Cyst with a Nodule - PEDS, you say JPA

I say Posterior Fossa Cyst with a Nodule - ADULT, you say Hemangioblastoma

Supratentorial - Most are Adults (DIG, DNET, PXA are exceptions).

Mets - The most common supratentorial mass -

Astrocytoma: Most common primary brain tumor in adults. Tumors fitting in the category include Pilocytic Astrocytoma (WHO1), Diffuse Astrocytoma (WHO 2), Anaplastic Astrocytoma (WHO 3), and GBM (WHO 4). Remember that low grade tumors don't typically enhance (WHO2) and higher grades do (GBM and some Anaplastics). The exception to this rule is the pilocytic astrocytoma which often has an enhancing nodule. GBM is the beast that cannot be stopped. It grows rapidly, it necrosis, it crosses the midline, and it can restrict on diffusion. Remember **Turcot Syndrome** (*that GI polyp thing*) is associated with GBMs.

Gliomatosis Cerebri: A diffuse glioma with extensive infiltration. It involves at least 3 lobes and is often bilateral. The finding is usually mild blurring of the gray-white differentiation of CT, with extensive T2 hyperintensity and little mass effect on MR. It's low grade, so it **doesn't typically enhance**.

Oligodendroglioma: Discussed under the cortical tumors - page 268.

Primary CNS Lymphoma: Seen in end stage AIDS patients, and those post-transplant. EB virus plays a role. Most common type in **non-hodgkin B cell**. *Classic picture would be an intensely enhancing homogeneous solid mass in the periventricular region, with **restricted diffusion**.* However, it can literally look like and do anything. Classic Multiple choice test question is that it is **Thallium Positive on Spect** (toxo is not).

I say restricting brain tumor, you say Lymphoma.

— These next 3 are most common in Peds PEDS —

PXA (Pleomorphic Xanthroastrocytoma): *Discussed under the cortical tumors - page 268.*

DNET :*Discussed under the cortical tumors - page 268.*

Desmoplastic Infantile Ganglioglioma / Astrocytoma "DIG": These guys are **large cystic tumors** that like to involve the superficial cerebral cortex and leptomeninges. Unlike the Atypical Teratoma / Rhabdoid, these have an ok prognosis. They **ALWAYS arise in the supratentorial location** usually involving more than one lobe (frontal and parietal most commonly), and usually present before the first birthday.

-Buzzword is "*rapidly increasing head circumference.*"

Skull Base:

Chordoma – This is a locally aggressive tumor that originates from the notochord.

WTF is the "notochord"? It's an embryology thing thats related to spine development.

The thing you need to know is that the notochord is a midline structure. Therefore all Chordomas are midline - either in the clivus, vertebral bodies (especially C2), or Sacrum. You can NOT get them in the hips, ribs, legs, arms, or any other structure that is not totally midline along the axis of the axial skeleton.

Things to know:
- It is most common in the sacrum (#2 is the clivus)
- When it involves the spine it's most common at C2 - but typically extends across a disc space to involve the adjacent vertebral body.
- It's T2 Bright
- It's ALWAYS Midline.

Chondrosarcoma – This is the main differential of the chordoma in the clivus. The thing to know is that it is **nearly always lateral to midline** *(chordoma is midline)*. These are also T2 bright, but will have the classic "arcs and rings" matrix on a chondrosarcoma. Obviously you'll need a CT to describe that matrix.

—

Dura:

Meningioma – As described above it is common and enhances homogeneously. The most common location is over the cerebral convexity and it has been known to cause hyperostosis.

Hemangiopericytoma – This is a soft tissue sarcoma that can **mimic an aggressive meningioma**, because they both enhance homogeneously. They also can mimic a dural tail, with a narrow base of dural attachment. They **won't calcify or cause hyperostosis, but will invade the skull.**

Mets – The most common met to the dura is from breast cancer. 80% will be at the gray-white junction. They will have more edema than a primary tumor of similar size.

Sella / Parasella - Adults

Pituitary Adenoma – The most common tumor of the sella. They are seen 97% of the time in adults. If they are greater than 1cm they are "macroadenomas." When functional, most are prolactin secreting (especially in women). Symptoms are easy to pick up in women (menstrual irregularity, galactorrhea). Men tend to present later because their symptoms are more vague (decreased libido). On MR, 80% are T1 dark and T2 bright. They take up contrast more slowly than normal brain parenchyma.

> **Pituitary Anatomy Refresher**
>
> FLAT - PEG
>
> FLAT is in the front
> -FSH, LSH, ADH, TSH
>
> PEG is back
> -Prolactin, Endorphins, GSH

Things to know (about Pituitary adenomas):

- *Microadenoma under 10mm,*
- *Macroadenoma over 10mm.*
- *Microadenomas typically form in the adenohypophysis (front 2/3).*
- *Prolactinoma is the most common functional type.*
- *Typically they enhance less than normal pituitary.*

Pituitary Apoplexy – Hemorrhage or Infarction of the pituitary, usually into an enlarged gland (either from pregnancy or a macroadenoma). Here are the multiple choice trivia association: taking **bromocriptine** (or other prolactin drugs), "**Sheehan Syndrome**" in pregnant woman, Cerebral Angiography. They will be **T1 bright** (remember adenoma is usually T1 dark). Supposedly this is an emergent finding because the lack of hormones can cause hypotension.

Rathke Cleft Cyst – Usually an incidental finding, that is rarely symptomatic. They are variable on T1 and T2, but are usually very bright on T2. They do NOT enhance.

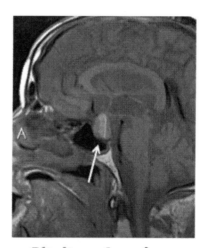

Pituitary Apoplexy
-Shown on T1
-T1 Bright Pituitary

Epidermoid - Discussed on page 274. Remember these guys restrict on diffusion.

Craniopharyngioma – They come in two flavors: (a) Papillary and (b) Adamantinomatous. The Papillary type is the adult type (Papi for Pappi). They are solid and do not have calcifications. They recur less frequently than the Adamantinomatous form (because they are encapsulated). They strongly enhance. The relationship to the optic chiasm is key for surgery. Pediatric type is discussed below (under on the next page with the peds tumors).

Sella / Parasella - Peds

Craniopharyngioma – As stated above, they come in two flavors: (a) Papillary and (b) Adamantinomatous. The kid type is the Adamantinomatous form. These guys are **calcified** (papillary is not). These guys recur more (Papillary does less – because it has a capsule). *Buzzword is "machinery oil."*

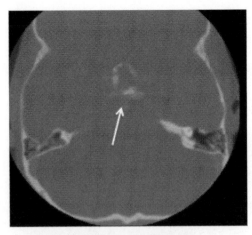

Craniopharyngioma
-Shown on bone window
-Calcifications in the Sella

Hypothalamic Hamartoma – A classic Aunt Minnie. This is a hamartoma of the tuber cinereum (part of the hypothalamus located between the mammillary bodies and the optic chiasm). They are T1 and T2 iso and they do NOT enhance.

The classic history is **gelastic seizures** (although precocious puberty is actually more common).

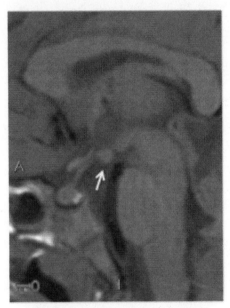

Hamartoma of the Tuber Cinereum

Pineal Region -

There are 3 main characters here, all of which can present with "vertical gaze palsy" (dorsal Parinaud syndrome).

Germinoma: The **more common of the 3**, and seen almost exclusively in boys (Germinomas in the suprasellar region are usually in girls). Precocious puberty may occur from secretion of hCG. Characteristic findings are a **mass containing fat and calcification** with variable contrast enhancement. It is heterogeneous on T1 and T2 (because of its mixed components).

Pineoblastoma: Does occur in childhood. Unlike the pineocytoma these guys are **highly invasive**. Some people like to think of these as PNETs in the pineal gland. They are **associated with retinoblastoma.** They are heterogeneous and enhance vividly.

Pineocytoma: Rare in childhood. Well-circumscribed, and **non-invasive**. Tend to be more solid, and the solid components do typically enhance.

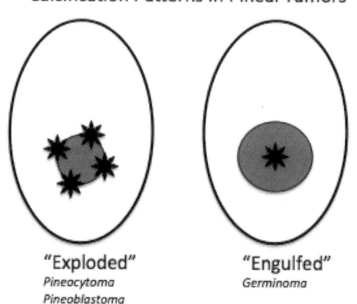

Calcification Patterns in Pineal Tumors

"Exploded"
Pineocytoma
Pineoblastoma

"Engulfed"
Germinoma

Pineal Cyst - An incidental findings that is meaningless… although frequently obsessed over.

Special Topics - A Few Extra Tips on Characterization:

"Restriction"

If they show a supratentorial case with restriction it's likely to be one of two things (1) **Abscess** or (2) **Lymphoma**. Technically any hypercellular tumor can restrict (**GBM, & Medulloblastoma**), but lymphoma is the one they classically show restricting.

If it's a CP angle case, then it's an **epidermoid**.

Lastly, a dirty move could be to show **Herpes** encephalitis restricting in the temporal horns.

"Midline Crossing"

If they show it crossing the midline its most likely going to be a **GBM or Lymphoma**. Alternatively sneaky things they could show doing this would be **radiation necrosis**, a big **MS** plaque in the corpus callosum, or Meningioma of the falx simulating a midline cross.

"Calcification"

If they show it in the brain it is probably an **Oligodendroglioma**. The trick is that Oligodendrogliomas calcify 90% of the time by CT (and 100% by histopathology), whereas astrocytoma only calcify 20% of the time. But astrocytoma is very common and oligodendroglioma is not. So in other words in real life it's probably still an astrocytoma.

"T1 Bright"

Most tumors are T1 dark (or intermediate). Exceptions might include a tumor that has bled (Pituitary apoplexy, or hemorrhagic mets). Hemorrhagic mets are classically seen on **MR** and **CT** (**M**elanoma, **R**enal, **C**arcinoid / **C**horiocarcinoma , **T**hyroid). Tumors with fat will also be T1 bright (Lipoma, Dermoid). Melanin is T1 bright (Melanoma). Lastly think about cholesterol in a colloid cyst.

T1 Bright:

Fat: Dermoid, Lipoma

Melanin: Melanoma

Blood: Bleeding Met or Tumor

Cholesterol: Colloid Cyst

Special Topic Syndromes:

NF-1	Optic Nerve Gliomas
NF-2	MSME: Multiple Schwannomas, Meningiomas, Ependymomas
VHL	Hemangioblastoma (brain and retina)
TS	Subependymal Giant Cell Astrocytoma, Cortical Tubers
Nevoid Basal Cell Syndrome (Gorlin)	Medulloblastoma
Turcot	GBM, Medulloblastoma
Cowdens	Lhermitte-Dulcos (Dysplastic cerebellar gangliocytoma)

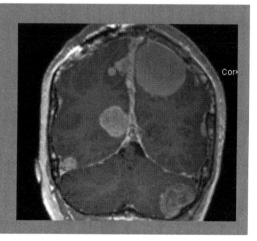

MSME

If you see tumors EVERYWHERE then you are dealing with <u>NF-2</u>. Ironically there are no neurofibromas in neurofibromatosis type 2 (obviously that would make a great distractor).

Just remember **MSME**
  Multiple **S**chwannomas,
  Meningiomas,
  Ependymomas

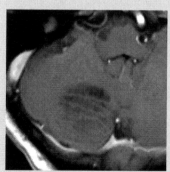

Lhermitte-Dulcos *(Dysplastic cerebellar gangliocytoma)* - This thing is very uncommon, but when you see it you need to have the following thoughts:

  Hey! Thats Lhermitte Dulcos....

  I guess she has Cowdens syndrome....

  I guess she has breast CA

Next Step? - Mammogram

The appearance is classic, with a "tiger stripe" mass, typically contained on one cerebellar hemisphere (occasionally crosses the vermis). It's not a "cancer", but actually a hamartoma - which makes sense since Cowdens is a hamartoma syndrome.

Trauma

Parenchymal Contusion: The rough part of the skull base can scrape the brain as it slides around in a high speed MVA. Typical locations include the anterior temporal lobes and inferior frontal lobes. The concept of coup (site of direct injury) and contre-coup (opposite side of brain along vector of force). Contusion can look like blood with associated edema in the expected regions.

Diffuse Axonal Injury/Shear Injury: There are multiple theories on why this happens (different density of white and gray matter etc…) they don't matter for practical purposes or for multiple choice.

Things to know:

- *Initial Head CT is often normal*
- *Favorite sites of DAI are the posterior corpus callosum, and GM-WM junction in the frontal and temporal lobes*
- *Multiple small T2 bright foci on MRI*

Subarachnoid Hemorrhage: Trauma is the most common cause. FLAIR is the most sensitive sequence. This is discussed in more detail below.

Subdural vs Epidural	
Epidural	**Subdural**
Trauma Patient – with a skull fracture	Old man or alcoholic with an atrophic brain who likes to fall a lot, and stretch / tear those bridging veins.
"Bi-convex" or Lenticular	"Bi-concave"
Can cross the midline	Does not cross the midline, may extend into interhemispheric fissure
Can NOT cross a suture	Can cross a suture
Usually arterial	Usually venous
Can rapidly expand and kill you	

The LeFort Fracture Pattern System: In the dark ages, Rene LeFort beat the skull of cadavers with clubs and threw them off buildings. He then described three facial fracture patterns that interns in ENT and people who write multiple test questions think are important. It can be overly complicated but the most common way a test question is written about these is either by asking the buzzword, or the essential component.

Buzzwords:

- LeFort 1: "The Palate Separated from the Maxilla" or "Floating Palate"
- LeFort 2: "The Maxilla Separated from the Face" or "Pyramidal"
- LeFort 3: "The Face Separated from the Cranium"

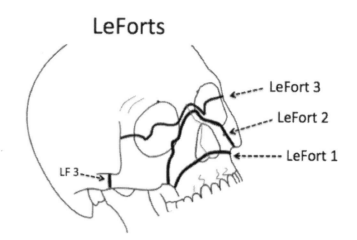

Essential Elements: All three fracture types share the pterygoid process fracture. If the pterygoid process is not involved, you don't have a LeFort. Each has a unique feature (which lends itself easily to multiple choice.

* LeFort 1: Lateral Nasal Aperture
* LeFort 2: Inferior Orbital Rim and Orbital Floor
* LeFort 3: Zygomatic Arch and Lateral Orbital Rim/Wall

Things to Know About Facial Fractures:

- Nasal Bone is the most common fracture
- Zygomaticomaxillary Complex Fracture (Tripod) is the most common fracture pattern, and involves the zygoma, inferior orbit, and lateral orbit.
- Le-Fort Fractures are both a stupid and a high yield topic in facial trauma – for multiple choice. Floating Palate = 1, Pyramidal = 2, Separated Face = 3
- Transverse vs Longitudinal Temporal Bone Fractures – this classification system is stupid and outdated since most are mixed and otic capsule violation is a way better predictive factor… but this is still extremely high yield – see chart on the next page (286).

Mucocele: If you have a fracture that disrupts the frontal sinus outflow tract (usually nasal-orbital-ethmoid types) you can develop adhesions, and obstruction of the sinus resulting in mucocele development. The **buzzword is "airless expanded sinus."** They are usually T1 bright, with a thin rim of enhancement (tumors more often have solid enhancement). The frontal sinus is the most common location – occurring secondary to trauma (as described above).

Temporal Bone Fractures: The traditional way to classify these is longitudinal and transverse and this is almost certainly how the questions will be written. In the real world that system is old and worthless, as most fractures are complex with components of both. The real predictive finding of value is violation of the otic capsule - as described in more modern papers.

Longitudinal	Transverse
Long Axis of T-Bone	Short Axis of T-Bone
More Common	Less Common
More Ossicular Dislocation	More Vascular Injury (Carotid / Jugular)
Less Facial Nerve Damage (around 20%)	More Facial Nerve Damage (>30%)
More Conductive Hearing Loss	More Sensorineural Hearing Loss

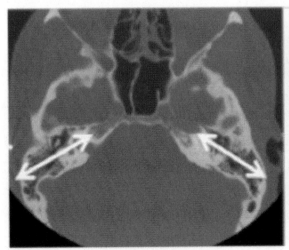
Longitudinal

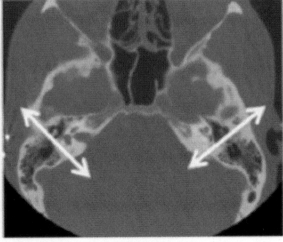
Transverse

How old is that blood?

This is an extremely high yield topic. Maybe the most high yield topic in all of neuro, with regard to multiple choice. The question can be asked with CT or MRI (MRI more likely). If they do ask the question with CT it's most likely to be the subacute subdural that is isointense to brain, with loss sulci along the margins. They could also show the "swirl sign" – see below.

Blood on CT	
Hyperacute Acute (< 1 hour)	Hypodense
Acute (1 hour – 3 days)	Hyperdense
Subacute (4 days – 3 weeks)	Progressively less dense, eventually becoming isodense to brain. **Peripheral rim enhancement may occur with contrast.**
Chronic (> 3 weeks)	Hypodense

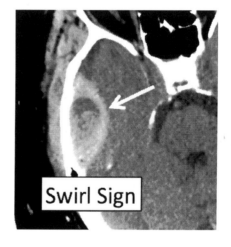

Swirl Sign – This is an ominous sign of active bleeding. The central low attenuation blood represents acute non-clotted blood, with surrounding more acute blood.

MRI is more difficult to remember. Some people use the mnemonic "IB, ID, BD, BB, DD" or "**It B**e **I**ddy **B**iddy, **BaB**y, **D**oo-**D**oo" which I find very irritating. I prefer mnemonics that employ known words (just my opinion). Another one with actual words is "**G**eorge **W**ashington **B**ridge" For T1 (Gray, White, Black), and Oreo Cookie for T2 (Black, White, Black).

Instead of memorizing baby babbling noises, I use this graph showing a clockwise movement. This thing may seem tricky and too much to bear, at first, but it does actually work and once you draw it twice, you'll have it memorized. You'll also notice a few things: (1) you won't feel like a dipshit for making baby noises, (2) you'll have a renewed sense of self-esteem, and (3) you are likely to notice marked improvement in your golf-swing.

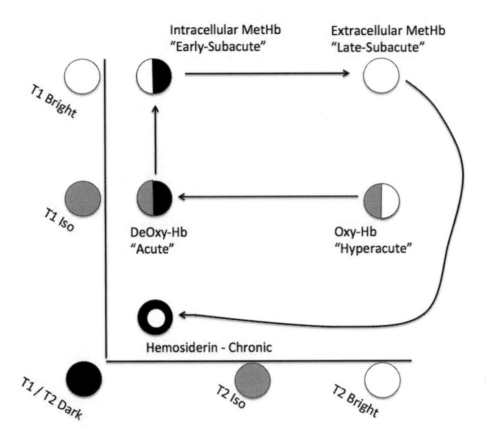

Another strategy is to actually try and understand the MRI changes (I strongly discourage this).

Hyperacute	< 24 hours	Oxyhemoglobin, Intracellular	T1- Iso, T2 Bright
Acute	1-3 days	Deoxyhemoglobin, Intracellular	T1 – Iso, T2 Dark
Early Subacute	> 3 days	Methemoglobin, Intracellular	T1 Bright, T2 Dark
Late Subacute	>7 days	Methemoglobin, Extracellular	T1 Bright, T2 Bright
Chronic	> 14 days	Ferritin and Hemosiderin, Extracellular	T1/ T2 Dark Peripherally, Center may be T2 bright

Hemorrhage (Non-Traumatic)

Subarachnoid Hemorrhage:

Yes, the most common cause is trauma. A common point of trivia is that the **most sensitive sequence on MRI for acute SAH is FLAIR** (because it won't suppress out - making it hyperintense). Be aware that **supplemental oxygen** (usually 50-100%) **can give you a fake out that looks like SAH on FLAIR**. When the blood is real, in the absence of trauma, there are a few other things to think about.

> **Sequella of SAH**
>
> (1) Hydrocephalus - Early
> (2) Vasospasm - 7-10 days
> (3) Superficial Siderosis - Late

- *Aneurysm* – Discussed below.

- **Benign Non-Aneurysm Perimesencephalic hemorrhage**: This is a well described entity (although not well understood). This is NOT associated with aneurysm (usually – 95%), and may be associated with a venous bleed. The location of the blood – around the midbrain and pons without extension into the lateral Sylvian cisterns or interhemispheric fissures is classic. **Just think anterior to the brainstem.** Re-bleeding and ischemia are rare- and they do extremely well.

- **Superficial Siderosis**: This is a side effect of repeated episodes of SAH. I like to think about this as *"staining the surface of the brain with hemosiderin."* The classic look is curvilinear **low signal on gradient coating the surface of the brain.** The classic history is **sensorineural hearing loss and ataxia.**

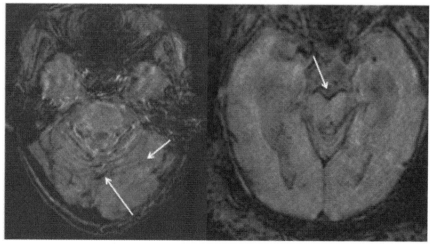

Superficial Siderosis – *Hemosiderin Staining*

Intraparenchymal Hemorrhage:

- **Hypertensive Hemorrhage:** Common locations are the basal ganglia, pons, and cerebellum. For the purpose of multiple choice tests the **basal ganglia is the most common location (specifically the putamen)**. You typically have intraventricular extension of blood.

- **Amyloid Angiopathy:** History of an old dialysis patient (or some other history to think Amyloid). *The classic look is multiple lobes at different ages with scattered microbleeds on gradient.*

- **Septic Emboli:** These are seen in certain clinical scenarios (**IV drug user**, organ transplant, cyanotic heart disease, AIDS patients, people with lung AVMs). **The classic look is numerous small foci of restricted diffusion. Septic emboli to the brain result in abscess, mycotic aneurysms (most commonly in the distal MCAs),** The location favors the gray-white interface and the basal ganglia. There will be surrounding edema around the tiny abscesses. The classic scenario should be parenchymal bleed in a patient with infection.

- **Other random causes:** This would include AVMs, vasculitis, brain tumors (primary and mets) - these are discussed in greater detail in various section of the text.

Intraventricular Hemorrhage:

- Not as exciting. Just think about trauma, tumor, hypertension, AVMs, and aneurysms – all the usual players.

Epidural / Subdural Hemorrhage:

- Obviously these are usually post-traumatic.

- **Dural AVFs and High Flow AVMs** can bleed causing subdurals / subarachnoid spaces. These are discussed further, later in the chapter.

Vascular

Stroke –

Stroke is a high yield topic. You can broadly categorize stroke into ischemic (80%) and hemorrhagic (20%). It's critical to remember that stroke is a clinical diagnosis and that imaging findings compliment the diagnosis.

WaterShed Zones: Below is a diagram showing the various vascular territories. The junction between these zones is sometimes referred to as a "Watershed". These areas are prone to ischemic injury, especially in the setting of hypotension or low oxygen states (near drowning or Roger Gracie's cross choke from the mount).

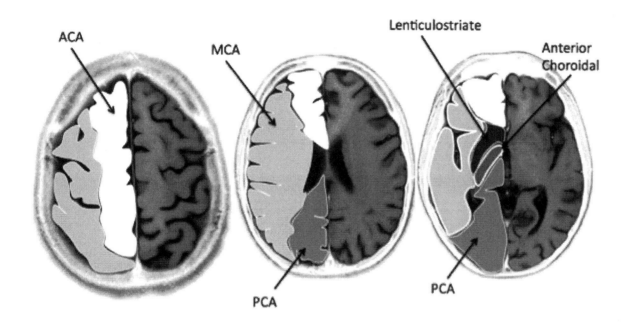

Gamesmanship: **Watershed Infarcts in a Kid = Moyamoya**

Imaging Signs on CT:

Dense MCA Sign	Intraluminal thrombus is dense, usually in the M1 and/or M2 segments
Insular Ribbon Sign	Loss of normal high density insular cortex from cytotoxic edema
Loss of GM-WM differentiation	Basal Ganglia / Internal Capsular Region and Subcortical regions
Mass Effect	Peaks to 3-5 days
Enhancement	Rule of 3s: Starts in 3 days, peaks in 3 weeks, gone by 3 months.

"Fogging" - This is a phase in the evolution of stroke when the infarcted brain looks like normal tissue. This is seen around 2-3 weeks post infarct. "Fogging" is classically described with non-contrast CT, but T2 MRI sequences have a similar effect (typically occurring around day 10). In the real world, you could give IV contrast to demarcate the area of infarct or just understand that fogging occurs.

Imaging Signs on MRI:

Restricted Diffusion: Acute infarcts usually are bright from about 30 mins after the stroke to about 2 weeks. **Restricted diffusion without bright signal on FLAIR should make you think hyperacute (< 6 hours).**

Not Everything That Restricts is a Stroke —
Bacterial Abscess, CJD (cortical), Herpes, Epidermoids, Hypercellular Brain Tumors (Classic is lymphoma), Acute MS lesions, Oxyhemoglobin, and Post Ictal States. Also artifacts (susceptibility and T2 shine through).

Enhancement: The rule of 3's is still useful. Enhancement starts around day 3, it peaks around 3 weeks, and is gone by 3 months.

	0-6 hours	6-24 hours	24 hours -1 week
Diffusion	Bright	Bright	Bright
FLAIR	**NOT BRIGHT**	Bright	Bright
T1	Iso	Dark	Dark, with Bright Cortical Necrosis
T2	Iso	Bright	Bright

Hemorrhagic Transformation – This occurs in about 50% of infarcts, with the typical time period between 6 hours and 4 days. If you got TPA it's usually within 24 hours of treatment. People break these into (1) tiny specs in the gray matter called "petechial" which is the majority (90%) and (2) full on hematoma – about 10%.

Who gets it? People on anticoagulation, people who get TPA, people with embolic strokes (especially large ones), venous infarcts.

Predictors of Hemorrhagic Transformation in Patients Getting TPA
Multiple Strokes, Proximal MCA occlusion, **Greater than 1/3 of the MCA territory**, Greater than 6 hours since onset "delayed recanalization", Absent collateral flow

Venous Infarct: Not all infarcts are arterial, you can also stroke secondary to venous occlusion (usually the sequelae of dural venous sinus thrombosis or deep cerebral vein thrombosis). In general, venous infarcts are at higher risk for hemorrhagic transformation. In little babies think dehydration, in older children think about mastoiditis, in adults think about coagulopathies (protein C & S def) and oral contraceptives. The most common site of thrombosis is the sagittal sinus, with associated infarct occurring 75% of the time.

Venous thrombosis can present as a dense sinus or "empty delta" on contrast. Venous infarcts tend to have *heterogeneous restricted diffusion*. Venous thrombosis can result in vasogenic edema that eventually progresses to stroke and cytotoxic edema.

- Arterial stroke = Cytotoxic Edema
- Venous Stroke = Vasogenic Edema + Cytotoxic Edema

Stigmata of chronic venous thrombosis include the development of a a dural AVF, or increased CSF pressure from impaired drainage.

Aneurysm

Who gets them? People who smoke, polycystic kidney disease, connection tissue disorders (Marfans, Ehlers-Danlos), people with aortic coarctation, NF, FMD, and AVMs.

Where do they occur? They occur at branch points (why do persistent trigeminals get more aneurysms ? – because they have more branch points). They favor the anterior circulation (90%) – with the **anterior communicating artery being the most common site**. As a piece of random trivia the basilar is the most common posterior circulation location (PICA origin is the second most common).

When do they rupture? Rupture risk is increased with size, a posterior location, history of prior SAH, smoking history, and female gender.

Which one did it? A common dilemma is SAH in the setting of multiple aneurysms. The things that can help you are location of the SAH/Clot, location of the vasospasm, size, and which one is the most irregular (*Focal out-pouching - "Murphy's tit"*)

Aneurysm Types:

Saccular (Berry): The most common type. They are commonly seen at bifurcations. The underlying pathology may be a congenital deficiency of the internal elastic lamina and tunica media (at branch points). Remember that most are idiopathic (with the associations listed above). They are multiple 15-20% of the time.

Fusiform Aneurysm – Associated with PAN, Connective Tissue Disorders, or Syphilis. These more commonly affect the posterior circulation. May mimic a CPA mass.

Pseudo Aneurysm – Think about this with an irregular (often sacular) arterial out-pouching at a strange / atypical location. You may see focal hematoma next to the vessel on non-contrast.

- *Traumatic* – Often distal secondary to penetrating trauma or adjacent fracture.

- *Mycotic* – Often distal (most commonly in the MCA), with the associated history of endocarditis, meningitis, or thrombophlebitis.

Pedicle Aneurysm – Aneurysm associated with an AVM. The trivia to know is that it's **found on the artery feeding the AVM** (75% of the time). *These may be higher risk to bleed than the AVM itself (because they are high flow).*

Blister Aneurysm – This is a sneaky little dude (the angio is often negative). It's broad-based at a non-branch point (supraclinoid ICA is the most common site).

Infundibular Widening – Not a true aneurysm, but instead a funnel-shaped enlargement at the origin of the Posterior Communicating Artery at the junction with the ICA. *Thing to know is "not greater than 3mm."*

Saccular (Berry)	Branch Points – in the Anterior Circulation
Fusiform	Posterior Circulation
Pedicle Aneurysm	Artery feeding the AVM
Mycotic	Distal MCAs
Blister Aneurysm	Broad Based Non-Branch Point (Supraclinoid ICA)

Maximum Bleeding – Aneurysm Location	
ACOM	Interhemispheric Fissure
PCOM	Ipsilateral Basal Cistern
MCA Trifurcation	Sylvian Fissure
Basilar Tip	Interpeduncular Cistern, or Intraventricular
PICA	Posterior Fossa or Intraventricular

Vascular Malformation:

There are 6 different kinds, and I will actually touch on all 6 – some in more detail than others.

(1) **High Flow AVMs:** This is the most common type of high flow lesion. They favor a supratentorial location and are the result of a congenital malformation in the development of the capillary bed. As the name "high flow" implies there is an arterial component (arterial component -> nidus -> draining veins). Hemorrhage is the most common complication, and has a bleeding incidence of about 3% per year. Seizure would be the second most common complication, and the adjacent brain may be atrophic and gliotic.

- *Increased Bleeding Risk: Small size of AVM (actually higher pressure), single draining vein, intranidal/perinidal aneurysm, basal ganglia/thalamic/ periventricular locations.*

(2) **Dural AVF:** These can be high flow or low flow. They are less common than the high flow AVMs. Unlike the AVM these are thought to be acquired secondary to dural sinus thrombosis. Unlike AVMs there is no nidus. This presents in the 50s-60s (AVMs present in 20s-30s). **Classic symptom is pulsatile tinnitus, when it involves the sigmoid sinus.** May have vision problems if the cavernous sinus is involved.

- *Increased Bleeding Risk: Direct cortical venous drainage.*
- *Can be occult on MRI/MRA - need catheter angio if suspicion high*
- *SPINAL AVFs are actually the most common type of AVFs - a helpful hint is the classic clinical history of "gradual onset LE weakness"*

(3) **DVA:** This is not actually a vascular malformation, just a variation in normal venous drainage. If you tried to resect one, you would end up with a nice venous infarct. Some buzzwords are "caput medusa" or "large tree with multiple small branches" – to describe its appearance. The big thing to remember is the **association with cavernous malformations.**

(4) **Cavernous Malformation:** These things are also called "cavernomas" and "cavernous angiomas." These are low flow lesions with a dilated capillary bed **without intervening normal brain tissue.** They can be single or multiple (more common in Hispanics). Buzzword is "popcorn-like" with "peripheral rim of hemosiderin." Look for them on gradient (because of the hemosiderin). They can ooze some blood, but typically don't have full-on catastrophic bleeds. As mentioned above, they may have a nearby DVA.

(5) **Capillary Telangiectasia:** This is another slow flow lesion, that unlike the cavernoma **does have intervening normal brain tissue**. They don't bleed and are usually totally incidental. The most common look for this is a single lesion in the pons. Again these are best seen on gradient (slow flow and deoxyhemoglobin). The buzzword is "brush-like" or "stippled pattern" of enhancement. Key high yield fact is that **these can develop as a complication of radiation therapy**.

(6) **Mixed** – This is a wastebasket term, most often used for DVA with AV shunting or DVAs with telangiectasias.

Vasospasm

Vessels do not like to be bathed in blood (SAH), it makes them freak out (spasm). The **classic timing for this is 4-14 days after SAH (NOT immediately)**. It usually looks like smooth, long segments of stenosis. It typically involves multiple vascular territories. It can lead to stroke.

Who gets it? It's usually for SAH and the more volume of SAH the greater the risk. In 1980 some neurosurgeon came up with this thing called the Fisher Score, which grades vasospasm risk. The gist of it is greater than 1mm in thickness or intraventricular / parenchymal extension is at higher risk.

Are there Non-SAH causes of vasospasm? Yep. Meningitis, PRES, and Migraine Headache.

Critical Take Home Point - Vasospasm is a delayed side effect of SAH. I does NOT occur immediately after a bleed. You see it 4-14 days after SAH.

Vascular Dissection

Vascular dissection can occur from a variety of etiologies (usually penetrating trauma, or a trip to the chiropractor). Penetrating trauma tends to favor the carotids, and blunt trauma tends to favor the vertebrals. This would be way too easy to show on CT as a flap, so if it's shown it's much more likely to be the T1 bright "crescent sign", or intramural hematoma.

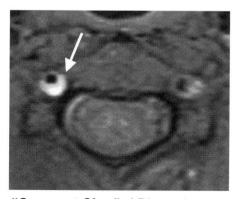

"Crescent Sign" of Dissection
- it's the T1 bright intramural blood.

Vasculitis

You can have a variety of causes of CNS vasculitis. One way to think about it is by clumping it into (a) Primary CNS vasculitis, (b) Secondary CNS vasculitis from infection, or sarcoid, (c) systemic vasculitis with CNS involvement, and (d) CNS vasculitis from a systemic disease.

Primary CNS vasculitis	Primary Angiitis of the CNS (PACNS)
Secondary CNS vasculitis from infection, or sarcoid	**Meningitis** (bacterial, TB, Fungal). Septic Embolus, Sarcoid,
Systemic vasculitis with CNS involvement	**PAN**, Temporal Arteritis, Wegeners, Takayasu's,
CNS vasculitis from a Systemic Disease	**Cocaine Use**, RA, SLE, Lyme's

They all pretty much look the same with multiple segmental areas of vessel narrowing, with alternating dilation ("beaded appearance"). You can have focal areas of vascular occlusion.

Trivia:

- *PAN is the Most Common systemic vasculitis to involve the CNS (although it is a late finding).*
- *SLE is the Most Common Collagen Vascular Disease*

Misc Vascular Conditions

Moyamoya – This non-atherosclerotic poorly understood entity (originally described in Japan – hence the name), is characterized by progressive stenosis of the supraclinoid ICA eventually leading to occlusion. The progressive stenosis results in an enlargement of the basal perforating arteries.

Things to know:

- *Buzzword = "Puff of Smoke" – for angiographic appearance*
- *Watershed Distribution*
- *In a child think sickle cell*
- *Other notable associations include: NF, prior radiation, Downs syndrome*
- *Bi-Modal Age Distribution (early childhood, and middle age)*
- *Children Stroke, Adults Bleed*

CADASIL *– (Cerebral Autosomal Dominant Arteriopathy with Subcortical Infarcts and Leukoencephalopathy).* Think about a 40 year old **presenting with migraine headaches**, then eventually dementia. The MRI will show severe white matter disease involving multiple vascular territories, in the frontal and **temporal lobe**. The occipital lobes are often spared.

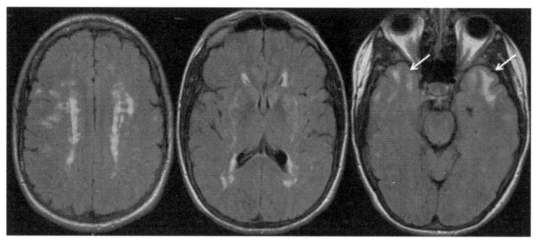

CADASIL – *Diffuse White Matter Disease, Hitting the Temporals, Sparing Occipitals*

NASCET Criteria: The North American Symptomatic Carotid Endarterectomy Trial (NASCET) criteria, is used for carotid stenosis.

The rule is: measure the degree of stenosis using the maximum internal carotid artery stenosis ("A") compared to a parallel (non-curved) segment of the distal, cervical internal carotid artery ("B").

You then use the formula [1- A/B] X 100%.

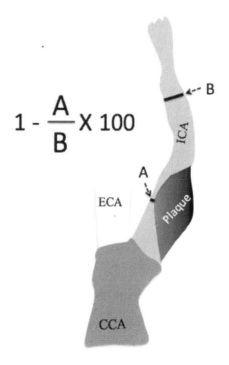

Developmental / Congenital

Congenital malformations is a very confusing and complicated topic, full of lots of long Latin and French sounding words. If we want to keep it simple and somewhat high yield you can look at it in 6 basic categories: (1) Failure to form, (2) Failure to cleave, (3) Failure to migrate, (4) Normal forming but massive insult makes you look like you didn't form (5) Herniation syndromes, and (6) Craniosynostosis.

Failure to Form:

A classic point of trivia is that the corpus callosum forms front to back (then rostrum last). Therefore hypoplasia of the corpus callosum is usually absence of the splenium (with the genu intact).

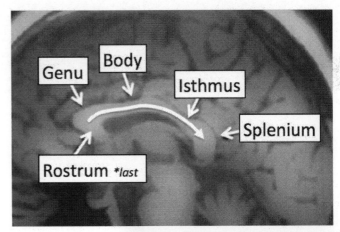

With agenesis of the corpus callosum, a common trick is to show colpocephaly (asymmetric dilation of the occipital horns).

When you see this picture you should say two things:

(1) Corpus Callosum Agenesis
(2) Pericallosal Lipoma

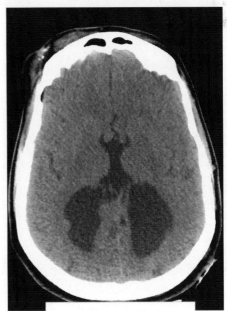

Colpocephaly
(asymmetric dilation of the occipital horns).

300

Callosal Dysgenesis / Agenesis: This is associated with lots of other syndromes/ malformations (Lipoma, heterotopias, schizencephaly, lissencephaly etc…). **"Most common anomaly seen with other CNS malformations."** If they ask this, it will either be the colpocephaly picture, the **steer horn** appearance of coronal, or the **vertical ventricles** widely spaced (racing car) on axial.

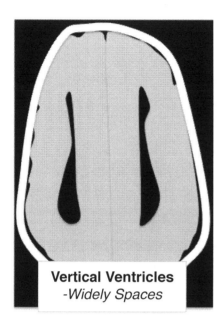
Vertical Ventricles
-Widely Spaces

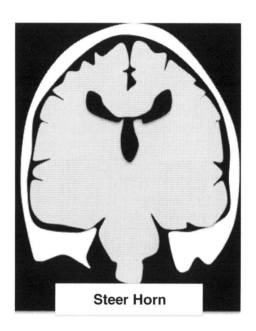
Steer Horn

Why are the lateral ventricles widely spaced when you have no Corpus Callosum ? There are these things called **"Probst bundles"** which are densely packed WM tracts - destined to cross the CC - but can't (because it isn't there). So instead they run parallel to the interhemispheric fissure -making the vents look widely spaced.

Intracranial Lipoma: Associated with callosal dysgenesis. 50% are found in the interhemispheric fissure and if they show it that's where is will be.

Trivia: CNS Lipomas are congenital malformations, not true neoplasms. The tubulonodular type frequently calcify.

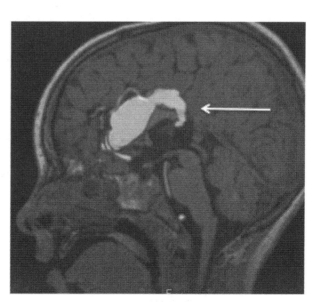
Intracranial Lipoma

Anencephaly: Neural tube fails to close on the cranial end leading to reduced or absent cerebrum and cerebellum. The hindbrain will be present. Obviously this is not compatible with life. Trivia: **AFP will be elevated**, **polyhydraminos** will be present (hard to swallow without a brain). If they show it, it will have to be antenatal ultrasound and will likely be polyhydramnios plus the incredibly creepy **"frog eye" appearance** on the coronal plane (due to absent cranial bone / brain with bulging orbits).

Iniencephaly: Rare neural defect with the main features including deficit of the occipital bones. This results in an enlarged foramen magnum. These guys also have really jacked up spines. **"Star Gazing Fetus"** is the buzzword because they are contorted in a way that makes their face turn upward (hyper-extended cervical spine, short neck, and upturned face).

Arhinencephaly: No olfactory bulbs and tracts. Seen with **Kallmann Syndrome** (hypogondaism, mental retardation).

Rhombencephalosynapsis: Congenital anomaly of the cerebellum, where the vermis doesn't develop and instead you just fuse your cerebellum. Classically a transversely oriented singe lobed cerebellum is shown (this is an Aunt Minnie).

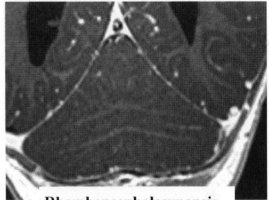

Rhombencephalosynapsis
-*Note the Vertical Line Across the Cerebellum*

Joubert Syndrome: OK so this is another Aunt Minnie, because of the **"Molar Tooth" appearance** of the superior cerebellar peduncles (they are elongated like the roots of a tooth). There is going to be a small or aplastic cerebellar vermis, and there will be absence of pyramindal decussation. It has a **strong association (50%) with retinal dysplasia.** There is also an association with multicystic dysplastic kidneys (30%). When you see it in combination with liver fibrosis it's a total zebra (near unicorn) called COACH syndrome.

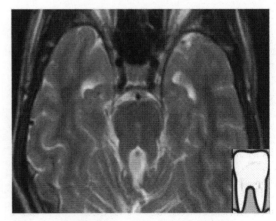

Joubert – Molar Tooth

Dandy Walker:

Radiologists love to nitpick and obsess over details. Usually, the more meaningless the detail the more ferocious the debate. Along those lines...

This is a "spectrum" that leads to much confusion and argument. For the purpose of the multiple choice tests I would just say that Dandy Walker = Absent Vermis. **The buzzword is "torcular-lambdoid inversion."** *The torcular is above the level of the lambdoid due to abnormally high tentorium.*

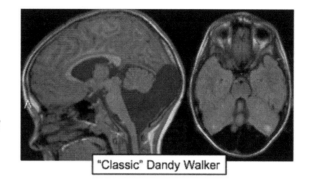

"Classic" Dandy Walker

The following chart is just for the sake of addressing the ridiculousness of this posterior fossa situation. It ought to be very low yield for the exam (which probably means it is high-yield). It may also be useful if you want to join in the debate.

Morphology (Most Severe -> Least Severe)	Features			
Ventriculocele" DWM Variant	Cystic Dilation of 4th	Complete or partial Agenesis of the Vermis	Enlarged Posterior Fossa PLUS erosion into the occipital bone -> encephalocele	
"Classic" DWM	Cystic Dilation of 4th	Complete or partial Agenesis of the Vermis	Enlarged Posterior Fossa	Superiorly rotated vermian remnant
"Variant" DWM	Partially obstructed 4th Ventricle	Variable Hypoplasia of the Vermis (*less severe*)	Posterior Fossa **NOT enlarged**	
Persistent Blake Pouch	Cyst below and posterior to the vermis	Normal Vermis	Posterior Fossa **NOT enlarged**	The tentorium is elevated
Mega Cisterna Magna	Retro-Cerebellar CSF Space > 10mm	Cerebellum Normal	Enlarged posterior fossa caused by enlarged cisterna magna	

Failure To Cleave

Holoprosencephaly (HPE): This is a midline cleaving problem with the brain failing to cleave into two separate hemispheres. The cleavage apparently occurs back to front (opposite of the formation of the corpus callosum), so in milder forms the posterior cortex is normal and the anterior cortex is fused.

It is classified as a spectrum:

Lobar → *Semilobar* → *Alobar (most severe)*

Lobar *(mild)*	Semi-Lobar	Alobar *(severe)*
Right and Left Hemispheres are separate (anterior/inferior frontal still sometimes fused)	Basic structure present but **fused at the thalami**. Posterior brain is normal.	There is a **single large ventricle**, with fusion of the thalami and basal ganglia.
May be limited to absent septum pellucidum	Olfactory tracts and bulbs are gone	No Falx. No corpus callosum.
Pituitary Problems are common		

The old saying "face predicts brain, but brain doesn't predict face" is actually mostly true. In other words, monster Cyclops babies usually have some midline defect (holoprosencephaly). There are several other associations that are frequently shown and often testable:

HPE Associations:

- Single Midline Monster Eye
- Solitary Median Maxillary Incisor (MEGA-Incisor)
- Nasal Process Overgrowth leading to Pyriform Aperture Stenosis

 : **Meckel-Gruber Syndrome:**
- Classic triad:
    - o Holoprosencephaly,
    - o Multiple Renal Cysts and
    - o Polydactyly

Anencephaly: This actually means "no –brain". This is basically the extreme end of the Holoprosencephaly spectrum. You are going to have no brain (only a brainstem), no skull, and no scalp. *See the reproductive chapter in Volume 1 for more on this.*

Failure to Migrate / Proliferate:

Hemimegalencephaly: Rare but unique (Aunt Minnie) malformation characterized by **enlargement of all or part/s of one cerebral hemisphere**. The cause of this condition is speculated to be problem of neuronal differentiation and cell migration in a single hemisphere. The affected hemisphere may have focal or diffuse neuronal migration defects, including areas of polymicrogyria, pachygyria, and heterotopia.

Here is the trick: Look at which side (the big side or the little side) has the ventriculomegaly.

- *Small Side + Big Ventricle = Atrophy (as might be seen with Rasmussen's Encephalitis)*
- *Big Side + Big Ventricle = Hemimegalencephaly*

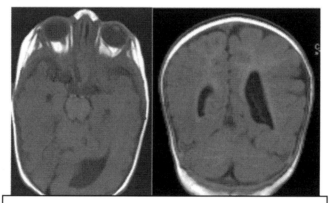

Hemimegalencephaly - *Big Side Big Ventricle*

Lissencephaly-Pachygyria Spectrum: The spectrum of diseases that cause relative smoothness of the brain surface. Vocabulary includes agyria (no gyri), pachygyria (broad gyri) and lissencephaly (smooth brain surface).

You can think about it as either:

- Type 1/Classic form = Smooth Brain. This results from arrest of migration. Buzzwords include **"figure 8"**, "**hours glass** appearance", "vertically oriented **shallow Sylvian fissures**". This one is associated with band heterotopias.

- Type II as a cobblestone brain. This results from over migration. There is not band heterotopia and the cortex is thinner than type I.

Grey Matter Heterotopias:
"Normal Neurons in Abnormal Locations" These guys can be grouped and then grouped and then subgrouped into groups.

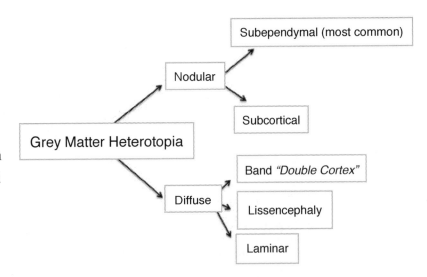

They are associated with other congenital neurologic conditions. A random point of trivia: if you are trying to compare subependymal heterotopias with the subependymal tubers of TS, the tubers are usually higher on T2 signal than gray matter and are often calcified (except in early childhood).

Schizencephaly: Migrational disorder that results in a grey matter lined cleft that will extend through the entire hemisphere. It comes in two main flavors: (1) Closed Lip (20%) and (2) Open Lip (80%).

Highly Testable Associations:
- *Optic Nerve Hypoplasia (30%)*
- *Absent Septum Pellucidum (70%)*
- *Epilepsy (demonic possession) 50-80%*

Classic THIS vs THAT: Porencephalic Cyst vs Open Lip Schizencephaly.

They look very similar, but the schizencephalic cleft should be lined with gray matter, and is a true malformation. The porencephalic cyst is a just a hole from a prior encephaloclastic event (ischemia). *Normal forming but massive insult makes you look like you didn't form.*

Hydranencephaly: Devastating condition characterized by destruction of the cerebral hemispheres. Basically this turns the skull into a bag of CSF. It is thought to be secondary to a vascular insult in utero (**think double MCA infarct**). This could be seen in the setting of a TORCH causing a necrotizing vasculitis (HSV does this). The key point is that you did have a normal brain, so you have a falx, but the cortical mantle is gone.

"Lots of CSF" - Brain Strategy

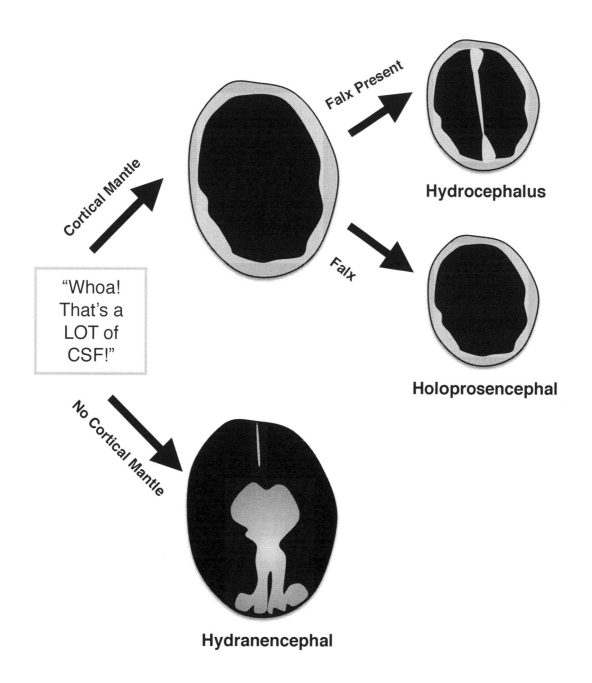

Herniation Syndrome Vocab

Cephaloceles – Herniation of the cranial contents through a defect in the skull.

- Meningoencephalocele – brain + Meninges
- Meningocele – just meninges (no brain)

Chiari Malformations:

Chiari malformation essentially occurs because of a mismatch between size and content of the posterior fossa.

Type 1: These guys have headaches. Criteria is one cerebellar tonsil **more than 5mm below the foramen magnum**. This is often accompanied by crowding of the posterior fossa and you should look for syringohydromyelia (seen in about 50% of cases). As you age, the tonsils ascend, so 3mm below the foramen in a 90 year old would be abnormal. There are several associations but the one that is most often asked is with Klippel-Feil syndrome (congenital C-spine fusion).

Type 2: This type is more complicated and there are like 20 findings. Hydrocephalus is found in more than 90% of cases. I'm going to try and pick the five I think they are most likely to ask or show.

- Myelomenigocele – Lumbar Spine
- Towering Cerebellum
- Tectal Plate Beaking
- Long Skinny 4th Ventricle (*elongated craniocaudally, short in other dimensions*) --- a normal 4th ventricle may suggest shunt malfunction
- Interdigitated Cerebral Gyri (most likely shown on axial CT, single image)

Type 3: Just think Chiari II + Encephalocele (either high cervical or low occipital)

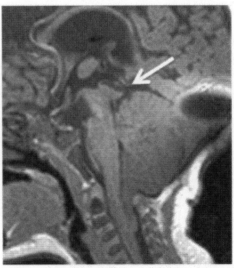

Tectal Beaking – Chiari 2

Craniosynostosis

Premature fusion of one or more of the cranial sutures can result in a weird shaped head. I have just a few high yield points regarding the subject. **S**caphocephaly (**S**agittal Suture) is the most common subtype and is often referred to a dolichocephaly. Brachycephaly (Coronal and/or Lambdoid) is often associated with syndromes.

Of course they are all zebras but a few are worth knowing:

- *Aperts:* Brachycephaly + Fused Fingers
- *Crouzons:* Usually Brachycepahly (but not always) + First Arch (Maxilla and Mandible Hypoplasia)
- *Cleidocranial Dysostosis*: Brachycephaly + Wormian Bones + Absent Clavicles

Plagiocephaly can result from unilateral coronal or lambdoid suture fusion (frontal or occipital plagiocephaly). **Ipsilateral coronal fusion can elevate the superior orbital wall and cause a harlequin eye.**

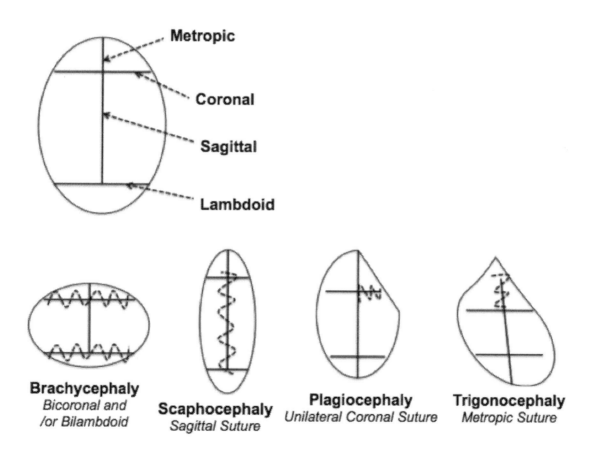

High Yield Trivia / Buzzwords for Craniosynostosis:

- Most common type = sagittal (dolichocephaly or scaphocephaly)
- Sagittal Suture craniosynostosis almost always (80%) affects boys
- Coronal Suture Craniosynostosis affects more girls.
- "Harlequin Eye" = Unilateral Coronal Suture Craniosynostosis (lifts supra-orbital margin).
- Lambdoid Craniosynostosis favors the right side (70%)
- Turricephaly (the tower) is from both coronal and lambdoid fusion

Misc Peds Brain Conditions:

Enlarged extra-axial fluid spaces: Extra-axial fluid spaces are considered enlarged if greater than 5mm. **BESSI** is the name people throw around for "**b**enign **e**nlargement of the **s**ubarachnoid **s**pace in **i**nfancy." The etiology is supposed to be immature villa (that's why you grow out of it).

> **BESSI vs Subdural Collection**
>
> **BESSI** - Cortical veins are adjacent to the inner table
>
> **Subdural** - Cortical veins are displaced away from the inner table.

BESSI Trivia: (1) It's the most common cause of macrocephaly, (2) it typically resolves after 2 years with no treatment, (3) there is an increased risk of subdural bleed - either spontaneous or with a minor trauma.

Trivia - Pre-mature kids getting tortured on ECMO often get enlarged extra-axial spaces. This isn't really the same thing as BESSI and more related to fluid changes / stress.

Choanal Atresia: This is a malformation of the choanal openings. Buzzwords are *"failure to pass NG tube"* and *"respiratory distress while feeding"* (neonates have to breath through their noses). It's usually unilateral (2/3). There are two different types: bony (90%), and membranous (10%). The appearance is a unilateral or bilateral posterior nasal narrowing, with thickening of the vomer. There are a bunch of syndromic associations: CHARGE, Crouzons, DiGeorge, Treacher Colins, and Fetal Alcohol Syndrome.

Piriform Aperture Stenosis – This can occur in isolation or with choanal atresia. The big thing to know is the **high association with hypothalamic-pituitary-adrenal axis dysfunction.**

MELAS – This is a mitochondrial disorder with lactic acidosis and stroke like episodes. The SPECT question is always: increased lactate, decreased NAA.

Leukodystrophies: These are zebra disorders that affect the white matter in kids. If you see a brain MRI on a kid with jacked up white matter, you should be thinking about one of these guys. The distinction between them is totally academic, since they are all untreatable and fatal.

Here are my tricks:
- *Canavans* is always shown with SPECT – with an elevated NAA.
- *Alexanders* has a big head (like Alexander the Great), and has frontal white matter involvement (frontal because of his personality disorder - metaphorically speaking).
- *Metachromatic* is the most common, and the buzzword is "tigroid." Tigroid refers to dark spots or stripes within the T2 bright demylinated periventricular white matter.

	Head Size	Age	Territory	Trivia
Metachromatic	Normal Head	Infantile form 1-2 yo. Juvenile form 5-7	Diffuse white matter involvement, with **tigroid appearance**.	**Most common Leukodystrophy**. Deficiency of the enzyme arylsulfatase A.
Adreno Leukodystrophy	Normal Head	5-10 yo.	Symmetric occipital and splenium of corpus callosum white matter involvement.	Sex-linked recessive condition (peroxisomal enzyme deficiency) **occurring only in boys.**
Leigh disease	Normal Head	Less than 5 yo.	Focal areas of subcortical white matter. Basal ganglia and periaquaductal gray matter involvement.	Also called subacute necrotizing encephalo-myelopathy. Mitochondrial enzyme defect.
Alexander disease	Big Head	Less than 1 yo.	**Frontal white matter** involvement.	
Canavan disease	Big Head	Less than 1 yo.	Diffuse Bilateral sub cortical U fibers.	Elevated NAA (MRS).

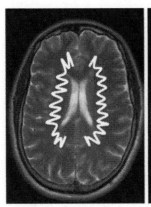
Metachromatic

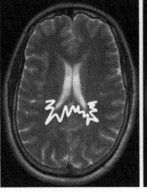
Adreno

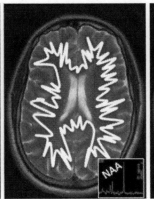
Canavans

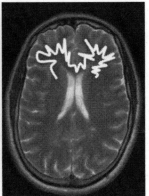
Alexander

High Yield MR SPECT Trivia:

- The highest normal peak is NAA.
- The NAA peak will be super high with Canavans.
- Choline is elevated in anything that causes cell turnover (tumor, infarct, or inflammation).
- Lactate and Lipid peaks superimpose - you need to use an intermediate TE (around 140) to causes an "inversion" of the lactate peak (so you can see it).
- Lactate-Lipid peak has a characteristic "double peak" at a long TE (around 280)
- A normal adult head should not have a lactate peak (it's a marker of aerobic metabolism) - so you see it in necrotic tumors (high grade) and infection (cerebral abscess).
- It's normal to see lactate elevated in the first hours of life. **Remember exceptions to rules are always high yield.*
- Myoinositol is elevated with Alzheimer's and low grade gliomas
- Alanine elevation is specific for Meningiomas
- Meningiomas do NOT have elevated NAA.
- Glutamine is elevated in Hepatic Encephalopathy
- High Grade Tumor = Choline Up, NAA down, Lactate and Lipids Up
- Low Grade Tumor = Choline Down, NAA down, Inositol Up
- Radiation Necrosis Pattern: Choline Down, NAA Down, Lactate Up

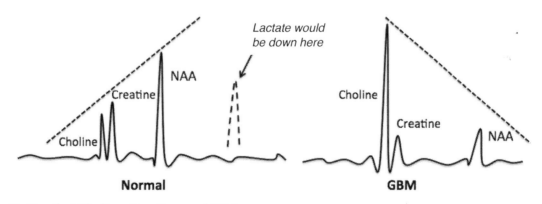

Notice that Choline, Creatine, and NAA fall in alphabetical order. That makes it easy to remember which is which

- *Vocab:* The normal dotted line is called "Hunter's Angle"

Section 2: Head and Neck

Temporal Bones:

Petrous Apex:

Anatomic Variation: Variation can occur in the amount of pneumatization, marrow fat, bony continuity, and vascular anatomy.

- *Asymmetric Marrow:* - Typically the petrous apex contains significant fat, closely following the scalp and orbital fat (T1 and T2 bright). When it's asymmetric you can have two problems (1) falsely thinking you've got an infiltrative process, when you don't and (2) overlooking a T1 bright thing (cholesterol granuloma) thinking it's fat. The key is to use STIR or some other fat saturating sequence.

- *Cephaloceles:* - A cephalocoele describes a herniation of CNS content through a defect in the cranium. In the petrous apex they are a slightly different animal. They don't contain any brain tissue, and simply represent cystic expansion and herniation of the posterolateral portion of Meckel's cave into the superomedial aspect of the petrous apex. Describing it as a **herniation of Meckel's Cave would be more accurate**. These are usually unilateral and are classically described as *"smoothly marginated lobulated cystic expansion of the petrous apex."*

- *Variant Anatomy of the Carotid Artery:* - The 2 main variants to be aware of are the persistent stapedial artery, and aberrant internal carotid. For the purpose of the exam the only things to know are **don't biopsy them** *(they aren't glomus tympanicum tumors),* and **they can give pulsatile tinnitus.**

Inflammatory Lesions:

- **Cholesterol Granuloma** – The **most common primary petrous apex lesion**. Mechanism is likely obstruction of the air cell, with repeated cycles of hemorrhage and inflammation leading to expansion and bone remodeling. The most common symptom is hearing loss. On CT the margins will be sharply defined. On MRI it's gonna be **T1 and T2 bright,** with T2 dark hemosiderin rim, and faint peripheral enhancement. The slow growing ones can be watched. The fast growing ones need surgery.

    o *Key Point; Cholesterol Granuloma = T1 and T2 Bright.*

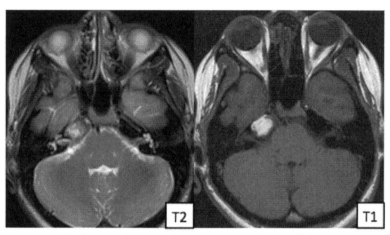

Cholesterol Granuloma = *T1 and T2 Bright.*

- **Cholesteatoma** - This is basically an epidermoid (ectopic epithelial tissue). They are congenital (not acquired) in the petrous apex. They are typically slow growing, and produce bony changes similar to cholesterol granuloma. The difference is their MRI findings; T1 dark, T2 bright, and restricted diffusion.

    o *Key Point; Cholesteatoma = T1 Dark, T2 Bright, Restricted Diffusion*

Cholesterol Granuloma	*Cholesteatoma*
T1 Bright	T1 Dark
T2 Bright	T2 Bright
Doesn't Restrict	**Does Restrict**
Smooth Expansile Bony Change	Smooth Expansile Bony Change

Apical Petrositis – Infection of the petrous apex is a rare complication of infectious otomastoiditis. It can have some bad complications if it progresses including osteomyelitis of the skull base, vasospasm of the ICA (if it involves the carotid canal), subdural empyema, venous sinus thrombosis, temporal lobe stroke, and full on meningitis. In children, it can present as a primary process. In adults it's usually in the setting of chronic otomastoiditis or recent mastoid surgery.

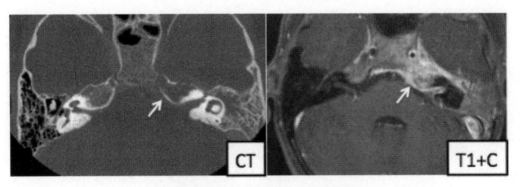

Apical Petrositis

- **Grandenigo Syndrome** – This is a complication of apical petrositis, when Dorello's canal (CN 6) is involved. They will show you (or tell you) that the patient has a **lateral rectus palsy**. The classic triad = otomastoiditis, face pain (trigeminal neuropathy), and lateral rectus palsy.

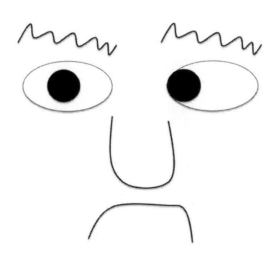

Tumors:

- **Endolymphatic Sac Tumor** – Rare tumor of the endolymphatic sac and duct. Although most are sporadic, when you see this tumor you should immediately think **Von-Hippel-Lindau**. They usually grow into the CPA. They almost always have **internal amorphous calcifications on CT**. There are T2 bright, with **intense enhancement**. They are **very vascular** often with **flow voids**, and **tumor blush** on angiography.

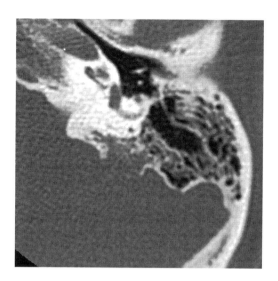

- **Paraganglioma** - On occasion, paraganglioma of the jugular fossa (glomus jugulare or jugulotympanic tumors) can invade the occipital bone and adjacent petrous apex. As much as **40% of the time it's hereditary, and they are multiple**. The **most common presenting symptom in hoarseness** from vagal nerve compression. They are very vascular masses - they enhance avidly with a **"salt and pepper" appearing on post contrast MRI, with flow voids**. They are FDG avid.

Please see the discussion of the subtypes on page 337.

Inner Ear

Congenital

Large Vestibular Aqueduct Syndrome - The vestibular aqueduct is a bony canal that connects the vestibule (inner ear) with the endolymphatic sac. When this becomes enlarged (> 1.5mm) it is associated with **progressive sensorineural hearing loss**. As a point of trivia, the large vestibular aqueduct syndrome is associated with an **absence of the bony modiolus in more than 90% of patients**. This has an Aunt Minnie appearance. Supposedly this is the result of failure of the endolymphatic sac to resorb endolymph, leading to endolymphatic hydrops and dilation.

Trivia:
- This is the most common cause of congenital sensorineural hearing loss
- The finding is often (usually) bilateral.
- There is an association with cochlear deformity - near 100%

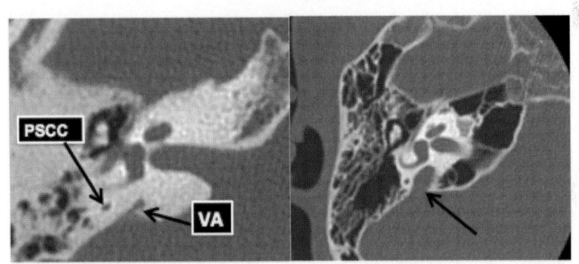

The normal VA is never larger than the adjacent PSCC **Enlarged Vestibular Aqueduct**

Infections

Labyrinthitis – This is an inflammation of the membranous labyrinth, most commonly the result of a viral infection. The cochlea and semicircular canals will be shown enhancing on T1 post contrast imaging.

Labyrinthitis Ossificans - This is the sequella of prior infection (typically meningitis). You see it in kids (ages 2-18 months). They will show this on CT – with ossification of the membranous labyrinth. They also get sensorineural hearing loss.

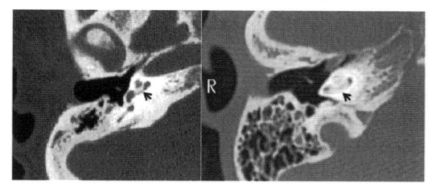

Otosclerosis (Fenestral and Retrofenestral): A better term would actually be "oto<u>spong</u>iosus," as the bone becomes more lytic (instead of sclerotic). When I say conductive hearing loss in an adult female, you say this.

- *Fenestral* – This is **bony resorption anterior to the oval widow** at the fissula ante fenestram. If not addressed, the footplate will fuse to the oval window.

- *Retro-fenestal* – This is a **more severe** form, which has progressed to have **demineralization around the cochlea**. This form usually has a sensorineural component, and is **bilateral and symmetric nearly 100% of the time**.

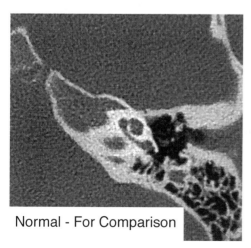

Middle Ear

Otitis Media (OM) – This is a common childhood disease with effusion and infection of the middle ear. It's more common in children and patients with Downs Syndrome because of a more horizontal configuration of the Eustacian tube. It's defined as chronic if you have fluid persisting for more than six weeks. The complications are more of an issue (and more amenable to multiple choice questions).

Complications of OM:

- *Coalescent Mastoiditis* – erosion of the mastoid septae with or without intramastoid abscess

- *Facial Nerve Palsy* – Secondary to inflammation of the tympanic segment (more on this below).

- *Dural Sinus Thrombosis* – Adjacent inflammation may cause thrombophlebitis or thrombosis of the sinus. This in itself can lead to complications:

    o *Venous Infarct:* This can occur secondary to dural sinus thrombosis
    o *Otitic Hydrocephalus:* Venous thrombosis can affect resorption of CSF and lead to hypdocephalus.

- *Meningitis, and Labyrinthitis* – can both occur

Cholesteatoma – This is a bunch of exfoliated skin debris growing in the wrong place. It creates a big inflammation ball which wrecks the temporal bone and the ossicles. The idea is basically this, you have two parts to the ear drum, a flimsy whimpy part "Pars Flaccida", and a tougher part "Pars Tensa." The flimsy Flacida is at the top, and the tensa is at the bottom. If you "acquire" a hole with some inflammation / infection involving the pars flaccida you can end up with this ball of epithelial crap growing and causing inflammation in the wrong place.

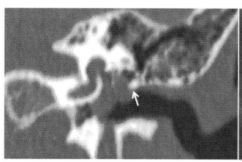
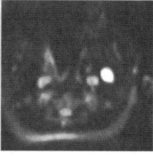

Pars Flaccida – Cholesteatoma
- *Typical location with erosion of scutum (arrow)*
- *They Restrict Diffusion*

Cholesteatoma Order of Destruction predictable (and testable):

(1) The Scutum
(2) The Ossicles (long process of the incus)
(3) The Lateral Segment of the Semi-Circular Canal.

Pars Flaccida Type	*Pars Tensa Type:*
• *Acquired Types are more common – typically involving the pars flaccida. They grow into* **Prussak's Space** • The **Scutum is eroded early** *(maybe first) – considered a very specific sign of acquired cholesteatoma* • *The Malleus head is displaced medially* • **The long process of the incus is the most common segment of the ossicular chain to be eroded.** • *Fistula to the semi-circular canal most commonly involves the lateral segment*	•*The inner ear structures are involved earlier and more often* •*This is less common than the Flaccida Type*

Labyrinthine Fistula: This is a potential complication of cholesteatoma (can also be congenital or iatrogenic), in which there is a bony defect between the inner ear and tympanic cavity. **The lateral semicircular canal is most often involved.**

Anatomy Blitz - Relevant Anatomy for the Cholesteatoma

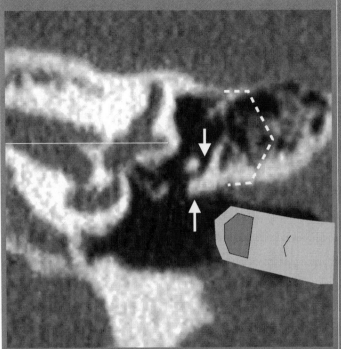

This is a coronal view of the T-Bone. To orient you I drew I cartoon finger in the ear. That finger is running right up to the ear drum (tympanic membrane). The membrane is usually too thin to see, but it's right around there. Remember the flimsy Flacida is at the top and the thicker Tensa is at the bottom.

There are two white arrows here.

The top arrow is pointing to a space between an ossicle (incus) and the lateral temporal bone. This is called **"Prussak's space"** and is the most common location of a pars flacida Cholesteatoma. Remember the incus was the most common ossicle eroded.

The bottom arrow is pointing to a bony shield shaped bone - "the **scutum**" which will be the first bone eroded by a pas flaccid

The white dotted bracket is showing where the **"attic"** is. This is also called the **"epitympanum"** by anatomists.

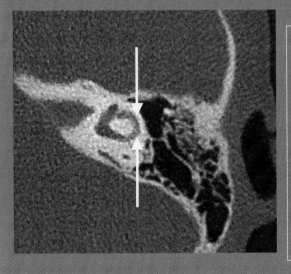

This is an axial through the level of that horizontal line on the coronal image above. The cut is right through the epitympanum.

There are two arrows, both of which are pointing to the **horizontal/lateral portion of the semi-circular canal (SCC)**. This is important because if the cholesteatoma eats the SCC - this is the part it will eat / fistula into.

Superior Semicircular Canal Dehiscence: This is an Aunt Minnie. It's supposedly from long standing ICP although the most likely way this will be asked is either (1) what is it? with a picture or (2) **"Noise Induced Vertigo"** or "Tulio's Phenomenon." You are probably wondering who "Tulio" was.

Pietro Tullio was some mad scientist who drilled holes in the semicircular canals of pigeons then observed that they became off balance when he exposed them to sound. He also created a "pigeon rat" like Hugo Simpson did in the 1996 Simpsons Halloween Special (this is not confirmed).

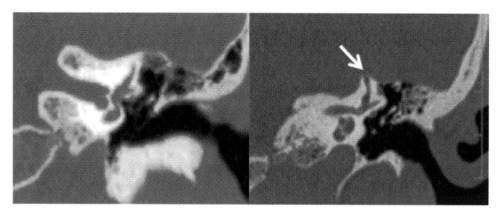

Normal Anatomy   Superior Semicircular Canal Dehiscence

External Ear

Necrotizing External Otitis: This is a raging terrible infection of the external auditory canal. You are going to see swollen EAC soft tissues, probably with a bunch of small abscesses, and adjacent bony destruction. They always (95%) have diabetes and the causative agent is always (98%) Pseudomonas.

The Facial Nerve

There are only 2 or 3 things that are likely to be tested regarding the facial nerve.

(1) *Which parts normally enhance?* - It's easier to remember what does NOT. The cisternal, canalicular, and labyrinthine segments should NOT enhance. The remainder of the nerve - the intratemporal course - can enhance (tympanic, mastoid). Normal enhancement is due to the perineural venous plexus.
(2) *What causes abnormal enhancement?* The big one is Bell's Palsy. Lymes, Ramsay Hunt, and Cancer can do it too.
(3) *When do you damage the facial nerve?* Usually the transverse T-Bone fracture (more than the longitudinal).

Skull Base

Pagets – This is discussed in great depth in the MSK chapter. Having said that, I want to remind you of the Paget skull changes. You can have osteolysis as a well-defined large radiolucent region favoring the frontal and occipital bones. The inner table is affected more than the outer table. The buzzword is **osteolysis circumscripta**.

Paget's Skull related complications:
- Deafness is the most common complication
- Cranial Nerve Paresis
- Basilar Invagination -> Hydrocephalus -> Brainstem Compression
- Secondary (high grade) osteosarcoma.

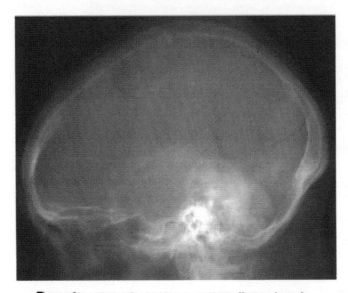

Pagets - *Osteolysis Circumscripta (lytic phase)* **Thickened Expanded Skull (Sclerotic Phase)**

Chordoma *(midline)* and **Chondrosarcoma** *(off midline) - discussed on page 278.*

Fibrous Dysplasia - The ground glass lesion. If you are getting ready to call it's Pagets stop and look at the age. Paget is typically an older person (8% at 80), where as fibrous dysplasia is usually in someone less than 30.

Trivia:
- Classically fibrous dysplasia of the skull spares the otic capsule
- McCune Albright Syndrome - Multi-focal fibrous dysplasia, cafe-au-lait spots, and precocious puberty.

Sinuses

Juvenile Nasal Angiofibroma (JNA) – Often you can get this one right just from the history. **Male teenager with nose bleeds** (obstruction is actually a more common symptom).

Antrochoanal Polyp – Also seen in young adults (30s-40s), this time with nasal congestion / obstruction symptoms. This one arises within the maxillary sinuses, and passes through and enlarges the sinus ostium (or accessory ostium). Buzzword is **"widening of the maxillary ostium."** Classically, there is no associated bony destruction but instead smooth enlargement of the sinus. The polyp will extend into the nasopharynx. This thing is basically a monster inflammatory polyp with a thin stalk arising from the maxillary sinus.

JNA Trivia to know:
- Mass is centered on the sphenoplatine foramen
- Expansion of the Pterygopalatine Fossa
- It's very vascular – and they may show an angiogram with a blush (during embolization therapy).
- Its primary vascular supply is from the ascending pharyngeal artery and/or internal maxillary artery

Inverting Papilloma: This uncommon tumor has distinctive imaging features (which therefore make it testable). The **classic location is the lateral wall of the nasal cavity – most frequently related to the middle turbinate.** Impaired maxillary drainage is expected. **A focal hyperostosis tends to occur at the tumor origin. The MRI buzzword is "cerebriform pattern"** – which sorta looks like brain on T1 and T2. **Another high yield pearl is that 10% harbor a squamous cell CA.**

Esthesioneuroblastoma - This is a neuroblastoma of olfactory cells so it's gonna start at the cribiform plate. It classically has a dumbbell appearance with growth up into the skull and growth down into the sinuses, with a waist at the plate. There are often cysts in the mass. There is a bi-modal age distribution.

Things to know:
- *Dumbbell shape with wasting at the cribiform plate is classic*
- *Intracranial posterior cyst is a "diagnostic" look*
- *Octreotide scan will be positive – since it is of neural crest origin*

Squamous Cell / SNUC: Squamous cell is the **most common head and neck cancer.** The maxillary antrum is the most common location. It's highly cellular, and therefore low on T2. Relative to other sinus masses it enhances less. *SNUC* (the undifferentiated squamer), is the monster steroided up version of a regular squamous cell. They are massive and seen more in the ethmoids.

Sinus Mass Summary

Path	Demographics	Typical Location	Trivia	Imaging Characteristics
Inverting Papilloma	40-70 M>F (4:1)	Lateral nasal wall centered at the middle meatus, with occasional extension into the antrum	40% show "entrapped bone" *Cerebriform Pattern* **10% Harbor a Squamous Cell CA**	Cerebriform Pattern May have focal hyperostosis on CT
Esthesioneuroblastoma	Bimodal 20s & 60s	Dumbbell shaped with waist at the cribiform plate		**AVID homogeneous enhancement**
SNUC	Broad Range (30s-90s)	Ethmoid origin more common than maxillary	<u>Large,</u> typically > 4cm on presentation	**Fungating and Poorly defined** Heterogeneous enhancement with necrosis
Squamous Cell CA	95% > 40 years old	Maxillary Antrum is involved in 80%	**Most Common Malignancy of Sino-Nasal track**	Aggressive Antral Soft Tissue Mass, with destruction of sinus walls **Low signal on T2 (highly cellular)** Enhances less than some other sinus malignancies
JNA *(Juvenile Nasopharyngeal Angiofibroma)*	**Nearly Exclusively Male Rare < 8 or > 25**	**Origin in the Spenopalantine Foramen (SPF)**	Radiation alone cures in 80%	**Enhancing mass arising from the SPF in adolescent male** Dark Flow Voids on T1 **Avidly Enhances**
Sinonasal Lymphoma	Usually older, peak is 60s	Nasal Cavity > Sinuses	Highly variable appearance	Homogeneous mass in nasal cavity with bony destruction **Low Signal on T2 (highly cellular)**

Epistaxis - This is usually idiopathic, although it can be iatrogenic (picking it too much - or not enough). They could get sneaky and work this into a case of HHT. The most common location is the anterior septal area (Kiesselbach plexus), but because these are anterior they tend to be easy to compress manually. The posterior ones are less common (5%) but tend to be the ones that "bleed like stink" (need angio). Most cases are given a trial of nasal packing. When that fails the N-IR team is activated. *The main supply to the posterior nose is the sphenopalatine artery (terminal internal maxillary artery) and tends to be the first line target.* Watch out for the variant anastomosis between the ECA and ophthalmic artery (you don't want to embolize the eye).

The Mouth

Floor of Mouth Dermoid / Epidermoid - There isn't a lot of trivia about these other than the buzzword and what they classically look like. The **buzzword is "sack of marbles"** - fluid sack with globules of fat. They are typically **midline**.

Ranula - This is a mucous retention cyst. They are typically **lateral**. There are two testable pieces of trivia to know: (1) **they arise from the sublingual gland / space**, and (2) use the word **"plunging" once it's under the mylohyoid muscle**.

Torus Palatinus - This is a normal variant that looks scary. Because it looks scary some multiple choice writer may try and trick you into calling it cancer. **It's just a bony exostosis** that comes off the hard palate in the midline. Classic history "Grandma's dentures won't stay in."

Sialolithiasis - Stones in the salivary ducts. The testable trivia includes: (1) **Most commonly in the submandibular gland duct (wharton's)**, (2) can lead to an infected gland "sialoadenitis", and (3) chronic obstruction can lead to gland fatty atrophy.

Odontogenic Infection – These can be dental or periodontal in origin. If I were writing a question about this topic I would ask three things. The first would be that infection is **more common from an extracted tooth** than an abscess involving an intact tooth.

The second would be that the **attachment of the mylohyoid muscle to the mylohyoid ridge dictates the spread of infection to the sublingual and submandibular spaces**. Above the mylohyoid line (anterior mandibular teeth) goes to the sublingual space, and below the mylohyoid line (second and third molars) goes to the submandibular space.

The third thing I would ask would be that an **odontogenic abscess is the most common masticator space "mass" in an adult.**

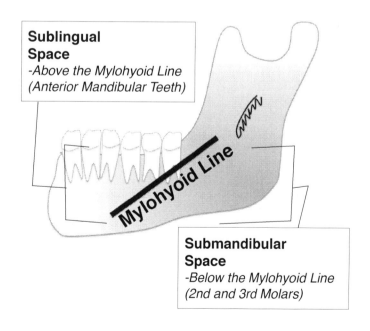

Sublingual Space
-Above the Mylohyoid Line (Anterior Mandibular Teeth)

Submandibular Space
-Below the Mylohyoid Line (2nd and 3rd Molars)

Ludwig's Angina - This is a super aggressive cellulitis in the floor of the mouth. If they show it, there will be gas everywhere. Trivia: most cases start with an odontogenic infection.

Osteonecrosis of the Mandible- The trivia is most likely gonna be etiology. Just remember it is related to prior radiation, licking a radium paint brush, or **bisphosphonate treatment**

Cancer - Squamous cell is going to be the most common cancer of the mouth (and head and neck). In an older person think drinker and smoker. In a younger person think **HPV**. HPV related SCCs tend to be present with large necrotic level 2a nodes (don't call it a brachial cleft cyst!). *Classic scenario = young adult with new level II neck mass = HPV related SCC.*

Thyroglossal Duct Cyst – This can occur anywhere between the foramen cecum (the base of the tongue) and the thyroid gland. They are usually found in the midline at or above the hyoid. It looks like a thin walled cyst. Further discussion in the endocrine chapter.

Classic Mouth Pictures:

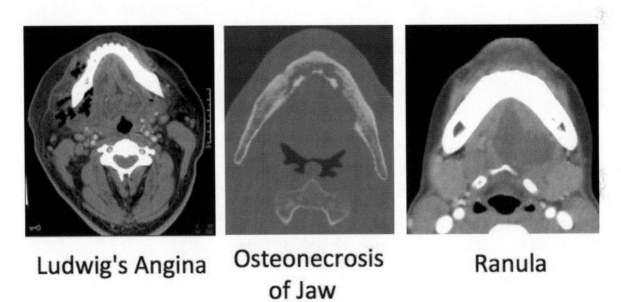

Ludwig's Angina | Osteonecrosis of Jaw | Ranula

Thyroid:

Anatomy: The thyroid gland is a butterfly shaped gland, with two lobes connected by an isthmus. The thyroid descends from the foramen cecum at the anterior midline base of the tongue along the thyroglossal duct. The posterior nodular extension of the thyroid (Zuckerkandl tubercle) helps give a location of the recurrent laryngeal nerve (which is medial to it).

Thyroid Nodules: Usually evaluated with ultrasound. Nodules are super super common and almost never cancer. This doesn't stop Radiologists from imaging them, and sticking needles into them. Ultrasound guided FNA of colloid nodules is a major cash cow for many body divisions, that on very rare occasions will actually find a cancer. Qualities that make them more suspicious include: more solid (cystic more benign), calcifications (especially microcalcifications). **Microcalcifications are supposed to be the buzzword for papillary thyroid cancer.** "Comet Tail" artifact is seen in Colloid Nodules. "Cold Nodules" on I-123 scans are still usually benign but have cancer about 15% of the time, so they actually deserve workup.

Thyroglossal Duct Cyst – This can occur anywhere between the foramen cecum (the base of the tongue) and the thyroid gland. They are usually found in the **midline at or above the hyoid**. It looks like a thin walled cyst.

Why care?
- They can get infected
- Rarely they can have papillary thyroid cancer (if you see an enhancing nodule)

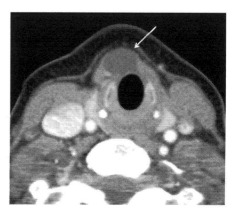

Thyroglossal Duct Cyst - *Midline*

Ectopic and Lingual Thyroid Similar to a thyroglossal duct cyst, this can be found anywhere from the base of the tongue through the central neck. The **most common location (90%) is the tongue base ("Lingual Thyroid")**. It will look hyperdense because of its iodine content (just like a normally located thyroid gland). If you find this, make sure you check for a normal thyroid (sometimes this is the only thyroid the dude has). As a point of trivia, the rate of malignant transformation is rare (3%).

Goiter – Thyroid that is too big. In North America it's gonna be a multi-nodular goiter or graves. In Africa it's low iodine. You can get compressive symptoms if it mashes the esophagus or trachea. These are often asymmetric - with one lobe bigger than the other.

Graves – Autoimmune disease that causes hyperthyroidism (most common cause). It's primary from an antibody directed at the TSH receptor. The actual TSH level will be low. The gland will be enlarged and "inferno hot" on Doppler.

- *Graves Orbitopathy*: Spares the tendon insertions, doesn't hurt (unlike pseudotumor). Also has increased intra-orbital fat.
- *Nuclear Medicine:* Increased uptake of I-123 %RAIU usually 50-80%. Visualization of pyramidal lobe is accentuated.

Hashimotos – The **most common cause of goitrous hypothyroidism** (in the US). It is an autoimmune disease that causes hyper then hypo thyroidism (as the gland burns out later). It's usually hypo – when it's seen. It has an **increased risk of primary thyroid lymphoma**. Step 1 trivia; associated with autoantibodies to thyroid peroxidase (TPO) and anti-thyroidglobulin.

On Ultrasound: There are two classic findings (a) the heterogeneous "giraffe skin" appearance, (b) white knights – uniform hyperechoic nodules – which are actually regenerative nodules.

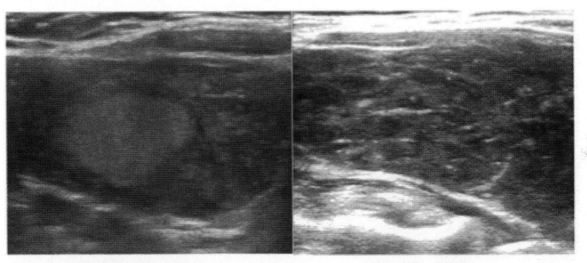

White Knight   **Giraffe Skin**

Level 6 Nodes - "Delphian Nodes"

- These are the nodes around the thyroid in the front of the neck. You can commonly see them enlarged with Hashimotos.
- However, for the purpose of multiple choice tests, a sick looking level 6 node - or "Delphian Node" is a laryngeal cancer met.

Subacute Thyroiditis / De Quervains Thyroiditis: The classic clinical scenario is a female with a painful gland after an upper respiratory infection. There is a similar subtype that happens in pregnant women, although this is typically painless. You get hyperthyroidism (from spilling the hormone) and then later hypothyroidism. As you get over your cold, the gland recovers to normal function. Radiotracer uptake will be decreased during the acute phase.

Reidels Thyroiditis - This is one of those IgG4 associated diseases (others include orbital pseudotumor, retroperitoneal fibrosis, sclerosing cholangitis). You see it in women in their 40s-70s. The thyroid is replaced by fibrous tissue and diffusely enlarges causing compression of adjacent structures (dysphagia, stridor, vocal cord palsy). On US there will be decreased vascularity. On an uptake scan you are going to have decreased values. A sneak trick would be to show you a MR (it's gonna be dark on all sequences - like a fibroma).

Acute Suppurative Thyroiditis: This is an actual bacterial infection of the thyroid. It is possible to develop a thyroid abscess in this situation. A unique scenario (highly testable) is that **in kids this infection may start in a 4th brachial cleft anomaly** (usually on the left), travel via a pyriform fistula and then infect the thyroid. Honestly, that is probably too much for the exam.

Colloid Nodules: These are super super common. Suspicious features include microcalcifications, and increased vascularity, solid size (larger than 1.5cm), and being cold on a nuclear uptake exam. **Comet artifact is the buzzword**.

Thyroid Adenoma: These look just like solid colloid nodules on ultrasound. They can be hyper functioning (hot on uptake scan). Usually if you have a hyper-functioning nodule, your background thyroid will be colder than normal (which makes sense).

Thyroid Cancer: You can get lots of cancers in your thyroid. There are 4 main subtypes of primary thyroid cancer (see chart on the next page). Additionally you can get mets to the thyroid or lymphoma in your thyroid – this is super rare and I'm not going to talk about it.

Papillary	The **Most Common** Subtype. *"Papillary is Popular"*	**Microcalcifications is the buzzword and key finding (seen in the cancer and nodes).**	Mets via the lymphatics. Has an overall excellent prognosis, and responds well to I-131.
Follicular	The second most common subtype.		**Mets hematogenously** to bones, lung, liver, etc.. Survival is still ok, (less good than papillary). Does respond to I-131.
Medullary	Uncommon	**Association with MEN II syndrome**. *Calcitonin production is a buzzword.*	Tendency towards local invasion, lymph nodes, and hematogenous spread. **Does NOT respond to I-131.**
Anaplastic	Uncommon	Seen in **Elderly**. Seen in people who have had **radiation treatment.**	Rapid growth, with primary lymphatic spread. **Does NOT respond to I-131.**
Hurthle Cell *(variant of Follicular)*	Uncommon	Seen more in Elderly.	**Does not take up I-131 as well as normal follicular.** *FDG-PET is the way to go for surveillance.*

Metastasis: The buzzword is going to be **microcalcifications in a node** (with papillary). The nodes are typically hyperechoic compared to regular nodes, hyperenhancing on CT, and T1 bright on MR. Remember that thyroid cancer is hyper vascular, and it can bleed like stink when it mets to the brain. If there are **mets to the lungs the classic pattern is "miliary."** The additional pearl with regard to lung mets is that they can be occult on cross sectional imaging, and only seen on whole body scintigraphy. For the purpose of multiple choice tests *pulmonary fibrosis is a risk of treating with I-131 if you have diffuse lung mets.*

Parathyroid

Anatomy: There are normally 4 parathyroid glands located posterior to the thyroid. The step 1 trivia is that the superior 2 are from the 4th branchial pouch, and the inferior 2 are from the 3rd branchial pouch. The inferior two are more likely to be in an ectopic location.

Parathyroid Adenoma - This is by far the **most common cause of hyperparathyroidism** (90%). On ultrasound these things look like hypoechoic beans posterior to the thyroid. A 4D-CT can be used to demonstrate early wash in and delayed wash out. Nuclear medicine can use two techniques (1) the single tracer, dual phase Sestamibi, or (2) the dual tracer Sestamibi + I-123 (or Pertechnetate).

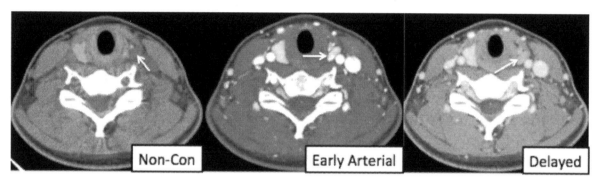

Parathyroid Adenoma - *4D CT shows early enhancement, and washout out*

Parathyroid Carcinoma - This is pretty uncommon, and only makes up about 1% of the causes of hyperparathyroidism. It looks exactly like an adenoma on imaging. The only way you can tell on imaging is if they show you cervical adenopathy or invasion of adjacent structures.

High Yield Parathyroid Trivia:

Q: What are the causes of hyperparathyroidism?
A: *Hyperfunctioning Adenoma (85-90%),* Multi-Gland Hyperplasia (8-10%), Cancer (1-3%).

Q: What factors does sestamibi parathyroid imaging depend on ?
A: Mitochondrial density, and blood flow

Suprahyoid Soft Tissue Neck

The suprahyoid neck is usually taught by using a "spaces" method. This is actually the best way to learn it. What space is it? What is in that space? What pathology can occur as the result of what normal structures are there. Example: lymph nodes are there – thus you can get lymphoma or a met.

Parotid Space:

The parotid space is basically the parotid gland, and portions of the facial nerve. You can't see the facial nerve, but you can see the retromandibular vein (which runs just medial to the facial nerve). Another thing to know is that the parotid is the only salivary gland to have lymph nodes, so pathology involving the gland itself, and anything lymphatic related is fair game.

Parotid Space Contains:
- The Parotid Gland
- Cranial Nerve 7 (Facial)
- Retro-mandibular Vein

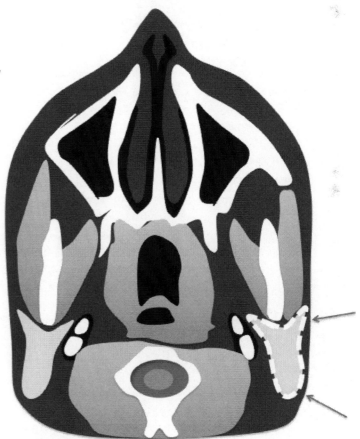

Pathology:

Pleomorphic Adenoma (benign mixed tumor) - This is the most common major *(and minor)* salivary gland tumor. It occurs most commonly in the parotid, but can occur in the submandibular, or sublingual glands. 90% of these tumors occur in the superficial lobe. They are commonly T2 bright, with a rim of low signal. **They have a small malignant potential** and are treated surgically.

- *Superficial vs Deep:* Involvement of the superficial (lateral to the facial nerve) or deep (medial to the facial nerve) lobe is critical to the surgical approach. A line is drawn connecting the lateral surface of the posterior belly of the digastric muscle and the lateral surface of the mandibular ascending ramus to separate superficial from deep.
- Apparently, if you resect these like a clown you can spill them, and they will have a massive ugly recurrence.

Warthins: This is the second most common benign tumor. This one ONLY occurs in the parotid gland. This one is **usually cystic, in a male, bilateral (15%), and in a smoker**. As a point of total trivia, this tumor **takes up pertechnetate** (it's basically the only tumor in the parotid to do it, *ignoring the ultra rare parotid oncocytoma*).

Mucoepidermoid Carcinoma – This is the **most common malignant tumor of minor salivary glands**. The general rule is – the smaller the gland the more common the malignant tumors, the bigger the gland the more common the benign tumors. There is a variable appearance based on the histologic grade. There is an association with radiation.

Adenoid Cystic Carcinoma – This is another malignant salivary gland tumor, which favors minor glands but can be seen in the parotid. The number one thing to know is perineural spread. This tumor likes perineural spread. **When I say adenoid cystic you say perineural spread**.

Pearl: I used to think that perineurial tumor spread would widen a neural foramen (foramen ovale for example). It's still might… but it's been my experience that a nerve sheath tumor (schwannoma) is much more likely to do that. Let's just say for the purpose of multiple choice that neural foramina widening is a schwannoma - unless there is overwhelming evidence to the contrary.

Lymphoma – Because the parotid has lymph nodes (it's the only salivary gland that does), you can get lymphoma in the parotid (primary or secondary). If you see it and it's bilateral, you should think Sjogrens. Sjogrens patients have a big risk (like 1000x) of parotid lymphoma. Like lymphoma is elsewhere in the body, the appearance is variable. You might see bilateral homogeneous masses. For the purposes of the exam, **just knowing you can get it in the parotid (primary or secondary) and the relationship with Sjogrens is probably all you need**.

Other Parotid Trivia:

- **Acute Parotitis:** Obstruction of flow of secretions is the most common cause. They will likely show you a stone (or stones) in Stensen's duct, which will be dilated. The stones are calcium phosphate. Post infectious parotitis is usually bacterial. Mumps would be the most common viral cause. As a point of trivia, sialography is contraindicated in the acute setting.

- **Benign Lymphoepithelial Disease:** You have **bilateral mixed solid and cystic lesions** with diffusely enlarged parotid glands. This is **seen in HIV**. The condition is painless (unlike parotitis – which can enlarge the glands).

- **Sjogrens** – Autoimmune lymphocyte induced destruction of the gland. "Dry eyes and Dry Mouth." Typically seen in women in their 60s. **Increased risk** (like 1000x) risk of non-Hodgkins MALT type **lymphoma**. There is a **honeycombed appearance of the gland**.

Carotid Space:

Carotid Space Contains:
- Carotid artery,
- Jugular vein,
- Portions of CN 9, CN 10, CN 11,
- Internal jugular chain lymph nodes

There are 3 Classic Carotid Space Tumors:
(1) Paraganglioma
(2) Schwannoma
(3) Neurofibroma

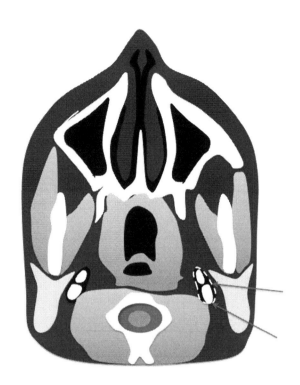

Paragangliomas: There are three different ones worth knowing about – based on location. The imaging features are the same. They are **hypervascular (intense tumor blush)**, with a **"Salt and Pepper" appearance on MRI** from all the heterogeneous stuff and flow voids. They can be multiple and bilateral in familial conditions. ^{111}**In- octreotide accumulates in these tumors** (receptors for somatostatin).

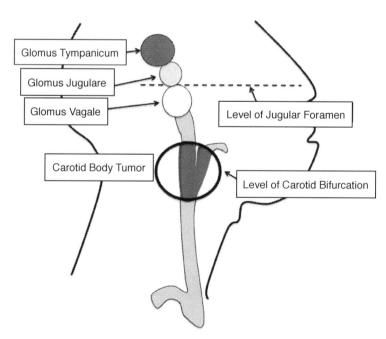

Carotid Body Tumor = Carotid Bifurcation (*Splaying ICA and ECA*)

Glomus Jugulare = Skull Base (*often with destruction of jugular foramen*)

Middle Ear Floor Destroyed = Glomus Jugulare.

Glomus Vagale = Above Carotid Bifurcation, but below the Jugular Foramen

Glomus Tympanicum = Confined to the middle ear. Buzzword is *"overlying the cochlear promontory."*

Middle Ear Floor Intact = Glomus Tympanum

Schwannoma – Can involve the 9, 10, 11, and even 12th CN.

Schwannoma	Paraganglioma
Not all that vascular on Angio	Hypervascular (tumor blush on angio)
No Salt and Pepper	Salt and Pepper Look on MRI
NOT ^{111}In- octreotide avid	^{111}In- octreotide avid
No Flow Voids (target sign)	Flow Voids

Lemierre syndrome – This is a thrombophlebitis of the jugular veins with distant metastatic sepsis (usually septic emboli in the lung). It's found in the setting of oropharyngeal infection (pharyngitis, tonsillitis, peri tonsillar abscess), or recent ENT surgery.

Lymph Nodes = Metastatic lesions from squamous cell cancer frequently involve this area.

Masticator Space:

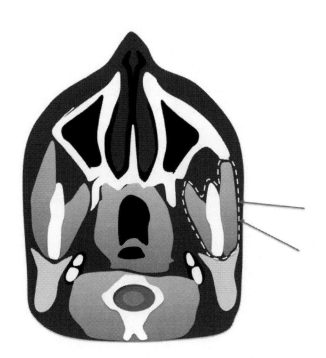

As the name implies this space contains the **muscles of mastication** (masticator, temporalis, medial and lateral pterygoids).

Additionally, you have the angle and **ramus of the mandible**, plus the **inferior aveolar nerve**.

A trick to be aware of is that the space extends superiorly along the side of the skull via the temporalis muscle. So, aggressive neoplasm or infection may ride right up there.

Odontogenic Infection – In an adult this is the most common cause of a masticator space mass. If you see a mass here, the next move should be to look at the mandible on bone windows. Just in general, you should be on the look out for spread via the pterygopalatine fossa to orbital apex and cavernous sinus. The relationship with the mylohyoid makes for good trivia - as discussed above.

Sarcomas – In kids, you can run into nasty angry masses like Rhabdomyosarcomas. You can also get sarcomas from the bone of the mandible (chondrosacroma favors the TMJ).

Cavernous Hemangiomas – These can also occur, and are given away by the presence of pleboliths. Venous or lymphatic malformations may involve multiple compartments / spaces.

*Congenital stuff and Aggressive Infection/Cancer tends to be trans-spatial.

Perineural Spread – You can have perineural spread from a head and neck primary along the 5th CN.

When I say "perineural spread" you should think two things:
(1) **adenoid cystic** minor salivary tumor and
(2) melanoma.

Nerve Sheath Tumors – Since you have a nerve, you can have a schwannoma or neurofibroma of V3. Remember the schwannoma is more likely to cause the foramina expansion vs perineurial tumor spread.

Retropharyngeal Space / Danger Space

Behind the middle layer of deep cervical fascia but anterior to the alar fascia, lives this midline space.

Danger Space - The so called "danger space", is actually just posterior to the "true" retropharyngeal space - <u>behind the alar</u> layer of fascia. It's a <u>potential space</u> - that you can't see unless it's distended. Certain Anatomists like to make the distinction that this space is separate from the "true retropharyngeal space," others lump them together. If forced to choose - simply read the mind of the question writer to decide which camp he/she falls into. I would pick them as separate entities because people who do academics / write questions tend to enjoy making things overly complicated.

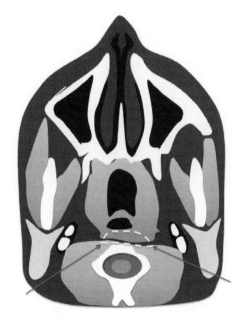

So what's the danger in infection in the danger space?? It tracts down into the mediastinum… so you can dump pus (or cancer) right into the mediastinum (that's bad).

Infection – Involvement of the retropharyngeal space most often occurs from spread from the tonsillar tissue. You are going to have enhancing soft tissue and stranding in the space. You should evaluate for spread of infection into the mediastinum.

Necrotic Nodes - **Squamous cell mets** or suppurative infection to the lateral retropharyngeal nodes of Rouviere. Papillary thyroid cancer can also met here. Lymphoma can involve these nodes, but won't be necrotic until treated.

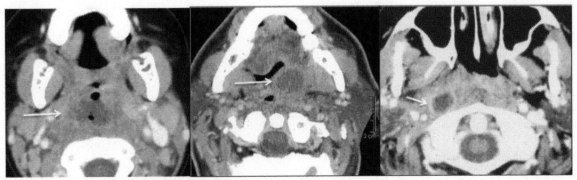

Retropharyngeal Abscess   Peritonsilar Abscess   Suppurative Node of Rouviere

> **Neck Infection Syndromes**
>
> **Grisel's Syndrome** - Torticollis with atlanto-axial joint inflammation seen in H&N surgery or retropharyngeal abscess
>
> **Lemierre's Syndrome** - URI / Neck injection or recent ENT surgery leads to jugular vein thrombosis and septic emboli. Buzzword bacteria ="Fusobacterium Necrophorum"

Parapharyngeal Space

The parapharyngeal space is primarily a ball of fat with a few branches of the trigeminal nerves, and the pterygoid veins. The primary utility of the space is when it is displaced (discussed below). Mets and infections can directly spread into this space (squamous cell cancer from tonsils, tongue, and larynx). Cancer and infection can spread rapidly in a vertical direction through this fat.

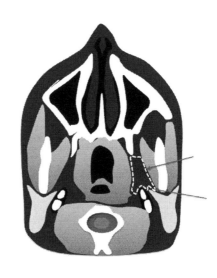

The parapharyngeal space is bordered on four sides by different spaces. If you have a mass dead in the middle, it can be challenging to tell where it's coming from. Using the displacement of fat, you can help problem solve. Much more important than that, this lends itself very well to multiple choice.

Parotid **M**ass **P**ushes **M**edially (PMPM)

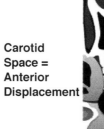 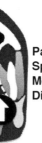 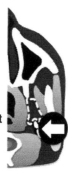

Carotid Space = Anterior Displacement

Parotid Space = Medial Displacement

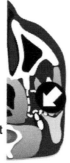 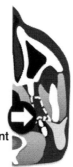

Masticator Space = Posterior Medial Displacement

Superficial Mucosal Space = Lateral Displacement

Squamous Cell Cancer

When you are talking about head and neck cancer, you are talking about squamous cell cancer. Now, this is a big complex topic and requires a fellowship to truly understand / get good at. Obviously, the purpose of this book is to prepare you for multiple choice test questions not teach you practical radiology. If you want to actually learn about head and neck cancer for a practical sense you can try and find a copy of Harnsberger's legendary handbook (which has been out of print for 20 years). A more modern alternative is probably Raghavan's Manual of Head and Neck Imaging. Now, for the trivia....

Lymph node anatomy:

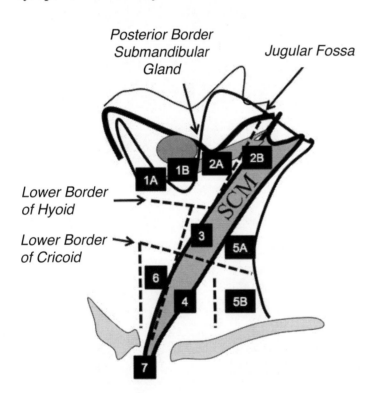

Testable Trivia:

Anterior Belly of Digastric separates 1A from 1B

Stylohyoid muscle *(posterior submandibular gland)* separates 1B from 2A

Spinal Accessory Nerve *(jugular)* separates 2A from 2B

Vertical borders:
2-3 = Lower Hyoid
3-4 = Lower Cricoid

Floor of the Mouth SCC: I touched on this once already. Just remember smoker/drinker in an old person. HPV in a young person. Necrotic level 2 nodes can be a presentation (not a brachial cleft cyst).

Nasopharyngeal SCC: This is more common in Asians and has a bi-modal distribution: group 1 (15-30) typically Chinese, and group 2 (> 40). Involvement of the parapharyngeal space results in worse prognosis (compared to nasal cavity or oropharynx invasion). The **most common location is the Fossa of Rosenmuller (FOR)**. If you see (1) a unilateral mastoid effusion, or (2) a pathologic retropharyngeal node look in the FOR. *The "earliest sign" of nasopharyngeal SCC is the effacement of the fat within the FOR.* If you see a supraclavicular node then you should look closely at the bones for mets (especially the clivus).

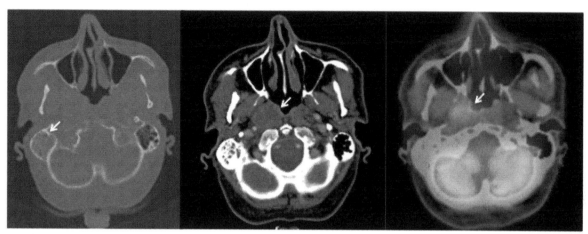

Unilateral Mastoid Effusion   Fossa of Rosenmuller Mass   PET Avid

Laryngeal SCC: The role of the Radiologist is not to make the primary cancer diagnosis here, but to assist in staging. Laryngeal cancers are subdivided into (a) supraglottic, (b) glottic, and (c) infraglottic types. "Transglottic" would refer to an aggressive cancer that crosses the laryngeal ventricle.

Things to know about laryngeal SCC:
- Glottic SCC has the best outcome (least lymphatics), and is the most common (60%)
- Subglottic is the least common (5%), and can be clinically silent till you get nodes
- Subglottic tumors are often small compared to nodal burden
- Fixation of the cords indicates at least a T3 tumor
- The only reliable sign of cricoid invasion is tumor on both sides of the cartilage (irregular sclerotic cartilage can be normal).
- Invasion of the cricoid cartilage is a contraindication to all types of laryngeal conservation surgery (cricoid cartilage is necessary for postoperative stability of the vocal cords).
- Paraglottic space involvement makes the tumor T3 and "transglottic." This is best seen in coronals.

Infrahyoid Soft Tissue Neck

Laryngocele: When the laryngeal saccule dilates with fluid or air you call it a laryngocele.

Why does it dilate ? Usually because its obstructed, and the testable point is that 15% of the time that obstruction is a tumor.

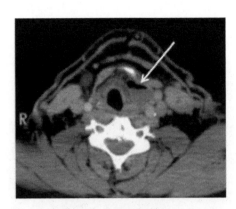

Laryngocele

Vocal Cord Paralysis: The **affected side will have an expanded ventricle** (it's the opposite side with a cancer). If you see it on the left, a good "next step" question would be to look at the chest (for recurrent laryngeal nerve involvement at the AP window).

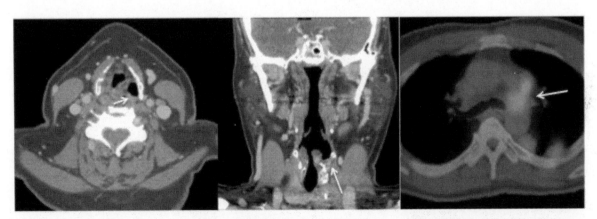

Vocal Cord Paralysis – Ipsilateral Expanded Ventricle   **AP Window PET Avid Node**

Orbit

Congenital

Coloboma: This is a focal discontinuity of the globe (failure of the choroid fissure to close). They are usually posterior. If you see a unilateral one - think sporadic. **If you see bilateral ones - think CHARGE** (coloboma, heart, GU, ears).

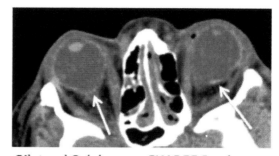
Bilateral Coloboma – CHARGE Syndrome

Persistent Hyperplastic Primary Vitreous (PHPV) - This is a failure of the embryonic ocular blood supply to regress. It can lead to retinal detachment. The classic look is a **small eye (microphthalmia) with increased density of the vitreous**. No calcification.

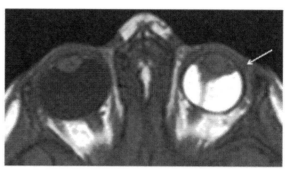
Retinal Detachment in the setting of PHPV

Coat's Disease - The cause of this is a retinal telangiectasis, that results in leaky blood and subretinal exudate. It can lead to retinal detachment. It's seen in young boys and typically unilateral. The key detail is that it is NOT CALCIFIED (retinoblastoma is).

Coats disease has a smaller globe. Retinoblastoma has a normal sized globe.

Retinal Detachment - This can occur secondary to PHPV or Coats. It can also be caused by trauma, sickle cell, or just old age. The imaging finding is a "V" or "Y" shaped appearance due to lifted up retinal leaves and subretinal fluid (as seen in the PHPV case above).

Globe Size - A Source of Possible Trivia

- *Retinoblastoma* - Normal Size
- *Toxocariasis* - Normal Size
- *PHPV* - Small Size *(Normal Birth Age)*
- *Retinopathy of Prematurity* - Bilateral Small
- *Coats* - Smaller Size

Orbital Tumors:

Optic Nerve Glioma: These almost always (90%) occur under the age of 20. You see expansion / enlargement of the entire nerve. If they are bilateral you think about **NF-1**. They are most often WHO grade 1 *Pilocystic Astrocytomas*. If they are sporadic they can be GBMs and absolutely destroy you.

Optic Nerve Sheath Meningioma: The buzzword is *"tram-track" calcifications*. Another buzzword is "doughnut" appearance, with **circumferential enhancement around the optic nerve**.

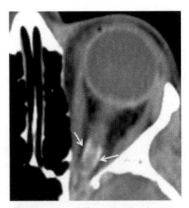
"Tram-Track" = Meningioma

IgG4 - Orbit

Orbital Pseudotumor: This is one of those IgG4 idiopathic inflammatory conditions that involves the extraoccular muscles. It looks like an expanded muscle. The things to remember are that this thing is **painful**, unilateral, it **most commonly involves the lateral rectus** and it **does NOT spare the myotendinous insertions**. Remember that Graves does not cause pain, and does spare the myotendinous insertions. It gets better with steroids. It's classically T2 dark.

Tolosa Hunt Syndrome: This is histologically the same thing as orbital pseudotumor but instead involves the cavernous sinus. It is painful (just like pseudotumor), and presents with multiple cranial nerve palsies. It responds to steroids (just like pseudotumor).

Lymphocytic Hypophysitis: This is the same deal as orbital pseudotumor and tolosa hunt, except it's the pituitary gland. Just think enlarged pituitary stalk, in a post partum / 3rd trimester woman. It looks like a pituitary adenoma, but it classically has a T2 dark rim.

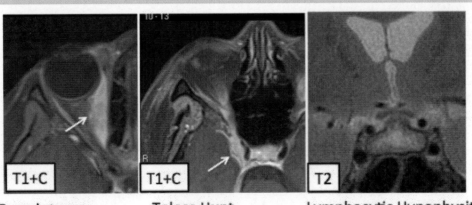

Pseudotumor - Involves Cavernous Sinus
Tolosa Hunt - Involves Cavernous Sinus
Lymphocytic Hypophysitis - Dark T2 Signal Around Gland

Dermoid: This is the most common benign congenital orbital mass. It's usually **superior and lateral,** arising from the frontozygomatic suture, and presenting in the first 10 years of life. It's gonna have fat in it (like any good dermoid). The location is classic.

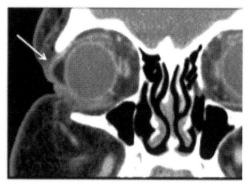

Orbital Dermoid – *Classic Location*

Rhabdomyosarcoma - *Most common extra-occular orbital malignancy in children* (dermoid is most common benign orbital mass in child). When they do occur - 40% of the time it's in the head and neck - and then most commonly it's in the orbit. It's still rare as hell.

Metastatic Neuroblastoma - This has a very classic appearance of **"Raccoon Eyes"** on physical exam. The *classic location is periorbital tumor infiltration with associated proptosis.* Don't forget a basilar skull fracture can also cause Raccoon Eyes... so clinical correlation is advised.

Metastatic Breast Cancer - This is classic gamesmanship here. The important point to know is that unlike primary orbital tumors that are going to cause proptosis, classically the **breast cancer met causes a desmoplastic reaction and enophthalmos**.

Lymphoma - There is an association with **Chlamydia Psittaci** (the bird fever thing) and MALT lymphoma of the orbit. It usually involves the upper outer orbit - closely associated with the lacrimal gland. It will enhance homogeneously and restricts diffusion - just like in the brain.

Globe Tumors:

Melanoma - This is the **most common intra-occular lesion in an adult.** If you see an enhancing soft tissue mass in the back of an adult's eye this is the answer. I can only think of three ways you could ask about this: (1) show a picture - what is it?, (2) ask what the most common intra-occular lesion in an adult is, or (3) ask the buzzword *"collar button shaped"* - which is related to Bruch's membrane.

Retinoblastoma - This is the most common primary malignancy of the globe. The step 1 question is RB suppressor gene (chromosome 13). That's the same chromosome osteosarcoma patients have issues with and why these guys are at increased risk of facial osteosarcoma after radiation. **If you see calcification in the globe of a child - this is the answer.** The globe should be normal in size (or bigger), where coats is usually smaller. It's **usually seen before age 3** (rare after age 6). The trivia is gonna be where else it occurs. They can be bilateral (both eyes - 30%), *trilateral* (both eyes, and the pineal gland), and *quadrilateral* (both eyes, pineal, and suprasellar).

Orbital Vascular Malformations:

Lymphangioma - These are actually a mix of venous and lymphatic malformations. They are ill-defined and lack a capsule. The usual distribution is infiltrative (**multi-spatial**) involving, pre septal, post septal, extraconal, and intraconal locations. **Fluid-Fluid levels** are the money shot, and the most likely finding to be shown by someone writing a multiple choice test question. They do NOT increase with valsalva.

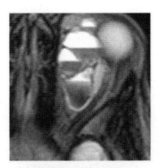

Lymphangioma – *Fluid Fluid Levels*

Varix - These occur secondary to weakness in the post capillary venous wall (gives you massive dilation of the valveless orbital veins). Most likely question is going to pertain to the fact that **they distend with provocative maneuvers** (valsalva, hanging head, etc...). Another piece of trivia is that they are the *most common cause of spontaneous orbital hemorrhage*. They can thrombose and present with pain.

Carotid-Cavernous Fistula: These come in two flavors: (1) Direct - which is secondary to trauma, and (2) Indirect - which just occurs randomly in post menopausal women. The direct kind is a communication between the intracavernous ICA and cavernous sinus. The indirect kind is usually a dural shunt between meningeal branches of the ECA and Cavernous Sinus.

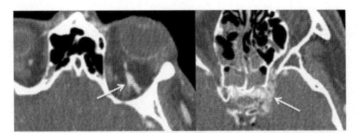

Carotid-cavernous Fistula – *Prominent left superior ophthalmic vein, prominent left cavernous sinus with proptosis.*

> **Pulsatile Exophthalmos**
> *The Buzzword*
>
> C-C Fistula is probably the most common cause.
>
> **NF-1** can also cause it, from *sphenoid wing dysplasia*.

Orbital Infection:

Pre-Septal/ Post Septal Cellulitis - The location of orbital infections are described by their relationship to the orbital septum. The testable trivia is probably (1) that the orbital septum originates from the periosteum of the orbit and inserts in the palpebral tissue along the tarsal plate, (2) that pre-septal infections usually start in adjacent structures likely teeth and the face, and that (3) post-septal infections are usually from paranasal sinusitis.

Dacryocystitis - This is inflammation and dilation of the lacrimal sac. It has an Aunt Minnie look, with a well circumscribed round rim enhancing lesion centered in the lacrimal fossa. The etiology is typically obstruction then bacterial infection (staph and strep).

Orbital Subperiosteal Abscess: If you get inflammation under the periosteum it can progress to abscess formation. This is usually associated with ethmoid sinusitis. This also has a very classic look.

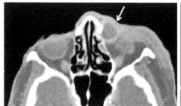
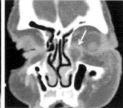
Dacroyocyctitis

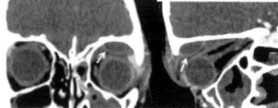
Orbital Subperiosteal Abscess

Misc:

Optic Neuritis: There will be **enhancement of the optic nerve**, *without enlargement* of the nerve/sheath complex. Usually (70%) unilateral, and painful. You will often see intracranial or spinal cord demyelination – in the setting of Devics (neuromyelitis optica). 50% of patient's with acute optic neuritis will develop MS.

Papilledema: This is really an eye exam thing. Having said that you can sometimes see dilation of the optic nerve sheath.

Thyroid Orbitopathy: This is seen in 1/4 of the Graves cases and is the most common cause of exophthalmos. The antibodies that activate TSH receptors also activate orbital fibroblasts and adipocytes.

Things to know:
- Risk of compressive optic neuropathy
- Enlargement of ONLY MUSCLE BELLY (spares tendon) - different than *pseudo tumor*
- NOT Painful - different than *pseudo tumor*
- Order of Involvement: IR > MR > SR > LR > SO "I'M SLOw"

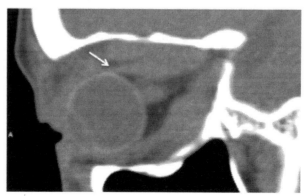
Thyroid Orbit – *Spares Tendon Insertion*

Section 3: Spine

Anatomy Trivia

Cord Blood Supply: There is an anterior blood supply and a posterior blood supply to the cord. These guys get taken out with different clinical syndromes.

- *Anterior spinal artery* - arises bilaterally as two small branches at the level of the termination of the vertebral arteries. These two arteries join around the level of the foramen magnum.

- *Artery of Adamkiewicz* – This is the most notable reinforcer of the anterior spinal artery. In 75% of people is **comes off the left side of the aorta between T8 and T1**. It supplies the lower 2/3 of the cord. This thing can get covered with the placement of an endovascular stent graft for aneurysm or dissection repair leading to spine infarct.

- *Posterior Spinal Artery* – arises from either the vertebral arteries or the posterior inferior cerebellar artery. Unlike the anterior spinal artery this one is somewhat discontinuous and reinforced by multiple segmental or radiculopial branches.

Conus Medullaris: This is the terminal end of the spinal cord. It usually terminates at around L1. Below the inferior endplate of the L2 / L3 body should make you think tethered cord (especially if shown in a multiple choice setting).

Which nerve is compressed?

There are 31 pairs of spinal nerves, with each pair corresponding to the adjacent vertebra – the notable exception being the "C8" nerve. Cervical disc herniations are less common than lumbar ones.

The question is most likely to take place in the lumbar spine (the same spot most disc herniations occur). In fact more than 90% of herniations occur at L4-L5, and L5-S1.

A tale of two herniations. It was the best of times, it was the worst of times...

Scenario 1:

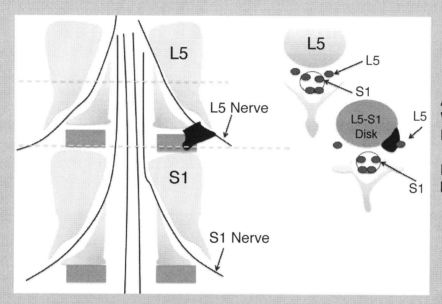

A Foraminal Disc Will Smash the Exiting Nerve.

In this case the L5 Nerve

Scenario 2:

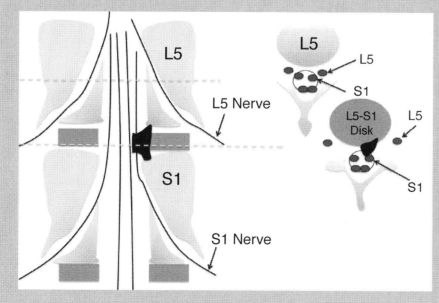

A Central or Paracentral Disc Will Smash the Descending Nerve.

In this case the S1 Nerve

Epidural Fat: The epidural fat is not evenly distributed. The epidural space in the cervical cord is predominantly filled with venous plexus (as apposed to fat). In the lumbar spine there is fat both anterior and posterior to the cord.

Degenerative Changes

Stenosis: Spinal stenosis can be congenital (associated with short pedicles) or be acquired. The Torg-Pavlov ratio can be used to call it (vertebral body width to cervical canal diameter < 0.85). Symptomatic stenosis is more common in the cervical spine (versus the thoracic spine or lumbar spine). You can get some congenital stenosis in the lumbar spine from short pedicles, but it's generally not symptomatic until middle age.

Disc Nomenclature: In order to "improve accuracy" with regard to the lumbar spine various administrative regulatory bodies have decided on the vocabulary you are allowed to use.

- *"Focal Herniation"* is a herniated disc less comprising than 90 degrees of the disc circumference.
- *"Broadbased Herniation"* is a herniated disc in between 90-180 degrees.
- *"Protrusion"* – is a term used when the distance between the edge of the disc herniation is less than the distance between the edges of the base
- *"Extrusion"* is a term used when the edges of the disc are greater than the distance of the base.

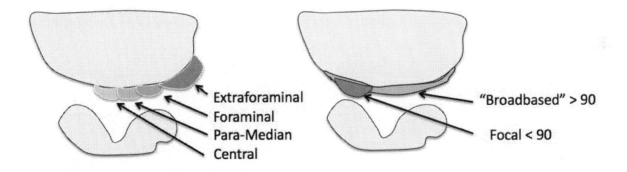

Schmorl Node: This is a herniation of disc material through a defect in the vertebral body endplate into the actual marrow.

Scheuermann's – This is multiple levels (at least 3) of Schmorl's nodes in the spine of a teenager, resulting in kyphotic deformity (40 degrees in thoracic or 30 degrees in thoracolumbar).

Limbus Vertebra – This is a fracture mimic, that is the result of herniated disc material between the non-fused apophysis and adjacent vertebral body.

Endplate Changes: Commonly referred to as "Modic Changes." There is a progression in the MRI signal characteristics that makes sense if you think about it. You start out with degenerative changes causing irritation / inflammation so there is edema (T2 bright). This progresses to chronic inflammation with leads to some fatty change – just like in the bowel of an IBD patient – causing T1 bright signal. Finally, the whole thing gets burned out and fibrotic and it's T1 and T2 dark. As a prominent factoid, Type 1 changes look a lot like Osteomyelitis (clinical correlation in recommended).

Modic – Endplate Marrow Changes Associated with Degenerative Disease	
Type 1 "Edema"	T1 Dark, T2 Bright
Type 2 "Fat"	T1 Bright, T2 Bright
Type 3 "Scar"	T1 Dark, T2 Dark

Annular Tears: You can have tears in your dorsal annulus. They are usually bright on T2 and have a curvilinear look. They are so bright that some people call them "high intensity zones." They may be a source of pain (radial pain fibers - trigger "discogenic pain") but are also seen as incidentals.

Myelogram Technique

Big point: Contrast should flow freely away from the needle tip gradually filling the thecal sac. The outlining of the the cauda equine is another promising sign that you did it right. If contrast pools at the needle tip or along the posterior or lateral thecal sac without free-flow, a subdural injection or injection in the fat around the thecal sac should be suspected.

Prior to the LP *(per ACR-ASNR recommendations)*

- STOP Coumadin 4-5 days
- STOP Plavix for 7 days
- Hold LMW Heparin for 12 hours
- Hold Heparin for 2-4 hours - document normal PTT
- Aspirin and NSAIDs are fine (not contraindicated)

Post Operative Back Trivia:

"Failed Back Surgery Syndrome" –Another entity invented by NEJM to take down the surgical subspecialties. Per the NEJM these greedy surgeons generally go from a non-indicated spine surgery, to a non-indicated leg amputation, to a non-indicated tonsillectomy on an innocent child. Text books will define it as recurrent or residual low back pain in the patient after disk surgery. This occurs about 40% of the time (probably more), since most back surgery is not indicated and done on inappropriate candidates. Causes of FBSS are grouped into early and late for the purpose of multiple choice test question writing:

	Complications of Spine Surgery
Recurrent Residual Disk	Will lack enhancement (unlike a scar – which will enhance on delays)
Epidural Fibrosis	Scar, that is usually posterior, and enhance homogeneously
Arachnoiditis	Buzzwords are *"clumped nerve roots"* and *"empty thecal sac"*, **Enhancement for 6 weeks post op is considered normal.** After 6 weeks may be infectious or inflammatory.
Conjoined Nerve Roots	Two adjacent nerve roots sharing an enlarged common sleeve – at a point during their exit from the thecal sac
12,000 Square Foot Mansion Syndrome	As spine surgeons perform more and more unnecessary surgeries they need something to spend all that money on.

Scar vs Residual Disc:

T1 Pre Contrast they will look the same… like a bunch of mushy crap.
T1 Post Contrast they disc will still look like mushy crap, but the scar will enhance.

Trauma to the Spine:

Jefferson	Burst Fracture of C1	Axial Loading
Hangman	Bilateral Pedicle or Pars Fracture of C2	Hyperextension
Teardrop	Can be flexion or extension	Flexion (more common)
Clay-Shoveler's	Avulsion of spinous process at C7 or T1	Hyperflexion
Chance	Horizontal Fracture through thoracolumbar spine ("seatbelt").	

Jefferson Fracture: This is an axial loading injury (jumping into a shallow pool) – with the blow typically to the top of the head. The anterior and posterior arches blow out laterally. They would most likely show it on a plain film open mouth odontoid view (the CT would be too easy). Remember the C1 lateral masses shouldn't slide off laterally.

Important trivia to remember: **Neurologic (cord) damage is rare**, because all the force is directed into the bones.

Odontoid Fracture Classification:
- Type 1: Upper part of Odontoid (maybe stable) – this is actually rare
- Type 2: Fracture at the base – unstable - and by far the most common.
- Type 3: Fracture through dens into the body of C2. This is unstable, but has the best prognosis for healing.

Os Odontoideum: A mimic for a type 1 Odontoid fracture. This is an ossicle located at the position of the normal odontoid tip (the orthotopic position). The base of the dens is usually hypoplastic. The thing to know are that **this is prone to subluxation and instability**. It's association with Morquio's syndrome.

Orthotopic vs Dystopic: Orthotopic is the position right on top of the dens. Dystopic is when it's fused to the clivus.

Hangman's Fracture: Seen most commonly when the chin hits the dashboard in an MVA ("direct blow to the face"). The **fracture is through the bilateral pars at C2** (or the pedicles – which is less likely). You will have anterior subluxation of the C2 body. Cord damage is actually uncommon with these, as the acquired pars defect allows for canal widening. There is often an associated fracture of the anterior inferior corner at C2 – from avulsion of the anterior longitudinal ligament.

Flexion Teardrop: This represents a teardrop shaped fracture fragment at the anterior-inferior vertebral body. Flexion injury is bad because it is associated with anterior cord syndrome (85% of patients have deficits). This is an unstable fracture, associated with posterior subluxation of the vertebral body.

> **Anterior Cord Syndrome:** The anterior portion of the cord is jacked. Motor function and anterior column sensations (pain and temperature) are history. The dorsal column sensations (proprioception and vibration) are still intact.

Extension Teardrop: Another anterior inferior teardrop shaped fragment with avulsion of the anterior longitudinal ligament. This is less serious than the flexion type.

Flexion Teardrop	Extension Teardrop
Impaction Injury	Distraction Injury
Unstable	Stable (maybe)
Hyperflexion	Hyperextension
Classic History: "Ran into wall"	Classic History" Hit from behind"

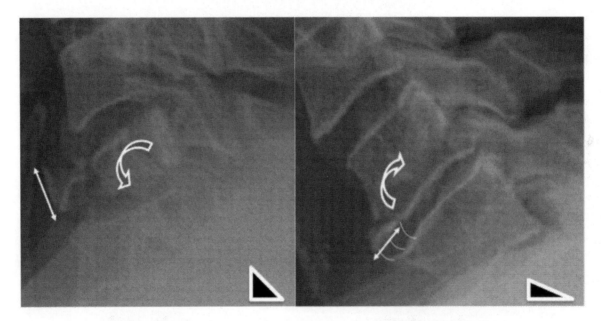

Flexion　　　　　　Extension

Clay-Shoveler's Fracture: This is an avulsion injury of a lower cervical / upper thoracic spinous process (usually C7). It is the result of a forceful hyperflexion movement (like shoveling). The "ghost sign" describes a double spinous process at C6-C7.

Facet Dislocation: This is a spectrum: Subluxed facets -> Perched -> Locked.

- Unilateral: If you have a unilateral facet (usually from hyperflexion and rotation) the superior facet slides over the inferior facet and gets locked. The unilateral is a stable injury. You will have the inverted hamburger sign on axial imaging on the dislocated side.

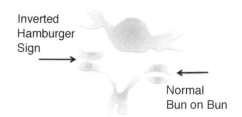

- Bilateral: This is the result of severe hyperflexion. You are going to have disruption of the posterior ligament complex. When this is full on you are going to have the dislocated vertebra displaced forward one –half the AP diameter of the vertebral body. This is highly unstable, and strongly associated with cord injury.

Atlantoaxial Instability - The articulation between C1 and C2 allows for lateral movement (shaking your head no). The transverse cruciform ligament straps the dens to the anterior arch of C1. The distance between the anterior arch and dens shouldn't be more than 5mm. The thing to know is the **association with Down syndrome and juvenile RA.** Rotary subluxation can occur in children without a fracture, with the kid stuck in a "cock-robbin" position – which looks like torticollis. Actually differentiating from torticollis is difficult and may require dynamic maneuvers on the scanner. This never, ever, ever happens in the absence of a fracture in an adult (who doesn't have Downs or RA). Having said that people over call this all the time in adults who have their heads turned in the scanner.

Benign Vs Malignant Compression Fracture: This is a high yield distinction and practical in the real world.

Malignant	Benign
Convex posterior vertebral body cortex	Retropulsed fragment
Involves Posterior Elements	Transverse T1 and T2 dark band
Epidural / Paraspinal Mass	
Multiple Lesions	

Trauma to the Cord: There is a known correlation between spinal cord edema length and outcome. Having said that, you need to know the **most important factor for outcome is the presence of a hemorrhagic spinal cord injury** (these do very very badly).

Spinal Cord Syndromes		
Central Cord	Old lady with spondylosis or young person with bad extension injury.	Upper Extremity Deficit is worse than lower (corticospinal tracts are lateral in lower extremity)
Anterior Cord	Flexion Injury	Immediate Paralysis
Brown Sequard	Rotation injury or penetrating trauma	One half motor, other half sensory
Posterior Cord	Uncommon – but sometimes seen with hyperextension	Proprioception gone

Congenital / Developmental

Pars Interarticularis Defects: This is considered a fatigue or stress fracture, probably developing in childhood (they are more common in athletic kids). They are usually not symptomatic (only 25% are). The most common level is L5-S1 (90%), with all the rest at L4-L5. They tend to have more spondylolisthesis and associated degenerative change at L4-L5 than L5-S1. They can be seen on the oblique plain film as a "collar on the scottie dog."

Pars Defects with Anteriorlithesis will have neuroforaminal stensosis, with spinal canal widening (when severe will have spinal canal stenosis as well).

Terminal Ventricle (ventricularis terminalis): This is a developmental variant. Normally, a large portion of the distal cord involutes in a late stage of spinal cord embryology. Sometimes this process is not uniform and you get stuck with a stupid looking cyst at the end of your cord. These things are usually small (around 4mm), and cause no symptoms. Sometimes they can get very big (like this example) and cause some neurologic symptoms.

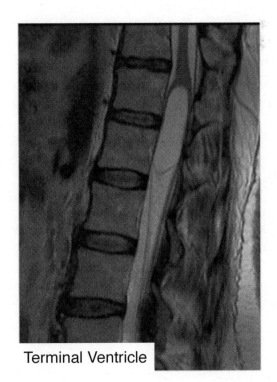

Terminal Ventricle

Spinal Dysraphism:

You can group these as open or closed (closed with and without a mass). Open means neural tissue exposed through a defect in bone and skin (spina bifida aperta). Closed means the defect is covered by skin (spina bifida occulta).

Open Spinal Dysraphisms: This is the result of a failure of the closure of the primary neural tube, with obvious exposure of the neural placode through a midline defect of the skin. You have a dorsal defect in the posterior elements. The **cord is going to be tethered.** There is an association with diastematomyelia and Chiari II malformations. Early surgery is the treatment / standard of care.

- *Myeloceles*: This is the more rare type where the neural placode is flush with the skin.

- *Myelomeningoceles:* This is the more common type (98%) where the neural placode protrudes above the skin. These are more common with Chiari II malformations.

Closed Spinal Dysraphisms with Subcutaneous Mass

- *Meningoceles*: This is herniation of a CSF filled sac through a defect in the posterior elements (spina bifida). It is most typical in the lumbar or sacral periods. Although they can occur in the cervical spine. They may be anterior (usually pre-sarcral). An important point is **that neural tissue is not present in the sac.**

- *Lipomyelocele / Lipomyelomeningoceles:* These are lipomas with a dural defect. On exam you are going to have a subcutaneous fatty mass above the gluteal crease. **These are 100% associated with tethered cord** (myelomeningocele may or may not).

- *Terminal Myelocystocele* – This is a herniation of the terminal syrinx into a posterior menigoccele via a posterior spinal defect.

Closed Spinal Dysraphisms without Subcutaneous Mass

- *Intradural lipomas* – Most common in the thoracic spine also the dorsal aspect. They don't need to be (but can be) associated with posterior element defects.

- *Fibrolipoma of the filum terminale* – This is often an incidental finding. There will be a linear T1 bright structure in the filum terminale. The filum is not going to be unusually thickened and the conus will be normally located.

- *Tight filum terminale* – This is a thickened filum terminale (> 2mm), with a low lying conus (below the inferior endplate of L2). You may have an associated terminal lipoma. The **"tethered cord syndrome"** is based on the clinical findings of low back pain and leg pain plus urinary bladder dysfunction. This is the result of stretching the cord with growth of the canal.

- *Dermal Sinus* – This is an epithelium lined tract that extends from the skin to deep soft tissues (sometimes the spinal canal, sometimes a dermoid or lipoma). These are T1 low signal (relative to the background high signal from fat).

Diastematomyelia – This describes a sagittal split in the spinal cord. They almost always occur between T9-S1, with normal cord both above and below the split. You can have two thecal sacs (or just one), and each hemicord has its own central canal and dorsal/ventral horns. Classification systems are based on the presence / absence of an osseous or fibrous spur and duplication or non-duplication of the thecal sac.

Caudal Regression: This is a spectrum of defect in the caudal region that ranges from partial agenesis of the coccyx to lumbosacral agenesis. The associations to know are VACTERL and Currarino triad. Think about this with maternal diabetes. "Blunted sharp" high terminating cord is classic, with a "shield sign" from the opposed iliac bones (no sacrum).

> **Currarino Triad:**
>
> *Anterior Sacral Meningocele,*
>
> *Anorectal malformation,*
>
> *Sacrococcygeal osseous defect (simitar sacrum).*

Spinal Vascular Disorders

AVFs / AVMs: There are 4 types. **Type 1 is by far the most common** (85%). **It is a Dural AVF**; the result of a fistula between the dorsal radiculomedullary arteries and radiculomedullary vein / coronal sinus – with the dural nerve sleeve. It is acquired and seen in older patients who present with progressive radiculomyelopathy. The most common location is the thoracic spine. If anyone asks the "gold standard for diagnosis is angiography", although CTA or MRA will get the job done. You will have T2 high signal in the central cord (which will be swollen), with serpentine perimedullary flow voids (which are usually dorsal).

	Spinal AVM / AVFs
Type 1	**Most Common Type** (85%). **Dural AVF** – with a single coiled vessel
Type 2	**Intramedullary Nidus** from anterior spinal artery or posterior spinal artery. Can have aneurysms, and can bleed. Most common presentation is SAH. Associated with HHT and KTS (other vascular syndromes).
Type 3	**Juvenile**, very rare, often complex and with a terrible prognosis
Type 4	Intradural **perimedullary** with subtypes depending on single vs multiple arterial supply. These tend to occur **near the conus.**

Foix Alajouanine Syndrome: This is a myelopathy association with a Dural AVF. The classic history is a 45 year old male with lower extremity weakness and sensory deficits. You have increased T2 signal (either at the conus, or lower thoracic spine), with associated prominent vessels. The underlying pathophysiology is venous hypertension - secondary to the vascular malformation.

Misc Disorders Affecting the Spine

Pagets – This is discussed in detail in the MSK chapter, but is such a high yield topic that it's worth touching on again. The incidence increases with age (around 8% at age 80). It's at increased risk for fracture, and has a 1% risk of sarcoma degeneration (usually high grade).

It's shown two ways in the spine:
(1) An enlarged "ivory vertebrae",
(2) Picture frame vertebrae (sclerotic border).

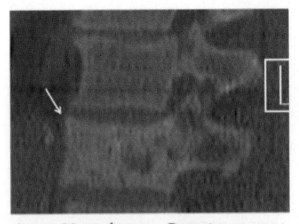

Ivory Vertebrae – Pagets *(or mets)*

Renal Osteodystrophy – Another high yield topic covered in depth in the MSK chapter. The way it's shown in the spine is the "Rugger Jersey Spine" – with sclerotic bands at the top and bottom of the vertebral body. You could also have paraspinous soft tissue calcifications

Osteopetrosis - Another high yield topic covered in depth in the MSK chapter. This is a genetic disease with impaired osteoclastic resorption. You have thick cortical bone, with diminished marrow. On plain film or CT it can look like a Rugger Jersey Spine or Sandwich vertebra. On MR you are going to have loss of the normal T1 bright marrow signal, so it will be T1 and T2 dark.

"H-Shaped Vertebra" – This is usually a **buzzword for sickle cell**, although it's only seen in about 10% of cases. It results from microvascular endplate infarct. If you see "H-Shaped vertebra" the answer is sickle cell. If sickle cell isn't a choice the answer is Gauchers. Another tricky way to ask this is to say which of the following causes **"widening of the disc space."** Widened disc space is another way of describing a "H Shape" without saying that.

Infectious

Discitis / Osteomyelitis:

Infection of the disc and infection of the vertebral body nearly always go together. The reason has to do with the route of seeding; which typically involves seeding of the vertebral endplate (which is vascular), subsequent eruption and crossing into the disc space, and eventual involvement of the adjacent vertebral body.

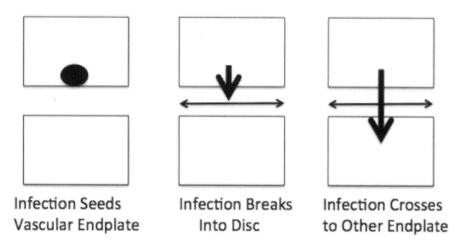

In adults, the source is usually from a recent surgery, procedure, or systemic infection. In children it's usually from hematogenous spread. For the Step 1 trivia: Staph A is the most common bug, and always think about an IV drug user. Almost always (80%) of the time the ESR and CRP are elevated.

Imaging: Early on it's very hard to see with plain films, you will need MRI. You are looking for paraspinal and epidural inflammation, T2 bright disc signal, disc enhancement

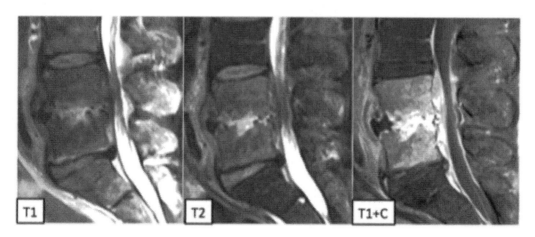

Vertebral Osteomyelitis

Pott's Disease: TB of the spine is more common in "developing" countries. It behaves in a few different ways, and that makes it easy to test on.

Things to know about TB in the spine:
- *It tends to **spare the disc space***
- *It tends to have multi-level thoracic "skip" involvement*
- *Buzzword "Calcified Psoas Abscess"*
- *Buzzword "Gibbus Deformity" – which is a destructive focal kyphosis*

Brucellosis: This is uncommon in the USA. It's somewhat unique feature make it testable. Just know that it **favors the lower lumbar spine & SI joints, and can spare the disk space (similar to TB).** Vertebral destruction and paraspinal abscess are actually less common. Step 1 buzzword was "cow's milk" or "farm exposure."

Epidural Abscess: This is an infected collection between the dura and periostium. Its usually MRSA and the patient usually has HIV or is a bad diabetic. This is most likely to be shown with diffusion. A collection that restricts is going be an abscess (in the spine and in the brain) – most of the time. It should also be T1 dark, T2 bright, with peripheral enhancement.

Cord Pathology

Syrinx – Also known as *"a hole in the cord"*. People use the word "syrinx" for all those fancy French / Latin words (hydromyelia, syringomyelia, hydrosyringomyelia, syringohydromyelia, syringobulbia etc…). They do this because they don't know what those words mean. Here is the way I do it… if there is a perfectly central high signal dilation in the middle of the cord, surrounded by totally normal cord I call it "central cord dilation" or "benign central cord dilation", if there is the same thing but the cord around it looks "sick" - its also got high signal, or the cord is atrophic, etc… then I use the word "myelia." Myelia is a word to use when you want to say it's pathologic.

Most (90%) cord dilations (healthy and sick ones) are congenital, and associated with Chiari I and II, as well as Dandy-Walker, Klippel-Feil, and Myelomeningoceles. The other 10% are acquired either by trauma, tumor, or vascular insufficiency.

Demyelinating:

Broadly you can think of cord pathology in 5 categories: Demyelinating, Tumor, Vascular, Inflammatory, and Infectious.

In the real world, the answer is almost always MS – which is by far the most common cause. The other three things it could be are Neuromyelitis Optica (NMO), acute disseminating encephalomyelitis (ADEM) or Transverse Myelitis (TM).

MS	Usually Short Segment	Usually Part of the Cord	Not swollen, or Less Swollen	Can Enhance / Restrict when Acute
TM	Usually Long Segment	Usually involves both sides of the cord	Expanded Swollen Cord	Can Enhance
NMO	Usually Long Segment	Usually involves both sides of the cord		Optic Nerves Involved
ADEM			Not swollen, or Less Swollen	
Infarct	Usually Long Segment			Restricted Diffusion
Tumor			Expanded Swollen Cord	Can Enhance

MS in the Cord: "Multiple lesions, over space and time." The lesions in the spine are typically short segment (< 2), usually only affect half / part of the cord. The cervical cord is the most common location. There are usually lesions in the brain, if you have lesions in the cord (isolated cord lesions occur about 10% of the time). The lesions can enhance when acute – but this is more common than in the brain. You can sometimes see cord atrophy if the lesion burden is large.

Transverse Myelitis: This is a focal inflammation of the cord. The causes are numerous (infectious, post vaccination – classic rabies, SLE, Sjogrens, Paraneolastic, AV-malformations). You typically have at least 2/3 of the cross sectional area of the cord involved, and focal enlargement of the cord. Spliters with use the terms "Acute partial" for lesions less than two segments, and "acute complete" for lesions more than two segments. The factoid to know is that the "Acute partials" are higher risk for developing MS.

ADEM: As described in the brain section, this is usually seen after a viral illness or infection typically in a child or young adult. The lesions favor the dorsal white matter (but can involve grey matter). As a pearl, the presence of cranial nerve enhancement is suggestive of ADEM. The step 1 trivia, is that the "anti-MOG IgG" test is positive in 50% of cases. Just like MS there are usually brain lesions (although ADEM lesions can occur in the basal ganglia and pons – which is unusual in MS).

NMO (Neuromyelitis Optica): This is also sometimes called Devics. It can be monophasic or relapsing, and favors the optic nerves and cervical cord. Tends to be longer segment than MS, and involve the full transverse diameter of the cord. Brain lesions can occur (more commonly in Asians) and are usually periventricular. If any PhDs ask the reason the periventricular location occurs is that the antibody (NMO IgG) attacks the Aquaporin 4 channels – which are found in highest concentration around the ventricles.

Subacute Combined Degeneration: This is a fancy way of describing the effects of a Vitamin B12 deficiency. The classic look is **bilateral symmetrically increased T2 signal in the dorsal columns**, without enhancement. The appearance has been described as an "inverted V sign." The signal change typically begins in the upper thoracic region with ascending or descending progression.

HIV Vacuolar Myelopathy: This has been described as a late finding in AIDS patients. You have spinal cord atrophy, and T2 high signal symmetrically involving the posterior columns. It looks like subacute combined degeneration.

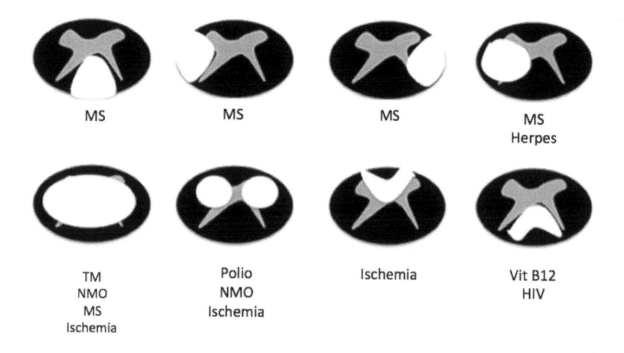

Spinal Cord Infarct: Cord infarct /ischemia can have a variety of causes. The most common cause is "idiopathic," although I'd expect the most common multiple choice scenario to revolve around treating an aneurysm with a stent graft, or embolizing a bronchial artery. Impairment involving the anterior spinal artery distribution is most common. With anterior spinal artery involvement you are going to have central cord / anterior horn cell high signal on T2 (because gray matter is more vulnerable to ischemia).

The "**owl eye appearance**" of anterior spinal cord infarct is a buzzword.

It's usually a long segment, being more than 2 segments. Diffusion using single shot fast spin echo or line scan can be used with high sensitivity (to compensate for artifacts from spinal fluid movement).

Inflammatory / Infectious:

Arachnoiditis: This is a general term for inflammation of the subarachnoid space. It can be infectious but can also be post-surgical. **It actually occurs about 10-15% of the time after spine surgery, and can be a source of persistent pain / failed back.**

It's shown two ways:

(1) **Empty Thecal Sac Sign** – Nerve roots are adherent peripherally, giving the appearance of an empty sac.

(2) *Central Nerve Root Clumping.* This can range in severity from a few nerves clumping together, to all of them fused into a single central scarred band.

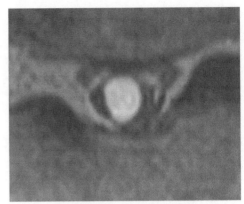

Empty Thecal Sac Sign

Guillain Barre Syndrome (GBS) - One of those weird auto-immune disorders that causes ascending flaccid paralysis. The step 1 trivia was **Campylobacter**, but you can also see it after surgery, or in patients with lymphoma or SLE.

The thing to know is **enhancement of the nerve roots of the cauda equina**.

Other pieces of trivia that are less likely to be asked are that the facial nerve is the most common cranial nerve affected, and that the anterior spinal roots enhance more than the posterior ones.

Chronic Inflammatory Demylinating Polyneuropathy (CIDP) - The chronic counterpart to GBS. Clinically this has a gradual and protracted weakness (GBS improves in 8 weeks, CIDP does not). The buzzword is thickened, enhancing, "onion bulb" nerve roots.

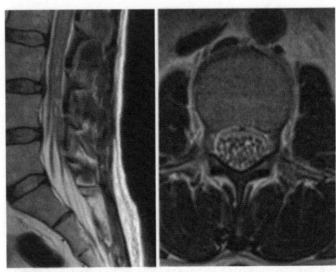

CIDP - Diffuse Thickening of the Nerve Roots

Tumor:

The classic teaching is to first describe the location of the tumor, as either (1) Intramedullary, (2) Extramedullary Intradural, or (3) Extradural. This is often easier said than done. Differentials are based on the location.

Intramedullary	Astrocytoma, Ependymoma, Hemangioblastoma
Extramedullary Intradural	Schwannoma, Meningioma, Neurofibroma, Drop Mets
Extradural	Disc Disease (most common), Bone Tumors, Mets, Lymphoma

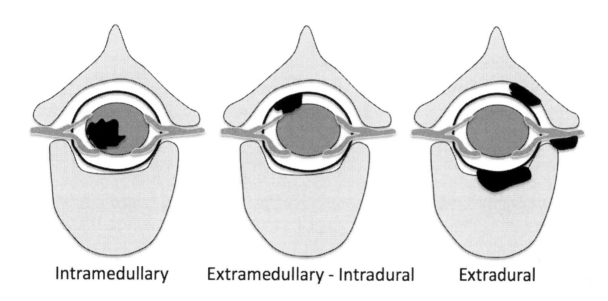

Intramedullary   Extramedullary - Intradural   Extradural

Intramedullary:

- **Astrocytoma** – This is the most common intramedullary tumor in peds. It favors the upper thoracic spine. There will be fusiform dilation of the cord over multiple segments. They are dark on T1, bright on T2, and they enhance. They may be associated with rostral or caudal cysts which are usually benign syrinx formation.

Astrocytoma	Ependymoma
More in Cervical Cord	More in Lower Cord
Eccentric	Central
Longer Segment	Shorter Segment
	More Often Hemorrhagic
Most common intramedullary in PEDS	Most common intramedullary in Adults

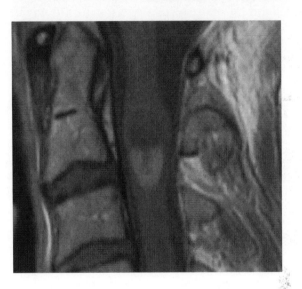

- **Ependymoma** – This is the most common primary cord tumor of the lower spinal cord, conus / filum terminale. This is the **most common intramedullary mass in adult**s. Although you can certainly see them in the cervical cord as well. The "**myxopapillary form**" is exclusively found in the conus /filum locations. They can be hemorrhagic, and have a **dark cap on T2.** They have tumoral cysts about ¼ of the time. They are a typically long segment (averaging 4 segments).

- **Hemangioblastoma** - These are associated with Von Hippel Lindau (30%). The thoracic level is favored (second most common is cervical). The classic look is a wide cord, with <u>considerable edema</u>. Adjacent serpinginous draining meningeal varicosities can be seen.

- **Intramedullary Mets:** This is very very rare, but when it does happen its usually lung (70%).

VHL Associations:

- Pheochromocytoma
- CNS Hemangioblastoma *(cerebellum 75%, spine 25%)*
- Endolymphatic Sac Tumor
- Pancreatic Cysts
- Pancreatic Islet Cell Tumors
- Clear Cell RCC

Extramedullary Intradural:

- **Schwannoma:** This is the most common tumor to occur in the Extramedullary Intradural location. The are benign, usually solitary, usually arising from the dorsal nerve roots. This can be multiple in the setting of NF-2 and the Carney Complex. The appearance is variable, but the classic look is a dumbbell with the skinny handle being the intraforaminal component. They are T1 dark, T2 bright, and will enhance. They look a lot like neurofibromas. If they have central necrosis or hemorrhage that favors a schwannoma.

- **Neurofibroma:** This is another benign nerve tumor *(composed of all parts of the nerve: nerve + sheath)*, that is also usually solitary. There are two flavors: solitary and plexiform. The plexiform is a multilevel bulky nerve enlargement that is pathognomonic for NF-1. Their lifetime risk for malignant degeneration is around 5-10%. Think about malignant degeneration in the setting of rapid growth. They look a lot like schwannomas. If they have a hyperintense T2 rim with a central area of low signal – "target sign" that makes you favor neurofibroma.

Schwannoma	Neurofibroma
Do NOT envelop the adjacent nerve root	Do envelop the adjacent nerve root (usually a dorsal sensory root)
Solitary	Solitary
Multiple makes you think NF-2	Associated with NF-1 (even when single)
Cystic change / Hemorrhage	T2 bright rim, T2 dark center "target sign"

- **Meningioma:** These guys adhere to but do not originate from the dura. They are more common in women (70%). They favor the posterior lateral thoracic spine, and the anterior cervical spine. They enhance brightly and homogeneously. They are often T1 iso to hypo, and slightly T2 bright. They can have calcifications.

- **Drop Mets:** Medulloblastoma is the most common primary tumor to drop. Breast cancer is the most common systemic tumor to drop (followed by lung and melanoma). The cancer may coat the cord or nerve root, leading to a fine layer of enhancement.

Extradural:

- **Vertebral Hemangioma:** These are very common – seen in about 10% of the population. They classically have thickening trabeculae appearing as parallel lineal densities "jail bar" or "corduroy" appearance. In the vertebral body they are T1 and T2 bright, although the extraosseuous components typically lack fat and are isointense on T1.

- **Osteoid Osteoma:** This is also covered in the MSK chapter, but as a brief review focusing on the spine they love to involve the posterior elements (75%), and are rare after age 30. They tend to have a nidus, and surrounding sclerosis. The nidus is T2 bright, and will enhance. The classic story is night pain, better with aspirin. Radiofrequency ablation can treat them (under certain conditions).

- **Osteoblastoma:** This is similar to an Osteoid osteoma but larger than 1.5cm. Again, very often in the posterior elements – usually of the cervical spine.

- **Aneursymal Bone Cyst:** These guys are also covered in the MSK chapter. They also like the posterior elements and are usually seen in the first two decades of life. They are expansile (as the name implies) and can have multiple fluid levels on T2. They can get big, and look aggressive.

- **Giant Cell Tumor:** These guys are also covered in the MSK chapter. These are common in the sacrum, although rare anywhere else in the spine. You don't see them in young kids. If they show this it's going to be a **lytic expansile lesion in the sacrum with no rim of sclerosis.**

- **Vertebral Plana** - The pancake flat vertebral body. Just say Eosinophilc Granuloma in a kid (could be neuroblastoma met), and Mets / Myeloma in an adult.

- **Chordoma:** This is **most common in the sacrum** (they will want you to say clivus – that is actually number 2). The thing to know is that vertebral primary tend to be more aggressive / malignant than their counter parts in the clivus and sacrum. The classic story in the vertebral column is "involvement of two or more adjacent vertebral bodies with the intervening disc. " Most are **very T2 bright**.

- **Leukemia:** They love to show it in the spine. You have loss of the normal fatty marrow – so it's going to be homogeneously dark on T1. More on this in the MSK chapter.

- **Mets:** The classic offenders are prostate, breast, lung, lymphoma, and myeloma. Think **multiple lesions, with low T1 signal**. Cortical breakthrough or adjacent paravertebral components are also helpful.

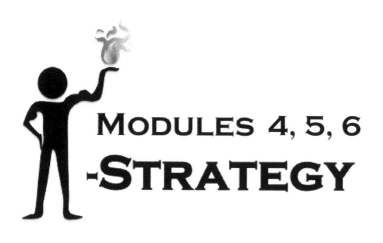
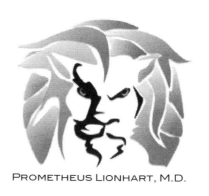
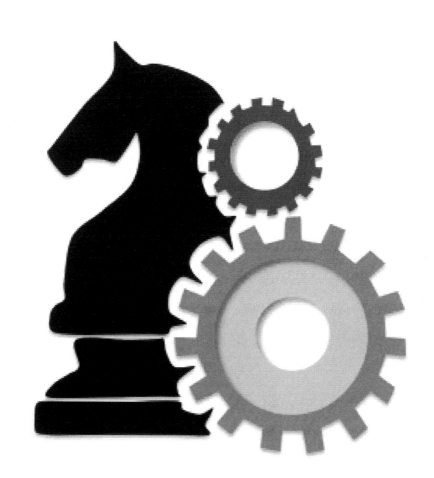

There are 3 kinds of questions on multiple choice tests

1. **The ones you know** – you want to get 100% of these right
2. **The ones you don't know** – you want to get 25% of these right (same as a monkey guessing)
3. **The ones you can figure out with some deep thought** – you want to get 60-70% of these right.

If you can do that you will pass the test, especially if you've read my books.

<u>My recommendations</u>:
- For the ones you know, just get them right.
- For the ones you don't know – just say to yourself *"this is one I don't know, Prometheus says just try and narrow it down and guess."*
- For the ones you think you can figure out, mark them, and go through the entire exam. If you follow my suggestion on the first two types of questions you will have ample time left over for head scratching. Other reasons to go ahead and do the whole exam before trying to figure them out is (a) you don't want to rush on the questions you can get right, and (b) sometimes you will see a case that reminds you of what the answer is. In fact it's not impossible that the stem of another question flat out tells you the answer to a previous question.

Let your plans be dark, and impenetrable as night, and when you move, fall like a thunderbolt.
　　　　　　　　　　　　　　　　　　　　　　　　　　　　　　　　　-Sun Tzu

Exploiting the "Genius Neuron"

Have you ever heard someone in case conference take a case and lead with "It's NOT this," when clearly "this" is what the case was? It happens all the time. Often the first thing out of people's mouths is actually the write answer, but many times you hear people say "it's not" first. Ever wondered why?

There is this idea of a "Genius Neuron." You have one neuron that is superior to the rest. This guy fires faster and is more reliable than his peers and because of this he is hated by them. He is the guy in the front row waving his hand shouting "I know the answer!" You know that guy, that guy is a notorious asshole. So, in your mind he shouts out the answer first, and then the rest of the neurons gang up on him and try and talk him out of it. So the end product is "It's NOT this."

For the purpose of taking cases in conference, this is why you should always lead with "this comes to mind," instead of "it's not." Now, the practical piece of advice I want to give you is to **trust your genius neuron**. Serious, there is a lot of material on this test. But if you read this book, there will be enough knowledge to pass the test existing somewhere between your ears. You just have to trust that genius neuron.

How?? - Do it like this:

(1) Read the entire question. Look at all the pictures.

(2) Read ALL the answer choices. Never stop at A thinking that is the answer.

(3) Look again at ALL the pictures – now that you see the choices.

(4) Choose the first answer your mind tells you is correct – the one your genius neuron thinks it correct.

(5) After you have finished the test, and you are re-reviewing your answers NEVER change the genius neuron's answer except for two criteria. (A) You read the question wrong. (B) You are 100% sure that it is another choice, and you can give a reason why. Never change based on your gut feelings. Those secondary gut feelings are the stupid neurons trying to gang up on the smart one. Just like in the real world the stupid people significantly outnumber the smart ones.

I know this sounds silly, but I really believe in this. This is a real thing. I encourage you to try it with some practice questions.

You either believe in yourself or you don't

    -Captain James T. Kirk.

It's Possible to Know Too Much

If you were to begin studying and begin taking multiple choice practice questions and you plotted your progress as you gained more knowledge you would notice something funny. At first you would begin to get more and more questions right… and then you would start to miss them.

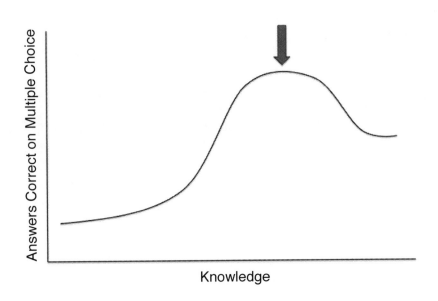

Well how can that be? I will tell you that once you know enough all choices on the exam become correction. Which of the following can occur?… well actually they can all occur - i've read case reports of blah blah blah. That is what happens.

The trick is to not over think things. Once you've achieved a certain level of knowledge, if they give you a gift — take it. It's usually not a trick (usually). Don't look for obscure situations when things are true. Yes… it's possible for you to know more than the person writing the questions. Yes… I said it and it's fucking true. These people don't know everything. You can out knowledge them if you study enough - and that is when you get yourself into trouble.

Take home point - once you've reached the peak (arrow on chart) - be careful over thinking questions past that point.

"Always remember: Your focus determines your reality"

-*Jedi Master Qui-Gon Jinn*

6 Promethean Laws For Multiple Choice

#1 - If you have a gut feeling - go for it ! (trust the genius neuron)

#2 - Don't over think to the extent that you veer from a reflexive answer - especially if choices seem equally plausible (you can know too much).

#3 - Read ALL the choices carefully

#4 - If it seems too obvious to be true (trickery), re-read it and then go with it (even if it seems to easy). Let it happen - it's usually not a trick… usually.

#5 - Add up what you know you know, and compare with what you think you know. Weight your answers by what you KNOW you KNOW.

#6 - Most Importantly - <u>Don't Panic</u>

Maybe I can't win, maybe the only thing I can do is just take everything he's got. But to beat me, he's gonna have to kill me, and to kill me, he's gonna have to have the heart to stand in front of me, and to do that, he's has to be willing to die himself

- *Rocky Balboa*

Section 1: Urinary

When I Say This..... You Say That.....

- When I say "bladder stones," you say neurogenic bladder
- When I say "pine cone appearance," you say neurogenic bladder
- When I say "urethra cancer," you say squamous cell CA
- When I say "urethra cancer - prostatic portion," you say transitional cell CA
- When I say "urethra cancer - in a diverticulum," you say adenocarcinoma
- When I say "vas deferens calcifications," you say diabetes
- When I say "calcifications in a fatty renal mass," you say RCC
- When I say "protrude into the renal pelvis," you say Multilocular cystic nephroma
- When I say "no functional renal tissue," you say Multicystic Dysplastic Kidney
- When I say "Multicystic Dysplastic Kidney," you say contralateral renal issues (50%)
- When I say "Emphysematous Pyelonephritis," you say diabetic
- When I say "Xanthogranulomatous Pyelonephritis," you say staghorn stone
- When I say "Papillary Necrosis," you say diabetes
- When I say "shrunken calcified kidney," you say TB
- When I say "big bright kidney with decreased renal function," you say HIV
- When I say "history of lithotripsy," you say Page Kidney
- When I say "cortical rim sign," you say subacute renal infarct
- When I say "history of renal biopsy," you say AVF
- When I say "reversed diastolic flow," you say renal vein thrombosis
- When I say "sickle cell trait," you say medullary RCC
- When I say "Young Adult, Renal Mass, + Severe HTN," you say Juxtaglomerular Cell Tumor
- When I say "squamous cell bladder CA," you say Schistosomiasis
- When I say "entire bladder calcified," you say Schistosomiasis
- When I say "urachus," you say adenocarcinoma of the bladder
- When I say "long stricture in urethra," you say Gonococcal
- When I say "short stricture in urethra," you say Straddle Injury

High Yield Trivia

- Calcifications in a renal CA - are associated with an improved survival
- RCC bone mets are "always" lytic
- There is an increased risk of malignancy with dialysis
- Horseshoe kidneys are more susceptible to trauma
- Most common location for TCC is the bladder
- Second most common location for TCC is the upper urinary tract
- Upper Tract TCC in more commonly multifocal (12%) - as opposed to bladder (4%).
- Weigert Meyer Rule - Upper Pole inserts medial and inferior
- Ectopic Ureters are associated with incontinence in women (not men)
- Leukoplakia is pre-malignant; Malakoplakia is not pre-malignant
- Extraperitoneal bladder rupture is more common, and managed medically
- Intraperitoneal bladder rupture is less common, and managed surgically
- Indinavir stones are the only ones not seen on CT.
- Uric Acid stones are not seen on plain film.

Section 2: OB GYN

When I Say This..... You Say That.....

- When I say "Unicornuate Uterus," you say Look at the kidneys
- When I say "T-Shaped Uterus," you say DES related or Vaginal Clear Cell CA
- When I say "Marked enlargement of the uterus," you say Adenomyosis
- When I say "Adenomyosis," you say thickening of the junctional zone (> 12mm)
- When I say "Wolffian duct remnant," you say Gartner Duct Cyst
- When I say "Theca Lutein Cysts," you say moles and multiple gestations
- When I say "Theca Lutein Cysts + Pleural Effusions," you say - Hyperstimulation Syndrome (patient on fertility meds).
- When I say "Low level internal echoes," you say Endometrioma
- When I say "T2 Shortening," you say - Endometrioma - "Shading Sign"
- When I say "Fishnet appearance," you say Hemorrhagic Cyst
- When I say "Ovarian Fibroma + Pleural Effusion," you say Meigs Syndrome
- When I say "Snow Storm Uterus, " you say Complete Mole - 1st Trimester
- When I say "Serum β-hCG levels that rise in the 8 to 10 weeks following evacuation of molar pregnancy," you say Choriocarcinoma
- When I say "midline cystic structure near the back of the bladder of a man," you say Prostatic Utricle
- When I say "lateral cystic structure near the back of the bladder of a man," you say Seminal Vesicle Cyst
- When I say "isolated orchitis," you say mumps
- When I say "onion skin appearance," you say epidermoid cyst
- When I say "multiple hypoechoic masses in the testicle," you say lymphoma
- When I say "cystic elements and macro-calcifications in the testicle," you say Mixed Germ Cell Tumor
- When I say "homogenous and microcalcifications," you say seminoma
- When I say "gynecomastia + testicular tumor," you say Sertoli Leydig
- When I say "fetal macrosomia," you say Maternal Diabetes
- When I say "one artery adjacent to the bladder," you say two vessel cord
- When I say "painless vaginal bleeding in the third trimester," you say placenta previa
- When I say "mom doing cocaine," you say placenta abruption
- When I say "thinning of the myometrium - with turbulent doppler," you say placenta creta

- When I say "mass near the cord insertion, with flow pulsating at the fetal heart rate," you say placenta chorioangioma
- When I say "Cystic mass in the posterior neck -antenatal period," you say cystic hygroma.
- When I say "Pleural effusions, and Ascites on prenatal US," you say hydrops.
- When I say "Massively enlarged bilateral kidneys," you say ARPKD
- When I say "Twin peak sign," you say dichorionic diamniotic

High Yield Trivia

- Endometrial tissue in a rudimentary horn (even one that does NOT communicate) increases the risk of miscarriage.
- Arcuate Uterus does NOT have an increased risk of infertility (it's a normal variant)
- Fibroids with higher T2 signal respond better to UAE
- Hyaline Fibroid Degeneration is the most common subtype
- Adenomyosis - favors the posterior wall, spares the cervix
- Hereditary Non-Polyposis Colon Cancer (NHPCC) – have a 30-50x increased risk of endometrial cancer
- Tamoxifen increases the risk of endometrial cancer, and endometrial polyps
- Cervical Cancer that has parametrial involvement (2B) - is treated with chemo/radiation. Cervical Cancer without parametrial involvement (2A) - is treated with surgery
- Vaginal cancer in adults is usually squamous cell
- Vaginal Rhabdomyosarcoma occurs in children / teenagers
- Premenopausal ovaries can be hot on PET (depending on the phase of cycle). Post menopausal ovaries should Never be hot on PET.
- Transformation subtypes: Endometrioma = Clear Cell, Dermoid = Squamous
- Post Partum fever can be from ovarian vein thrombophlebitis
- Fractured penis = rupture of the corpus cavernosum and the surrounding tunica albuginea.
- Prostate Cancer is most commonly in the peripheral zone, - ADC dark
- BPH nodules are in the central zone
- Hypospadias is the most common association with prostatic utricle
- Seminal Vesicle cysts are associated with renal agenesis, and ectopic ureters
- Cryptorchidism increases the risk of cancer (in both testicles), and is not reduced by orchiopexy
- Immunosuppressed patients can get testicular lymphoma -hiding behind blood testes barrier
- Most common cause of correctable infertility in a man is a varicocele.

- Undescended testicles are more common in premature kids.
- Membranes disrupted before 10 weeks, increased risk for amniotic bands
- The earliest visualization of the embryo is the "double bleb sign"
- Hematoma greater than 2/3 the circumference of the chorion has a 2x increased risk of abortion.
- Biparietal Diameter - Recorded at the level of the thalamus from the outermost edge of the near skull to the inner table of the far skull.
- Abdominal Circumference - does not include the subcutaneous soft tissues
- Abdominal Circumference is recorded at the the level of the junction of the umbilical vein and left portal vein
- Abdominal Circumference is the parameter classically involved with asymmetric IUGR
- Femur Length does NOT include the epiphysis
- Umbilical Artery Systolic / Diastolic Ratio should NOT exceed 3 at 34 weeks - makes you think pre-eclampsia and IUGR
- A full bladder can mimic a placenta previa
- Nuchal lucency is measured between 9-12 weeks, and should be < 3mm. More than 3mm is associated with downs.
- Lemon sign will disappear after 24 weeks
- Aquaductal Stenosis is the most common cause of non-communicating hydrocephalus in a neonate

Section 3: Breast

When I Say This..... You Say That.....

- When I say "shrinking breast," you say ILC
- When I say "thick coopers ligaments," you say edema
- When I say "thick fuzzy coopers ligaments - with normal skin," you say blur
- When I say "dashes but no dots," you say Secretory Calcifications
- When I say "cigar shaped calcifications," you say Secretory Calcifications
- When I say "popcorn calcifications," you say degenerated fibroadenoma
- When I say "breast within a breast," you say hamartoma
- When I say "fat-fluid level," you say galactocele
- When I say "rapid growing fibroadenoma," you say Phyllodes
- When I say "swollen red breast, not responding to antibiotics," you say Inflammatory breast CA
- When I say "lines radiating to a single point," you say Architectural distortion.
- When I say "Architectural distortion + Calcifications," you say IDC + DCIS
- When I say "Architectural distortion without Calcifications," you say ILC
- When I say "Stepladder Sign," you say Intracapsular rupture on US
- When I say "Linguine Sign," you say Intracapsular rupture on MRI
- When I say "Residual Calcs in the Lumpectomy Bed," you say local recurrence
- When I say "No cacls in the core," you say milk of calcium (requires polarized light to be seen).

High Yield Trivia

- No grid on mag views.
- Nipple enhancement can be normal on post contrast MRI - don't call it Pagets.
- Upper outer quadrant has the highest density of breast tissue, and therefore the most breast cancers.
- Majority of blood (60%) is via the internal mammary
- Majority of lymph (97%) is to the axilla
- The sternalis muscle can only be seen on CC view
- Most common location for ectopic breast tissue is in the axilla
- The follicular phase (day 7-14) is the best time to have a mammogram (and MRI).
- Breast Tenderness is max around day 27-30.
- Tyrer Cuzick is the most comprehensive risk model, but does not include breast density.
- If you had more than 20Gy of chest radiation as a child, you can get a screening MRI
- BRCA 2 (more than 1) is seen with male breast cancer
- BRCA 1 is more in younger patients, BRCA 2 is more is post menopausal
- BRCA 1 is more often a triple negative CA
- Use the LMO for kyphosis, pectus excavatum, and to avoid a pacemaker / line
- Use the ML to help catch milk of calcium layering
- Fine pleomorphic morphology to calcification has the highest suspicion for malignancy
- Intramammary lymph nodes are NOT in the fibroglandular tissue
- Surgical scars should get lighter, if they get denser - think about recurrent cancer.
- You CAN have isolated intracapsular rupture.
- You CAN NOT have isolated extra (it's always with intra).
- If you see silicone in a lymph node you need to recommend MRI to evaluate for intracapsular rupture
- The number one risk factor for implant rupture is the age of the implant
- Tamoxifen causes a decrease in parenchymal uptake, then a rebound.
- T2 Bright things - these are usually benign. Don't forget colloid cancer is T2 bright.

Section 4: Peds

When I Say This..... You Say That.....

- When I say "Subglottic Hemangioma," You Say PHACES Syndrome
- When I say "PHACES Syndrome," You say Cutaneous Hemangioma
- When I say "Ropy Appearance," You say Meconium Aspiration
- When I say "Post Term Delivery," You Say Meconium Aspiration
- When I say "Fluid in the Fissures," You say Transient Tachypnea
- When I say "History of c-section", You say Transient Tachypnea
- When I say "Maternal sedation", You say Transient Tachypnea
- When I say "Granular Opacities + Premature", You say RDS
- When I say "Granular Opacities + Term + High Lung Volume," You say Pneumonia
- When I say "Granular Opacities + Term + Low Lung Volume," You say B-Hemolytic Strep
- When I say "Band Like Opacities", You say Chronic Lung Disease (BPD)
- When I say "Linear Lucencies", You say Pulmonary Interstitial Emphysema
- When I say "Pulmonary Hypoplasia," You say diaphragmatic hernia
- When I say "Lung Cysts and Nodules," You Say LCH or Papillomatosis
- When I say "Lower lobe bronchiectasis," You Say Primary Ciliary Dyskinesia
- When I say "Upper lobe bronchiectasis," You Say CF
- When I say "Posterior mediastinal mass (under 2)," You Say Neuroblastoma
- When I say "No air in the stomach", You say Esophageal Atresia
- When I say "Excessive air in the stomach", You say "H" Type TE fistula
- When I say "Anterior Esophageal Impression," You say pulmonary sling
- When I say "Pulmonary Sling," You say tracheal stenosis.
- When I say "Single Bubble," You say Gastric (antral or pyloric) atresia
- When I say "Double Bubble," You say duodenal atresia
- When I say "Duodenal Atresia", You say Downs
- When I say "Single Bubble with Distal Gas," You say maybe Mid Gut Volvulus
- When I say "Non-bilious vomiting", You say Hypertrophic Pyloric Stenosis
- When I say "Paradoxial aciduria" You say Hypertrophic Pyloric Stenosis
- When I say "Bilious vomiting - in an infant", You say Mid Gut Volvulus
- When I say "Corkscrew Duodenum" You say Mid Gut Volvulus
- When I say "Reversed SMA and SMV" You say Malrotation
- When I say "Absent Gallbladder" You say biliary atresia
- When I say "Triangle Cord Sign" You say biliary atresia
- When I say "Asplenia", You say "cyanotic heart disease"
- When I say "Infarcted Spleen," You say Sickle Cell
- When I say "Gall Stones," You say Sickle Cell

- When I say "Short Microcolon," You say Colonic Atresia
- When I say "Long Microcolon," You say Meconium ileus or distal ileal atresia
- When I say "Saw tooth colon," You say Hirschsprung
- When I say "Calcified mass in the mid abdomen of a newborn", you say Meconium Peritonitis
- When I say "Meconium ileus equivalent," you say Distal Intestinal Obstruction Syndrome (CF).
- When I say "Abrupt caliber change of the aorta below the celiac axis", You say Hepatic Hemangioendothelioma.
- When I say "Cystic mass in the liver of a newborn," you say Mesenchymal Hamartoma
- When I say "Elevated AFP, with mass in the liver of a newborn," you say Hepatoblastoma
- When I say "Common Bile Duct measures more than 10mm", You say Choledochal Cyst
- When I say "Lipomatous pseudohypertrophy of the pancreas," You say CF
- When I say "Unilateral Renal Agenesis" You say unicornuate uterus
- When I say "Neonatal Renal Vein Thrombosis," You say maternal diabetes
- When I say "Neonatal Renal Artery Thrombosis," You say Misplaced Umbilical Artery Catheter
- When I say "Hydro on Fetal MRI," You say Posterior Urethral Valve
- When I say "Urachus," You say bladder Adenocarcinoma
- When I say "Nephroblastomatosis with Necrosis," you say Wilms
- When I say "Solid Renal Tumor of Infancy," you say Mesoblastic Nephroma
- When I say "Solid Renal Tumor of Childhood," you say Wilms
- When I say "Midline pelvic mass, in a female," you say Hydrometrocolpos
- When I say "Right sided varicocele," you say abdominal pathology
- When I say "Blue Dot Sign," you say Torsion of the Testicular Appendages
- When I say "Hand or Foot Pain / Swelling in an Infant", You say - sickle cell with hand foot syndrome.
- When I say Extratesticular scrotal mass, you say embryonal rhabdomyosarcoma
- When I say "Narrowing of the interpedicular distance," you say Achondroplasia
- When I say "Platyspondyly (flat vertebral bodies)," you say Thanatophoric
- When I say "Absent Tonsils after 6 months" You say "Immune Deficiency"
- When I say "Enlarged Tonsils well after childhood (like 12-15)" You say "Cancer"… probably lymphatic
- When I say "Mystery Liver Abscess in Kid, "You say "Chronic Granulomatous Disease"

High Yield Trivia:

- Pulmonary Interstitial Emphysema (PIE) - put the bad side down
- Bronchial Foreign Body - put the lucency side down (if it stays that way, it's positive)
- Papillomatosis has a small (2%) risk of squamous cell CA
- Pulmonary sling is the only variant that goes between the esophagus and the trachea. This is associated with trachea stenosis.
- Thymic Rebound – Seen after stress (chemotherapy) – Can be PET-Avid
- Lymphoma – Most common mediastinal mass in child (over 10)
- Anterior Mediastinal Mass with Calcification – Either treated lymphoma, or Thymic Lesion (lymphoma doesn't calcify unless treated).
- Neuroblastoma is the most common posterior mediastinal mass in child under 2 (primary thoracic does better than abd).
- Hypertrophic Pyloric Stenosis - NOT at birth, NOT after 3 months (3 weeks to 3 months is easiest for me to remember)
- Criteria for HPS - 4mm and 14mm (4mm single wall, 14mm length).
- Annular Pancreas presents as duodenal obstruction in children and pancreatitis in adults.
- Most common cause of bowel obstruction in child over 4 = Appendicitis
- Intussusception - 3months to 3 years is ok, earlier or younger think lead point
- Gastroschisis is ALWAYS on the right side
- Omphalocele has associated anomalies (gastroschisis does not).
- Physiologic Gut Hernia normal at 6-8 weeks
- AFP is elevated with Hepatoblastoma
- Endothelial growth factor is elevated with Hemangioendothelioma
- Most Common cause of pancreatitis in a kid = Trauma (seatbelt)
- Weigert Meyer Rule - Duplicated ureter on top inserts inferior and medial
- Most common tumor of the fetus or infant - Sacrococcygeal Teratoma
- Most common cause of idiopathic scrotal edema - HSP
- Most common cause of acute scrotal pain age 7-14 - Torsion of Testicular Appendages
- Bell Clapper Deformity is the etiology for testicular torsion.
- SCFE is a Salter Harris Type 1
- Physiologic Periostitis of the Newborn doesn't occur in a newborn - seen around 3 months
- Acetabular Angle should be < 30, and Alpha angle should be more than 60.

Section 5: Neuro

When I Say This..... You Say That.....

- When I say "cervical kyphosis", you say NF-1
- When I say "lateral thoracic meningocele," you say NF-1
- When I say "bilateral optic nerve gliomas," you say NF-1
- When I say "bilateral vestibular schwannoma," you say NF-2
- When I say "retinal hamartoma," you say TS
- When I say "retinal angioma," you say VHL
- When I say "brain tumor with restricted diffusion," you say lymphoma
- When I say "brain tumor crossing the midline," you say GBM (or lymphoma)
- When I say "Cyst and Nodule in Child," you say Pilocystic Astrocytoma
- When I say "Cyst and Nodule in Adult," you say Hemangioblastoma
- When I say "multiple hemangioblastoma," you say Von Hippel Lindau
- When I say "Swiss cheese tumor in ventricle," you say central neurocytoma
- When I say "CN3 Palsy," you say posterior communicating artery aneurysm
- When I say "CN6 Palsy," you say increased ICP
- When I say "Ventricles out of size to atrophy," you say NPH
- When I say "Hemorrhagic putamen," you say Methanol
- When I say "Decreased FDG uptake in the lateral occipital cortex," you say Lewy Body Dementia
- When I say "TORCH with Periventricular Calcification," you say CMV
- When I say "TORCH with hydrocephalus," you say Toxoplasmosis
- When I say "TORCH with hemorrhagic infarction," you say HSV
- When I say "Neonatal infection with frontal lobe atrophy," you say HIV
- When I say "Rapidly progressing dementia + Rapidly progressing atrophy," you say CJD
- When I say "Expanding the cortex," Oligodendroglioma
- When I say "Tumor acquired after trauma (LP)," you say Epidermoid
- When I say "The Palate Separated from the Maxilla / Floating Palate," you say LeFort 1
- When I say "The Maxilla Separated from the Face" or "Pyramidal" you say LeFort 2
- When I say "The Face Separated from the Cranium," you say LeFort 3
- When I say "Airless expanded sinus," you say mucocele
- When I say "DVA," you say cavernous malformation nearby
- When I say "Single vascular lesion in the pons," you say Capillary Telangiectasia
- When I say "Elevated NAA peak," you say Canvans
- When I say "Tigroid appearance," you say Metachromatic Leukodystrophy
- When I say "Endolymphatic Sac Tumor," you say VHL
- When I say "T1 Bright in the petrous apex," you say Cholesterol Granuloma
- When I say "Restricted diffusion in the petrous apex," you say Cholesteatoma

- When I say "Lateral rectus palsy + otomastoiditis," you say Grandenigo Syndrome
- When I say "Cochlea and semicircular canal enhancement," you say Labrinthitis
- When I say "Conductive hearing loss in an adult," you say Otosclerosis
- When I say "Noise induced vertigo," you say Superior Semicircular Canal dehiscence
- When I say "Widening of the maxillary ostium," you say Antrochonal Polyp
- When I say "Inverting papilloma," you say squamous cell CA (10%)
- When I say "Adenoid cystic," you say perineural spread
- When I say "Left sided vocal cord paralysis," you say look in the AP window
  When I say "Bilateral coloboma," you say CHARGE syndrome
- When I say "Retinal Detachment + Small Eye" you say PHPV
- When I say "Bilateral Small Eye," you say Retinopathy of Prematurity
- When I say "Calcification in the globe of a child," you say Retinoblastoma
- When I say "Fluid-Fluid levels in the orbit," you say Lymphangioma
- When I say "Orbital lesion, worse with Valsalva," you say Varix
- When I say "Pulsatile Exophthalmos," you say NF-1 and CC Fistula
- When I say "Sphenoid wing dysplasia," you say NF-1
- When I say "Simitar Sacrum," you say Currarino Triad
- When I say "bilateral symmetrically increases T2 signal in the dorsal columns," you sat B12 (or HIV)
- When I say "Owl eye appearance of spinal cord," you say spinal cord infarct
- When I say "Enhancement of the nerves root of the cauda equina," you say Guillain Barre
- When I say "Subligamentous spread of infection," you say TB

High Yield Trivia

- The order of tumor prevalence in NF2 is the same as the mnemonic MSME (schwannoma > meningioma > ependymoma).
- Maldeveloped draining veins is the etiology of Sturge Weber
- All phakomatosis (NF 1, NF -2, TS, and VHL) EXCEPT Sturge Weber are autosomal dominant - family screening is a good idea.
- Most Common Primary Brain Tumor in Adult = Astrocytoma
- "Calcifies 90% of the time" = Oligodendroglioma
- Restricted Diffusion in Ventricle = Watch out for Choroid Plexus Xanthogranuloma (not a brain tumor, a benign normal variant)
- Pituitary - T1 Bright = Pituitary Apoplexy
- Pituitary - T2 Bright = Rathke Cleft Cyst
- Pituitary – Calcified = Craniopharyngioma
- CP Angle – Invades Internal Auditory Canal = Schwannoma
- CP Angle - Invades Both Internal Auditory Canals = Schwannoma with NF2
- CP Angle – Restricts on Diffusion = Epidermoid
- Peds – Arising from Vermis = Medulloblastoma
- Peds- 4th ventricle "tooth paste" out of 4th ventricle = Ependymoma
- Adult myelination pattern: T1 at 1 year, T2 at 2 years
- Brainstem and posterior limb of the internal capsule are myelinated at birth.
- CN2 and CNV3 are not in the cavernous sinus
- Persistent trigeminal artery (vertebral to carotid) increases the risk of aneurysm
- Subfalcine herniation can lead to ACA infarct
- ADEM lesions will NOT involve the calloso-septal interface.
- Marchiafava-Bignami progresses from body -> genu -> splenium
- Post Radiation changes don't start for 2 months (there is a latent period).
- Hippocampal atrophy is first with Alzheimer Dementia
- Most common TORCH for CMV
- Toxo abscess does NOT restrict diffusion
- Small cortical tumors can be occult without IV contrast
- JPA and Ganglioglioma can enhance and are low grade
- Nasal Bone is the most common fracture
- Zygomaticomaxillary Complex Fracture (Tripod) is the most common fracture pattern and involves the zygoma, inferior orbit, and lateral orbit.
- Supplemental oxygen can mimic SAH on FLAIR
- Putamen is the most common location for hypertensive hemorrhage
- Restricted diffusion without bright signal on FLAIR should make you think hyperacute (< 6 hours) stroke.
- Enhancement of a stroke; Rule of 3s - starts at day 3, peaks at 3 weeks, gone at 3 months
- PAN is the Most Common systemic vasculitis to involve the CNS
- Scaphocephaly is the most common type of crainosynostosis

- Piriform aperture stenosis is associated with hypothalamic pituitary adrenal axis issues.
- Cholesterol Granuloma is the most common primary petrous apex lesion
- Large vestibular aqueduct syndrome has absence of the bony modiolus in 90% of cases
- Octreotide scan will be positive for esthesioneuroblastoma
- The main vascular supply to the posterior nose is the sphenopalatine artery (terminal internal maxillary artery).
- Warthins tumors take up pertechnetate
- Sjogrens gets salivary gland lymphoma
- Most common intra-occular lesion in an adult = Melanoma
- Enhancement of nerve roots for 6 weeks after spine surgery is normal. After that it's arachnoiditis
- Hemorrhage in the cord is the most important factor for outcome in a traumatic cord injury.
- Currarino Triad: Anterior Sacral Meningocele, Anorectal malformation, Sarcococcygeal osseous defect
- Type 1 Spinal AVF (dural AVF) is by far the more common.
- Herpes spares the basal ganglia (MCA infarcts do not)

I'VE POURED ALL MY KNOWLEDGE INTO YOU. WHEN YOU TAKE THE EXAM, MY SPIRIT WILL TAKE THE EXAM WITH YOU.

THERE IS NO STOPPING US NOW
WE START, AND WE DON'T STOP

ALL YOUR STRENGTH
ALL YOUR POWER
ALL YOUR LOVE

EVERYTHING YOU GOT

—-

What's Next For Prometheus Lionhart ? Check out TitanRadiology.com for updates

—Register for free at TitanRadiology.com to get my weekly multiple choice quiz

—Physics Review Course - Video Series - January 2016

—Expanded Stand Alone Physics Book - "The War Machine" - January 2016

—"TOP 100" - Rapid Review Book - February 2016

—"Titan Radiology Video Lecture Series" - The Magnum Opus - April 2016